SPORTS MEDICINE
Problems and
Practical Management

*"I just had to get up and do it.
At the 500m I felt tired, but I could see the lead I had gained
and I didn't care if one of my arms fell off."*

(Kierin Perkins at time of 2nd gold medal,
1500m, swimming, Atlanta 1996)

SPORTS MEDICINE
PROBLEMS AND
PRACTICAL MANAGEMENT

Eugene Sherry
MB ChB, MD, MPH, FRACS
Senior Lecturer
Orthopaedic Surgery
University of Sydney

Des Bokor
MB, BS(Hons), FRACS, FAOrthA
Orthopaedic Surgeon
Western Sydney
Orthopaedic Associates
Sydney

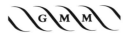

© 1997

GREENWICH MEDICAL MEDIA LTD.
219 The Linen Hall
162-168 Regent Street
London
W1R 5TB

ISBN 1 900151 553

First Published 1997

British Library Cataloguing in Publication Data
A catalogue record for this book is available from the British Library

Distributed worldwide by
Oxford University Press

Designed and Produced by
Derek Virtue, DataNet

Printed in UK

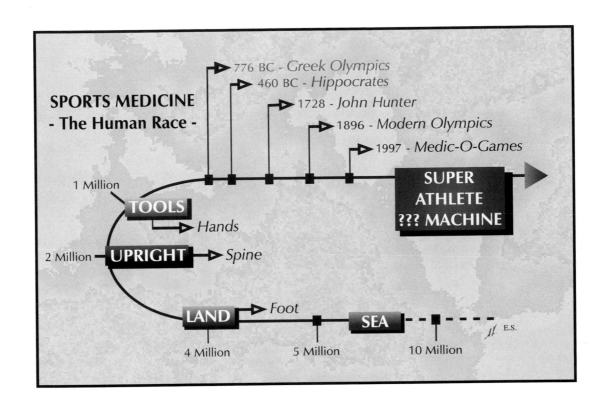

Dedicated to our wives Patricia and Sandy and our children Conor, Declan, Tom, David, Jacqueline and Peter and inspired by our Teachers Geoffrey Cocker, Ronald Huckstep and Bruce Shepherd (ES) and Mervyn Cross and Richard Hawkins (DJB).

Acknowledgements

This book would have been impossible without the work of Margaret Kenny and staff (illustrations and preparation of manuscript) of JadaArt Pty Ltd, Penrith, Sydney; the generous support of Jamison and Hills Private Hospitals (Health care of Australia), Castlereagh Radiology, Sydney (in particular, Dr Quentin Reeves) and Drs Barratt and Smith, Pathologists, a division of Sonic Healthcare Limited, Sydney. The authors would like to thank Churchill Livingstone for permission to use photographs and drawings from 'Sports Medicine in the Colour Guide Series' (1996) in this text (Fig. page v, Chap. 2 (Figs. 10, 26), Chap. 4 (Figs. 3, 4, 6, 11, 12, 15, 18, 22), Chap. 6 (Fig. 2), Chap. 7 (Fig. 14), Chap. 9 (Figs. 1, 2, 8, 14, 17, 35, 40), Chap. 10 (Figs. 12, 14, 18, 28, 32, 36, 40), Chap. 11 (Figs. 10, 14, 28, 30), Chap. 12 (Figs. 26, 29, 30, 34, 36, 39), Chap. 13 (Figs. 3, 4, 6, 7, 8, 11, 12, 14-19, 22, 24, 32, 35, 36), Chap. 14 (Figs. 1-3, 7,14, 15, 19, 25), Chap. 15 (Figs. 10, 12, 13, 18, 21, 23, 27, 40,-42), Chap. 16 (Fig. 18) Chap.17 (Figs. 17, 22, 23), Chap. 18 (Figs. 30, 31, 35, 36, 42), Chap. 19 (Figs. 4, 10, 14), Chap.20 (Figs. 1, 3), Chap. 21 (Fig. 4)

CONTENTS

PART II

APPENDIX

INDEX

CONTRIBUTORS

Des J Bokor,
MB, BS(Hons), FRACS, FAOrthA

Orthopaedic Surgeon
Western Sydney Orthopaedic
Associates
Sydney
Member of the International Baseball
Association Medical Commission

Philip M Boyce,
MD, F.R.A.N.Z.C.P.

Professor Psychiatry
Clinical Sciences Building,
Nepean Hospital
University of Sydney

Carolyn Broderick,
MB, BS, Dip SPORT, Sc FA CSP

Sports Physician
Sydney

Grace Bryant,
MBB GRAD, Dip Sport Sc., SASMS, FACSP

Sports Physician
Sydney
Australian Netball Medical Officer
Newtown Rugby League Med Officer
Consulting Medical Officer
Aust Atlanta Olympic Team

Jeffrey S Compton,
MB, BS, BSC(HONS), FRACS

Neurosurgeon
Nepean, Westmead and
Liverpool Hospitals
Sydney

Michael R Cox,
MS, FRCAS

Staff Specialist Surgeon
Upper Gastro Intestinal Surgery
Senior Lecturer
University of Sydney
Nepean Hospital

David Dilley,
MB, BS, FRCAS

Hand Surgeon
Westmead Hosptital
Sydney

David G Duckworth,
MB, BS, FRACS

Orthopaedic Surgeon
Western Sydney Orthopaedic
Associates
Sydney

Ian D Farey,
MB, BS, FRACS, FAOrthA
**Orthopaedic Surgeon and Spinal
Surgeon**
Royal North Shore Hospital
Sydney

Michael Foster
MBBS

Intern
University of Sydney

Mark Freeman
BSc (Hons)
Medical School
University of Sydney

Kerwyn Y Foo
BSc

Orthopaedic Research Associate
Medical School
University of Sydney

Peter C Gray
MBBS, FRACS, FAOrthA

Orthopaedic Surgeon
Western Sydney Orthopaedic
Associates
Sydney

I-Van Ho
MB, BS

Orthopaedic Research Associate
Nepean Hospital
Sydney

Eugene Hollenbach
MB, BS

Eye Registrar
Westmead Hospital
Sydney

Can Huynh
Dept Surgery
Medical School
University of Sydney

Talal Ibrahim
Medical School
University of Sydney

John E Ireland,
MB, BS, FRACS, (OrthA)
Orthopaedic Surgeon
Nepean and Liverpool Hospitals
Sydney

Vincent Lam
Medical School
University of Sydney

Lydia Lim
BDS (Hons), MDSC, SRACDS, FRACS (OMS)
**Oral and Maxillo-Facial
Surgeon**
Sydney

Cindy H Mak
Orthopaedic Research Associate
Nepean Hospital
Sydney

Donald Kuah
MB, BS, FACSP
Sports Physician
Sydney

Eugene Sherry
MD, MPH, FRACS
**Senior Lecturer Orthopaedic
Surgery**
University of Sydney
Nepean Hospital

Robert Standen
BSc (ANAT), GRAD. Dip.Sports PHTY
Sports Physiotherapist
Penrith

Stuart G Stapleton
MB, BS, FACEM
**Emergency Room
Physician**
Nepean Hospital
Sydney

James A Sullivan
MB, BS, FRACS
Orthopaedic Surgeon
Western Sydney Orthopaedic
Associates
Sydney

Beverley Trevithick
Dip. Phys.
Hand Therapist
Woorabinda Hand Therapy Centre

Vanessa Tung,
MB, BS
Surgical Resident
Sydney

INTRODUCTION

S ports Medicine is an exciting specialty dedicated to the medical care of athletes (injuries, illness, training needs and performance parameters).

There is little doubt that sports, properly supervised, has significant health benefits for all sectors of the community including Olympic athletes and mentally challenged children. It is our charge to understand and care for the particular needs and problems of all athletes.

This book represents our skill and accumulated experience in the care of the athlete. It evolved from our experiences on the ski fields as a general practitioner (ES) in the early 1980's (before becoming an orthopaedic surgeon) surrounded by injuries but with little texts to guide; from our orthopaedic training in Australia and Canada (DJB) where we were exposed to many excellent teachers in orthopaedic sports medicine; and from our current practices as orthopaedic surgeons caring for a variety of sports problems.

It is intended as a practical guide with scant use of references but a list of recommended further reading is included in the appendix.

Enjoy this text and let us know how we can improve it.

E.S.
D.J.B.
Sydney 1997

Part I

General

1

HISTORY OF SPORT AND MEDICINE

Eugene Sherry

The urbanised sophisticate of today sits with laptop computer on knee, mobile phone by ear, digtal phone in hand, cable TV in view, yearning for the open sports field. Sport fulfils our primitive biological need to **hunt, fight, use tools (and gather food)** (Fig.1).

Sport has, in fact, come to play an increasingly important role in modern society, though its origins date bsck to the dawn of man (Fig. 2).

Planet Earth is 4,600 million years old. Initially there was no oxygen; UV radiation (not blocked by an ozone barrier) stimulated photosynthesis to produce **organic molecules** (from H_2O, CO_2, NH_3). 3,500 million years ago, **anaerobic metabolism** developed. The original organisms released O_2 into the atmosphere and eventually aerobic metabolism developed (2,600 million years ago).

Nucleated unicellular organisms appeared 1,500 million years ago (**the eukaryote**). It contained the ATP-ADP energy system.

Large animals appeared at 700 million years; with the first primate at 60–70 million years. When the dinosaurs disappeared, mammals, flowering plants and birds appeared.

Evolution (modified Darwinian theory) is the gradual accumulation of genetic variants (from mutations and chromosomal re-arrangements) with nature selecting the "best" variants.

Hominids arrived 5 to 20 million years ago and Australopithecus at 4 million. This was a major step as an upright posture with bipedal gait freed the hands to use tools (and so the brain expanded). Then followed **H. Habilis, H. erectus** (hunters, food gatherers, the use of fire), **H. sapiens. Neanderthalensis** (tribes and common language) and modern man (**H. sapiens** – 50,000 years ago).

Modern man's success is due to his brain, upright posture, use of tools (opposition of the thumb) and speech. Unfortunately the same mind has an urge to **self-destruction**.

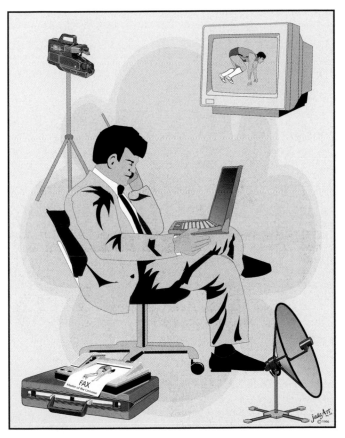

Figure 1 –The urban sophisticate surrounded by high technology yearns for the open sports field

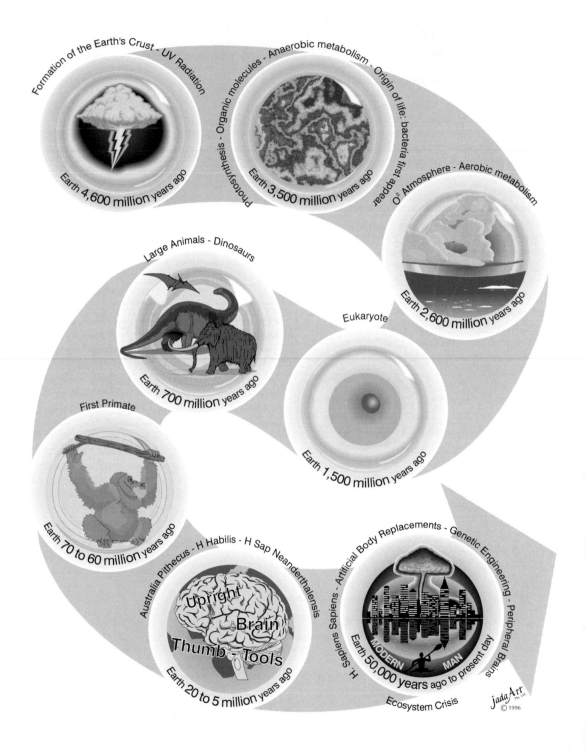

Figure 2 – Development of the Earth.

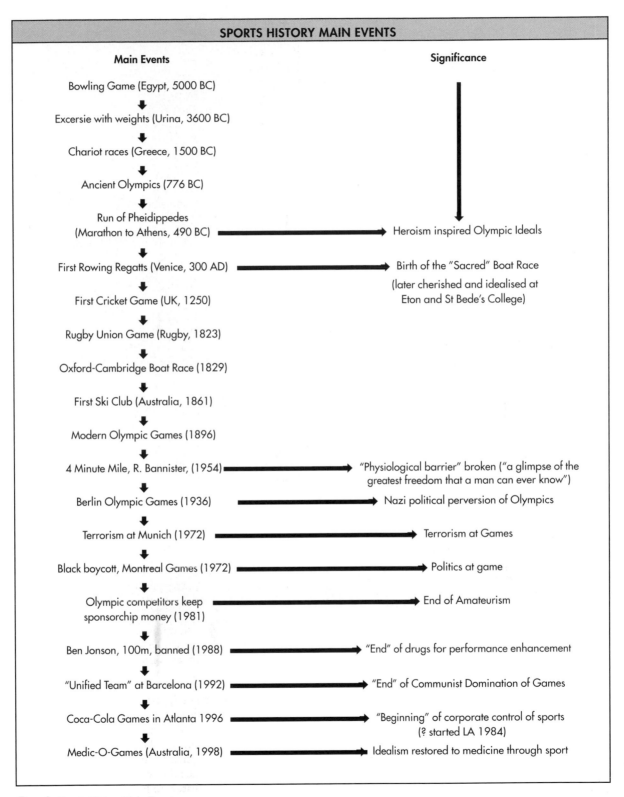

SPORTS HISTORY MAIN EVENTS

| Main Events | Significance |

Bowling Game (Egypt, 5000 BC)

Excersie with weights (Urina, 3600 BC)

Chariot races (Greece, 1500 BC)

Ancient Olympics (776 BC)

Run of Pheidippedes
(Marathon to Athens, 490 BC) ⟶ Heroism inspired Olympic Ideals

First Rowing Regatts (Venice, 300 AD) ⟶ Birth of the "Sacred" Boat Race
(later cherished and idealised at
Eton and St Bede's College)

First Cricket Game (UK, 1250)

Rugby Union Game (Rugby, 1823)

Oxford-Cambridge Boat Race (1829)

First Ski Club (Australia, 1861)

Modern Olympic Games (1896)

4 Minute Mile, R. Bannister, (1954) ⟶ "Physiological barrier" broken ("a glimpse of the
greatest freedom that a man can ever know")

Berlin Olympic Games (1936) ⟶ Nazi political perversion of Olympics

Terrorism at Munich (1972) ⟶ Terrorism at Games

Black boycott, Montreal Games (1972) ⟶ Politics at game

Olympic competitors keep ⟶ End of Amateurism
sponsorchip money (1981)

Ben Jonson, 100m, banned (1988) ⟶ "End" of drugs for performance enhancement

"Unified Team" at Barcelona (1992) ⟶ "End" of Communist Domination of Games

Coca-Cola Games in Atlanta 1996 ⟶ "Beginning" of corporate control of sports
(? started LA 1984)

Medic-O-Games (Australia, 1998) ⟶ Idealism restored to medicine through sport

Figure 3 – Sports History Main Events

Outdoor activities (hunting, food gathering) have been an essential part of our development for millions of years and so constitute an important part of even modern man's emotional, social and intellectual well-being.

Organised sporting competition has **three major milestones** and **several main events** (Fig. 3). **Firstly**, in the Ancient Calender, there is evidence that the Egyptians exercised (5000 BC) and had running rituals at Memphis (3800 BC); also the Chinese Emperors encouraged their subjects to exercise daily with weights (3600 BC). **Secondly the Olympic Games**; the Ancient (Greek) Games (776 BC) and the Modern Games (1896). Olympic competition introduced idealism (with devotion to Zeus) into sport with a celebration of mind and body (by the Greeks) and the ability to rise above politics (Modern Games). Sport not only served a fundamental biological need of man but also to elevate us to a higher plane of idealistic behaviour. **Thirdly** the great English public Schools recognised (before Baron Pierre de Coubertin) the civilising influence of organised sport. In the eighteenth and early nineteenth centuries their school pupils (the future masters of the British Empire) often behaved violently towards their headmasters and teachers with school riots not uncommon. (Lord Byron, with co-conspirator school-mates, laid explosives at Harrow to blow-up the new headmaster Butler, in 1805). Organised sports diverted their energies into enterprises of co-operation and heroicism on the football field (Eton Wall Game) and the water (rowing). Squash was first played at Harrow School (1817) and Rugby at Rugby School (1823). The same schoolboys went up to university and sport continued (First Oxford Cambridge Boat Race 1829).

British Colonies, existing and former, developed sporting prowess to maintain status and as a means of successful competition with mother England (US Football, NZ Rugby Champions, West Indies Cricket, Australian swimming and tennis).

All schools and universities now have organised athletic events as an important part of the curriculum.

In the Third World, improved standards of nutrition and overall health are leading teenagers to sport (First Asian Games, 1951).

The International Federation of Sports Medicine (FIMS) was initially founded in 1928 in St Mori It serviced as a catalyst for other groups despite the difficulties of the World Wars. The American College

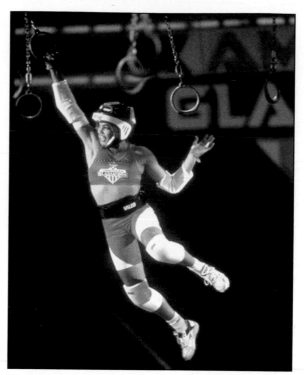

Figure 4 –The gladiators of the Classical Era were cared for by the famous second century Roman physician, Claudius Galen; todays gladiators are looked after by Modern Sports Medicine Physicians

of Sports Medicine was established in 1954 and one of the first Sports Medicine Departments at the Lake Placid (USA) in 1982.

Various interest and special groups have either their own Olympic Games (First Paraplegic Games 1948, Veterans Games, Fireman's Games, Doctor's Games (Medic-O-Games, 1998s).

The care of the sick and injured athlete was initially left to interested orthopaedic surgeons (O'Donoghue and Hughston) and general practitioners. In 1983 when the author was treating thousands of injured and sick downhill snow skiers there was little written to guide me in the particular care of skiers. A Ski Injury Clinic was therefore established in Perisher Valley, Australia in 1983.

Today the discipline of Sports Medicine has evolved as a specialty with dedicated associations and literature, Colleges of Sports Medicine and Sports Specific Institutes in most countries. The care of athletes is now in the hands of physicians dedicated to their needs almost 1800 years since the work of Claudius Galen as physician to the gladiators in Pergamum (Fig. 4).

THE FUTURE

The ultimate goal of competition is the breaking of world records. Despite supposed physiological barriers to better performance, records continue to fall. Roger Bannister in 1954 broke the 4 minute mile barrier and crashed through the "physiological limits" to his performance but it was really a psychological barrier he overcame. (Glenn Cunningham, the miler of the 1930s, had regularly run sub-4 minute miles in practice sessions).

The basic structure of the human machine coupled with improved training techniques and tactics, rules, equipment, numbers and nutrition of competitors will ensure an endless breaking of records.

Here are our predictions for 2020 and beyond: future sports trainers will be training their athletes in environmental cocoons to minimise adverse effects of ecosystem pollutants on performance; techniques for extending anaerobic and aerobic potential will be developed by genetic bio-engineers; athletes will undergo biomechanical alterations to their bodies to enhance performance (lengthen femurs and create metatarsus adductus (pigeon toes); peripheral brains (bio-computers) will be implanted to alter personality (and psychological barriers), and to enhance neuro-muscular and cardio-respiratory performance) and design engineers will improve sporting equipment and facilities to better performances and limit injuries (faster cycles, safer helmets, better splints, spring-loaded basketball courts to minimise impact. These advances will be based on sound science and a commitment to the study of performance parameters.

These bio-advantages will be available and only regulations will determine their use. Human beings may be cloned and developed for sporting spectacles (much the same as ancient schools of gladiators) or "ordinary" athletes will have their bodies adjusted (much the same way we have plastic surgery, or artificial joint surgery) to enhance their enjoyment of sport as an adjunct to their daily living. Already the All Blacks (NZ Rugby) are, in practice, pre-selecting a genetic prototype for successful competition (large players of Polynesian extraction). We will adjust to these varying standards and levels of competition in much the same way we abandoned the absolute necessity of amateurism in sporting competition (Fig. 3). Our philosophical acceptance will depend upon whether they will, in general, improve the "human lot".

The future of sports medicine, although daunting, will truly be spectacular.

2

BASIC SPORTS MEDICINE SCIENCE

Eugene Sherry

INTRODUCTION

Milon of Croton became a five times wrestling champion in the Ancient Greek Olympics by training every day. He picked up a calf and carried it about. With time his strength became prodigious, so was established progressive resistance training (bigger calf – bigger loads) – the basis of modern sports medical science.

It is important to understand the structure and function of the athlete's powered (heart, lung, nutrition, fluid) musculo-skeletal system (bones, joints, muscles, nerves).

BONE

Normally lamellar (stress-oriented) and either cortical (80% skeleton, tightly packed, made up of Haversian system) or cancellous (less dense, higher turnover, more elastic).

Bone is composed of cells and matrix (Figs. 1 and 2)

Bones may fail under breaking loads (fracture) or submaximal breaking loads (stress fracture). Fractures heal in an orderly way (Figs. 3 and 4)

Complications of fractures are not common but may be serious (Fig. 5).

Growth of bone occurs at the growth plates (physis and epiphysis) and under the periosteum. Fractures in children usually involve these growth plates and may disturb subsequent bone growth since growth arrests with shortening and angulation, (Salter-Harris classification I-VI).

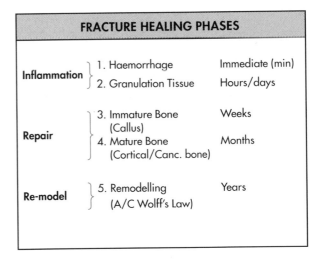

Figure 2 – Basic long bone structure

BONE STRUCTURE	
Cells	**Matrix**
• Osteoblasts - make bone	• Organic part (collagen type I, proteo glycans, glyco proteins, phospho-lipids, phosphoproteins, growth factors and cytokines)
• Osteocyte - regulate bone	
• Osteoclasts	• Non-organic part (crystal) calcium hydroxy apatite, osteocalcium.

Figure 1 – Essential elements of bone structure

FRACTURE HEALING PHASES		
Inflammation	1. Haemorrhage	Immediate (min)
	2. Granulation Tissue	Hours/days
Repair	3. Immature Bone (Callus)	Weeks
	4. Mature Bone (Cortical/Canc. bone)	Months
Re-model	5. Remodelling (A/C Wolff's Law)	Years

Figure 3 – Orderly sequence of fracture healing

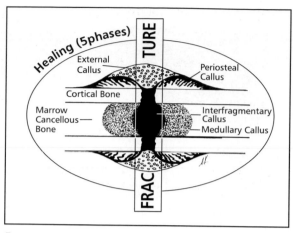

Figure 4 – Diagram of fracture healing

COMPLICATIONS OF FRACTURES	
Healing :	Delayed union (slow), non-union (not healed), mal-union (crooked)
Blood supply :	Avascular necrosis
Infections :	Osteomyelitis (usually where surgery)
Soft tissue :	Arterial entrapment, compartment syndrome (muscles), nerve injuries
General :	ARDS, Fat Embolism, DVT

Figure 5 – Common fracture complications

JOINTS

There are three types (Fig. 6)

Joint–cartilage (hyaline) is made up of water (65%), collagen (Type II, 10-20%, tensile-strength), proteo-glycans (10-15%) compressive strength), chondrocytes

1. **Synarthroses:**	As in skull (bone/cartilage/bone)
2. **Amphiarthrodial:**	As in symphysis pubis (bone/cartilage/disc/cartilage/bone)
3. **Diarthrodial:**	Synovial

Figure 6 – The three main types of joins

(5%) and other proteins (fibronectin) (Fig. 7).

Hyaline cartilage ages and stiffens (fewer chondro-cytes/proteoglycens, increased protein, less water) and heals (deeply with fibro cartilage, and superficially by proliferation) aided by continuous passive motion (Figs. 7 and 8). Sport (activity) probably wears out joints. Intensive sporting activity results in a 4.5× increased incidence of osteoarthritis (OA) of the hip (called skier's hip) which goes up to 8.5× when combined with occupational exposure.

Synovium regulates the composition of the synovial joint fluid (an ultra-filtrate). Synovial fluid nourishes (by diffusion) and **lubricates** hyaline cartilage.

Meniscus deepens the articular surface and so broadens the area of contact. The knee meniscus is composed of fibro-cartilage (network of collagen/proteoglycans/glycoproteins cells). The outer ¼ has a blood supply and thus will heal.

Joints can be damaged by osteoarthritis (post fracture), rheumatoid arthritis, avascular necrosis (secondary to steroids), infections and haemorrhage.

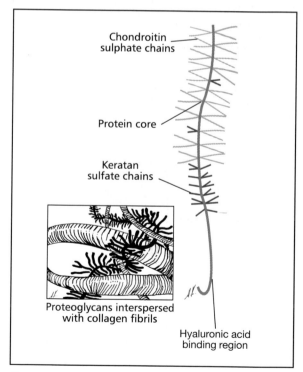

Figure 7 – Hyaline cartilage (microscopically) is made up of proteoglycans (chondroitin/Keratin sulphate chains/protein core/hyaluronic acid links) mixed with collagen.

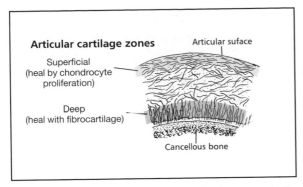

Articular cartilage zones   Articular suface

Superficial
(heal by chondrocyte
proliferation)

Deep
(heal with fibrocartilage)

Cancellous bone

Figure 8 – Hyaline cartilage (macroscopically) is composed of a superficial and deep layer.

SKELETAL MUSCLES

Composed of muscle fibres (muscle cells/endomysium/muscle fascicles/perimysium/muscle bundles/epimysium). The basic unit of work (contraction) is the sarcomere, made up of thick and thin filaments which slide by each other (Fig. 9). Muscle action follows the tension/length curve (Fig. 10). The motor unit (muscle fibres, 10 to 1000, per α–motor neuron) is the functional unit which varies with velocity/force and maintenance of contraction.

TYPES OF MUSCLE CONTRACTION

- Isotonic - constant tension (resistance), either concentric (muscle shortens) or eccentric contraction (lengthens). **Variable resistance** is where there is changing external load during weight lifting.

- Isometric - tension changes but no shortening of muscle (constant length), causes muscle hypertrophy but no endurance benefit. Improved by stretching.

- Isokinetic (dynamic) - maximum tension at constant speed. Increases muscle strength.

- Functional - dynamic exercises which allow rapid rehabilitation (as in jump ropes).

MUSCLE METABOLISM

Muscle fibres are either **Type I** or **Slow Red Ox** (red, slow twitch, oxidative, aerobic metabolism, endurance activities) or **Type II** (white, fast twitch glycolytic, anaerobic metabolism, sprinting, fine motor control).

Genes determine the relative distribution of fast twitch (FT) to slow twitch (ST) fibres. Sprinters and weight-lifters have more FT (Type II); endurance athletes ST (Type I). Training techniques can determine the relative efficiency of FT/ST fibres (endurance versus strength).

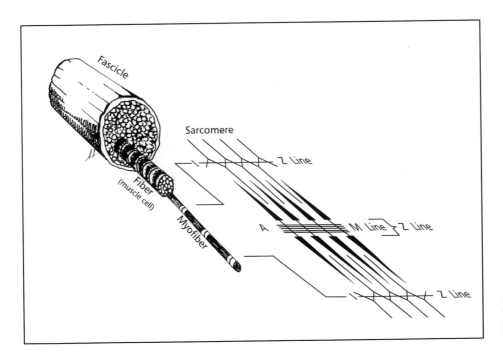

Fascicle

Sarcomere

Z Line

Fiber
(muscle cell)

Myofiber

A

M Line   Z Line

Z Line

Figure 9 – Basic structure of muscle which includes the "work-horse" - the sarcomere

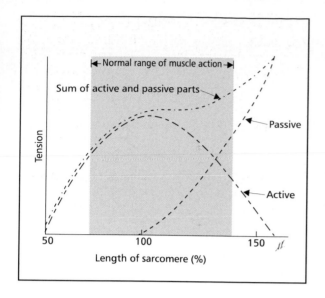

Figure 10 – Muscle action follows the length – tension curve

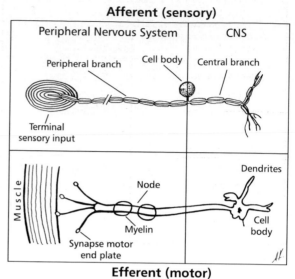

Figure 11 – Essential structure of the nervous system (excluding the brain)

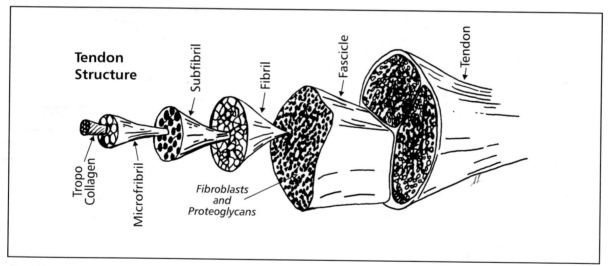

Figure 12 – Essential tendon structure

SPORTS TENDON OVERLOAD	
Site	**Sport**
Tendo achilles	Tennis
Iliotibial band	Running
Patellar tendon	Basketball
Patello-femoral pain	Running
Plantar fasciitis	Running
Shin splints	Running
Rotator cuff	Swimming
ECRB	Tennis
(EPB/APL)	Rowing

Figure 13 – Tendons commonly overloaded in sport

CAUSES OVERUSE INJURIES LOWER LIMB (60% OF ALL)		
1.	Training Errors	– Sudden increase mileage (>64 km/week)/ inadequate stretching/wrong scheduling.
2.	Anatomical factors	– Equinus foot/varus/ LLD/hyper pronations/ psychological
3.	Training surfaces	– Hills/tracks/wrong surfaces
4.	Running shoes	– Worn out/wrong size/ poor care

Figure 14 – Look carefully for the cause of tendon overload

NERVES

Peripheral nerves are made up of bundles of axons (cell body/axon/dendrites/synapse) wrapped in a sheath of Schwann (myelinated/unmyelinated) cells, and are either afferent (sensory) or efferent (motor) (Fig. 11). They heal after Wallerian degeneration (neuropraxia/ stingers, axonotmesis, neurotmesis). There is little direct evidence of the adaptive modification of motor neurons by exercise.

TENDONS

Tendons attach muscle to bone (by Sharpcy's fibres) and are composed of collagen (Type I) bundles (fascicles) in a bed of proteoglycans with fibroblasts, encased in endotenon/epitenon/paratenon (tendon sheath) (Fig 12). Tendons may be injured in sport acutely or through tensile overload overuse (Fig. 13).

Injuries occur at the muscle-tendon junction and in muscles crossing two joints (hamstrings, tendo-achilles). Most involve the lower limb and a cause should be sought (Fig. 14). Other overuse injuries of the lower limb also occur and need to be considered (Fig. 15).

A good rehabilitation programme is important (Fig. 16). Steroid injections have a limited but well-defined role (Fig. 17).

** OTHER COMMON OVERUSE INJURIES OF THE LOWER LIMB
Stress fractures
•
Chronic (exertional) compartment syndrome
•
Shin splints

Figure 15 – Other overuse injuries may mimic tendon overload

Where tendons are ruptured and repaired, it should be remembered that tendon repair is weakest at 7 days and restored at 6 months (improved by immobilisation, however this causes decreased range of movement ROM).

LIGAMENTS

Ligaments stabilise joints and are composed of Type I collagen (higher elastin content). Extra-articular ligaments, such as the MCL, heal in three phases; Firstly, haemorrhage and inflammation with fibroblasts; secondly, type I collagen formation; thirdly, maturation). Intra-articular (ACL) ligament healing is soon stalled by synovial fluid. Immobilisation adversely affects ligament repair, whilst exercise helps.

REHABILITATION REGIME			
Stage	**Pathology**	**Treatment**	**Progress**
Acute	Tissue damage	Rest/NSAID/Physical Therapy Protected ROM Isometrics/Isotonic	▼ pain ▲ ROM ▼ swelling
Recovery	Overload	Careful loading/ ROM/Resistive + functional exercises	No pain, 80% strength; Normal ROM
Follow-up	Biomechanical deficit	Strength/flexibility maintenance	Normal strength/ balance/ROM

In general:
Rest/cross-train/ice massage/stretching/resistance exercises/physical/NSAID/correct biomechanical problems/
correct training errors/assess running shoes.

Figure 16 – Essential rehabilitation programme

CORTICOSTEROID INJECTION USE

Use

1. After 6 week trial physical therapy
2. Discrete inflammatory lesion
3. Only 3 injections

Do not use

1. For acute injury
2. Where infection is present
3. Into tendon
4. Before competition

Figure 17 – Strict criteria for steriod use

AEROBIC EXERCISE PROGRAMME	
• Mode	Use large muscle groups
• Intensity	40-85% VO_2 max * 55-90% HR max (age predicted, 220-age ±15)
• Duration	15-60 min sessions
• Frequency	3 to 5/week
• Progression	Systematically increase intensity
• Individualise programme	
• Specify training according to metabolic and neuromuscular requirements.	

* (Max capacity to extract O_2 to make ATP; = Cardiac
output, CO (Heart rate, HR × Stroke volume, SV)
x O_2a-v; genetically determined; can be increased by 5%
(in fit) to 25% (in unfit) over 8-12 weeks

Figure 18 – Aerobic Exercise Program (from Am. College Sports
Med.)

TRAINING

The goal of exercise is to improve fitness and general well-being. Fitness means improved cardiovascular (aerobic, measured by VO_2 max) capacity and strength by rhythmic exercise of large muscle groups. Cardiac output (CO)is consequently increased.

A proper aerobic exercise programme (from Am College of Sports Medicine) should consider several variables (Fig. 18).

STRENGTH TRAINING (WEIGHT-TRAINING)

This is gained by variation of intensity (load, resistance lifted per repetition), volume (weight lifted), frequency (every other day) and rest periods (< 60 secs is optimal). Beneficial (when supervised) for young athletes (prevents injury, aids rehabilitation, improves self-esteem). Should include warm-up (15-20 min, calisthenics, stretching), lifting session and cool-down (as for warm-up).

PHYSIOLOGIC RESPONSE TO EXERCISE

The human condition is maintained by genetic reproduction, adaptive capability and metabolism. There are 65 billion body cells, about 50% are muscle cells which require delivery of nutrients and removal of waste products (increased demand with exercise). This is met by the cardiovascular (CO which is SV (Stroke Volume) × HR (Heart Rate) (and arterio venous oxygen difference) and pulmonary (O_2 uptake in lungs) systems.

CARDIOVASCULAR RESPONSE

Summarised in Figure 19 is the static (isometric) and dynamic exercise (from OKU - Sports Medicine, 1996).

Cardiovascular response: **the athlete's heart** is typified by biventricular cardiac enlargement, soft ejection murmur, extra heart sounds, resting sinus bradycardia and increased cardiac output.

The heart (ventricular hypertrophy) enlarges from pressure load in static exercise (concentric hypertrophy) and volume overload in dynamic/exercise (eccentric hypertrophy). Endurance athletes may have up to 45% larger left ventricular mass than non-athletes.

Variable	❏ Static Exercise	*Dynamic Exercise
Heart Rate (HR)	▲	▲▲
Cardiac Output (CO)	▲	▲▲
Blood Pressure (BP) systolic	▲	▲
Blood Pressure (BP) diastolic	▲	▼
Blood Pressure (BP) mean	▲	○
Systemic Vascular Resistance	▲	▼▼
V Return	○	
Ejection fraction	○/▲	
Stroke Volume (SV)	○	▲▲
O_2 Consumption	▲	▲▲

* ▲ Cardiac output by ▲ left ventricular volume and muscle vasodilation

❏ ▲ Cardiac output by ▲ heart rate.

Figure 19 – The cardiovascular response to static and dynamic exercise.

Overall, **maximum exercise capacity** is mainly determined by increased O_2 delivered from increased cardiac stroke volume and cardiac output, vasodilation and, to a lesser extent, by increased mitochondrial volume. This decreases with age (from ↓ max HR and ↓ SV), however, training may maintain it.

PULMONARY RESPONSE

Exercise increases total lung capacity by reducing residual volume, increasing vital capacity and improved respiratory muscle efficiency. The fit athlete is therefore able to process larger volumes of air at maximum exertion (from 6 litres per min at rest to 120 l/min max).

The pulmonary system may determine the athletes full metabolic potential; with champions being those with the largest 'vital capacities'.

Overall, exercise (regular) decreases: HR, BP, insulin requirements (in diabetics), cardiovascular risk and increases lean body mass. HDL (high density lipoprotein) which is anti-atherosclerotic is increased (and LDL low density lipoprotein and triglycerides decreased).

SPORTS NUTRITION

Food contains the chemically-bonded energy necessary for life and movement. This energy is stored in the body as ATP (adenosine tri phosphate).

The Dietary Guidelines for Americans (five basic principles) provides a foundation for athletes everywhere. In general, keep training diet high in carbohydrates, moderate in fat and protein (Figs. 20 and 21).

Daily energy requirements are calculated according to level of activity, (Fig. 22), as follows

Weight (in pounds) × 11 (female), or × 12 (male) + calories burnt in training

It is important to follow a well-planned nutritional programme for competition (Fig. 23).

Carbohydrates are the athletes most essential food source. Stored in liver and muscle as glycogen and are the main fuel for high intensity, short duration events, (sprinting) and the only source in the first few min of exercise (though possibly depleted within 60 min).

Athletes will "slow down" as glycogen is depleted (sudden weight loss independent of fluid status). Complex carbohydrates are necessary (simple sugar <12% total carbohydrate intake) and should make up 60–70% of total calories. Carbohydrate requirement for non-endurance exercise is 5 g/kg/day and for endurance 8–10 g/kg/day.

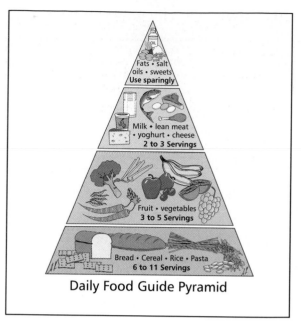

Figure 21 – The daily food pyramid provides a practical guide to nutrition for all

PROTEINS

Protein requirements are controversial. Generally, 1–1.5 g protein per kg body weight is adequate but can depend on type, intensity and duration of exercise (body-builders and endurance athletes require more protein). Female and amenorrhoeic athletes especially may not get enough protein.

PRINCIPLES OF ATHLETIC NUTRITION
• Eat variety foods
• Maintain body weight
• Keep diet low in fat/saturated fat/cholesterol
• Eat vegetables, fruits, grain products
• Use in moderation (Sugar/Salt/Alcohol)

Figure 20 – Principles of athletic nutrition

DAILY ENERGY REQUIREMENTS

Level of Activity	Men	Women
Light	17*	16
Moderate	19	17
Heavy	23	20

* Kilocalories per pound body weight per day from Nat Res Council, USA, 1989.

Figure 22 – Daily energy requirements

EATING STRATEGY FOR COMPETITION	
Pre-competition	
1 week prior	➡ build up glycogen stores (50 to 70% CHO)
1 day prior	➡ keep up glucose + fluid levels
In competition	
Events > 60 min	➡ CHO supplements (240 ml 5 to 8% CHO drank every 15 min)
Recovery	
Replace glycogen/fluids ➡	Replace (fluids) 1-lb weight loss with 500 ml fluid glucose. Consume 1.5 g CHO/kg wgt/every 2 hours for 24 hrs afterwards

Figure 23 – Eating strategy for competition

High protein diets, although popular, carry a risk of increased body fats, blood lipids, dehydration, incidence of gout and calcium excretion.

Amino–acid supplements probably play only a minor role in enhancing performance.

Vitamin and mineral supplements do not enhance performance and are supplied in a good diet. Female athletes should supplement diet with iron and calcium.

FAT

Fat is used at rest and low to moderate exercise levels. It is called upon as a source of energy in endurance sports (especially for females). It should be close to 20% of total calorie intake.

Caffeine at a level of 5 mg/kg enhances performance (by increasing the level of free fatty acids in blood), however it is illegal.

HYDRATION

This is the single most important nutrient for athlete. Correct hydration determines athletic performance. It is important to maintain weight during exercise. Work capacity, temperature regulation and performance all fall-off with fluid loss (Fig. 24).

Fluid (replacement) Guidelines
(Measure weight; monitor urine output)

In general: 0.45 kg weight loss requires 500 ml fluid over 24 hours)

- Events < 60 min ➡ Cool water
- Events > 60 min ➡ Drink beverage with 6–10% Carbohydrate (No Fructose)

- Sports Drinks with 6–10% CHO + electrolytes are good (do not need complex sugars)

Do not use salt tablets.

- Drink 600 ml 1-2 hrs pre exercise; 300-450 ml 15 min before exercise; 90-180 ml every 10-20 min of exercise; replace lost fluids immediately post exercise (500 ml for every pound lost).

- Urine output is normally 840 ml/day. If no urine for several hours, or if urine dark ➡ drink more fluid.

EFFECTS OF FLUID LOSS	
% Loss Body Weight	**Effect**
1%	Feel thirsty, decreased work capacity.
2%	Sense of oppression/loss appetite
3%	Dry mouth, ▼ urine output
4%	20 to 30% ▼ work capacity
5%	Headache, sleepiness, ▼ concentration
6%	▼ Temp regulation, ▲ resp. rate
7%	Imminent collapse
In general: For every 100 ml fluid lost:	Rectal temp ▲ by 0.3°C C.O. ▼ by 1 l/min H.R. ▲ 8 beats/min

Figure 24 – Effects of fluid loss quantified

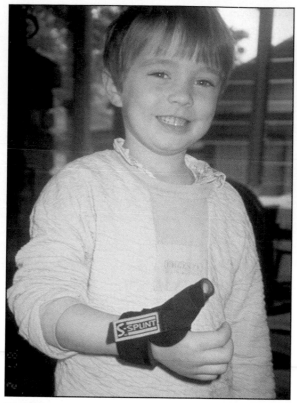

Figure 25 – The S-Thumb splint can protect the thumb from damaging abduction/hyper extension in sport

SPLINTS

Splints or braces are intended to prevent and treat (with or without corrective surgery) joint injuries. It is difficult to scientifically test their effectiveness, so often their use is empirical.

KNEE BRACES

Prophylactic knee braces may or may not prevent MCL/ACL injuries of the knee. There is no strong evidence to support their use; in fact some suggest they may increase the chance of injury. Use/Decision to be made on individual basis.

Functional knee braces are used to provide stability for unstable knees but in young and high-level athletes, surgical reconstruction is better.

Rehabilitative knee braces are useful for protection after reconstructive surgery (ACL/MCL) of the knee.

Patellar bracing or taping may be useful for an unstable/maltracking patella.

ANKLE BRACES

Taping, although initially effective, is expensive and loosens in competition. A well designed, light-weight, easy to apply ankle splint (S-Ankle) will prevent and treat lateral ligament sprains of the ankle (see Fig. 13 Chapter 15). There is increasing evidence of the effectiveness of prophylactic ankle splinting.

THUMB SPLINTS

UCL/MCL (Skier's Thumb) injury is difficult to immobilise. No good splint/brace exists; studies suggest the effectiveness of the S-Splint to limit abduction of the thumb MCP joint (Fig. 25).

FOOT

Orthotics are available for the foot with the most common indication being a hyper pronated indication foot and heel pain. Stress fractures may also be treated with soft-impact relieving orthotics. It is important that orthotics be comfortable and soft/firm (seldom rigid). Turf toe may respond to strapping of the 1st MTP joint.

HELMETS

Advisably worn in most contact (person-to-person, person-to-ground) sports (US football, ice hockey, skiing, cycling, cricket). In closed head injuries there is

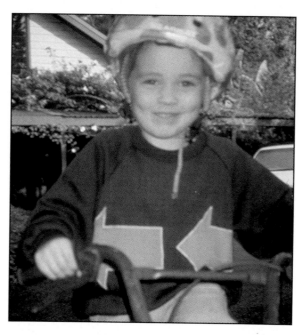

Figure 26 – Helmets (hard outer shell with energy absorbing inner lining) are now mandatory for children on bicycles in many parts of the world (protect brain from shearing injuries)

shearing of brain tissue from angular acceleration imparted to the semifluid brain tissue. A football helmet should be made of a hard, polycarbonate outer shell (to deflect blows) and adjustable (energy absorbing) inner air-filled cells or web liners and face-mask.

Where suspected neck injury, remove face mask **on field** (with cutters) and helmet **in hospital** (with a practised routine) (Fig. 26).

OTHER BRACES

Neck braces are used in US football. A tennis elbow counterforce brace is said to help.

MOUTH GUARDS

Should be used by US footballers (and other football/rugby codes) to protect the teeth and jaw (reduces impact of chin blows to prevent concussion and/or neck injuries).

PERFORMANCE AND EQUIPMENT (SURFACES)

Equipment affects performance and (inter-related) safety. This is obvious for sports such as rowing (boat and blade design) and cycling (aerodynamic considerations) and less obvious or documented for track and field events (sports shoe design is not clearly proven to enhance performance or reduce likelihood of injury, although there is increasing evidence for prophylactic bracing to prevent ankle injuries). Recently, a water cooling jacket has been used by the Australian Olympic team to prevent illness cause by excessive heat.

The interaction of equipment with injury has been carefully documented for downhill snow skiing. Improving the design and function of bindings has reduced the incidence of tibial shaft fractures over the last 20 years; better ski foot design has reduced the likelihood of ankle fractures and sprains. The adoption of ski breaks (rather than sharps) reduced the incidence of lacerations to limbs and the face, however conundrums remain. The incidence of knee and upper body injuries appears to continue to increase. Changes in a behaviour (fall technique) may influence these patterns.

There is evidence that certain sports surfaces have higher injury rates (artificial turf, made of polyvinyl chloride/urethane plastic, causes more injuries) and that although synthetic surfaces have better wear characteristics, wood is still an excellent all-round playing surface. Considerations include wear, maintenance, impact characteristics, safety and slip. Dance and aerobics require impact relieving surfaces with no slip and bounce; tennis surfaces have to consider the ball bounce. In track and field it is better to use polyurethane or latex-bound surfaces.

3

SPORT WITHIN OUR ECOSYSTEM

Eugene Sherry

INTRODUCTION

This chapter introduces a concept not previously recognised in sports medicine texts - the relationship between sport and the eco-environment.

As we enter the next millennium, it seems we have all but **destroyed our environment** (Fig. 1). Doctors may soon be standing helplessly by as our children exercise and play sport in the disease-ridden scrap yards of the planet.

John Hunter, the intrepid eighteenth century surgeon/scientist, set the pace for development and research in medicine but we have lagged behind. The initial successes with anaesthesia, infectious diseases, antibiotics, open heart surgery, artificial joint surgery and vaccinations have fallen short with unrealistic expectations of the Human Genome Project. We should be ashamed of our failure to cure cancer and HIV disease (despite the resources available) and to confront environmental problems.

Rapid population (Fig. 2) **and industrial growth** with associated pollution and resource exhaustion are precipitating a global disaster. Increased life expectancy has resulted from higher living and social standards, public health measures, education and biomedical advances. Recently, this has been achieved by the education of young women and family planning. However, this success is pushing us towards a global population of 11 billion by 2100. We must face-up to the resulting tropical forest destruction, soil erosion, water and air pollution and global re-warming. We can no longer reign supreme over the environment thinking that technology and science will fix the problems.

ENVIRONMENT PROBLEMS	
Effect	**Result**
Urban air pollution	Caused by oxides of sulphur and nitrogen, Carbon monoxide (CO), particulates and metals, secondary formation of acids and ozone. Greater incidence of heart and respiratory illness.
Drinking water pollution	Chemicals such as nitrates, nitrites, metals, pesticides and radioactive products. The wars of the 21st century will be fought over this scarce resource.
Food contamination	Pesticide, carcinogens, radioactive fall-out, PCB's, heavy metals.
Adverse working environments	
Nuclear weaponry	Plutonium (carcinogen/teratogen/mutagen) is now incorporated into all living organisms.
Wars	Biological/chemical/nuclear agents have devastated ecosystems.
Loss of ozone and hazards	Skin cancer, cataracts, plant toxicity, increased UV radiation
Climatic changes	Global re-warming will increase vector-borne disease (malaria, schistosomiasis, Ebola virus). Heat stress in major cities. Starvation and injury from droughts, floods and storms.
Uncontrolled population growth (Fig. 2)	Reaching 10 billion by 2050 and possibly 11 billion by 2100 we will be responsible for 80% of the world's deforestation and eventual exhaustion of food supplies.
Unnatural rates of extinctions	*Homo sapiens* has been here for 100,000 years but is causing extinction of other life-forms at a rate of 1000 times the natural rate.
Deforestation	Causing rainfall to drop and epidemics of infectious diseases as vectors leave their natural hosts in the destroyed forests and move on to man (eg. in malaria).
Failure of Modern City	Urban homelessness/poverty/underclass/collapse of public health infrastructure. Old diseases (Tuberculosis, bubonic plague, malaria) re-emerge.

Figure 1 – The environmental problems facing us and about to destroy us

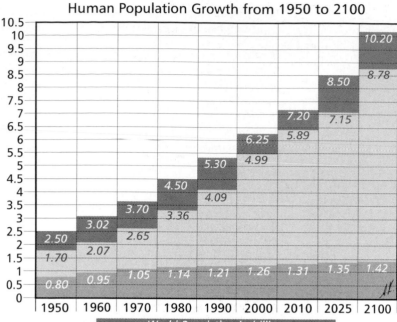

Figure 2 – The world population is growing to unsustainable levels

Recent civilisation (last 50-150 years) has led to the **Modern City** - with its dense urban population, homelessness, poverty and the creation of an unhealthy "underclass" from the rapid movement between countries and the collapse of public health infrastructure. The 'Big City' is merely a military citadel (creating an urban hell within) and squandering vital resources. The "top" echelons are well but the "underclass" are as sick as the Irish city dwellers of the 1830s and not much better off than the hunter-food gatherers of the Stone Age.

The old diseases have re-emerged; tuberculosis is at the highest rate in history (one-third of the world's population), the bubonic plague is present in major US cities and an extra 50 to 80 million cases of malaria are expected each year.

Just as the Battle of Waterloo was won on the playing fields of Eton so might the problems of the environment be solved at Olympia. Perhaps not entirely unre-

alistic. After all, the Olympic Games are the highlight of sport and are dedicated to idealism and the Glory of Zeus, (**the mind, body and spirit of man**). Baron Pierre de Coubertin said "The Olympic movement tends to bring together in a radiant union all the qualities which guide mankind to perfection". Athletes, their trainers and health carers and their spectators should care about not only their bodies but their environs. There seems little sense in a perfect performance in a planetary junk-yard (Fig. 3). The culture of sport needs a new creed.

THE CREED ...

for the athlete of the
next millennium will be:

- I will protect my body
- I will protect my environment

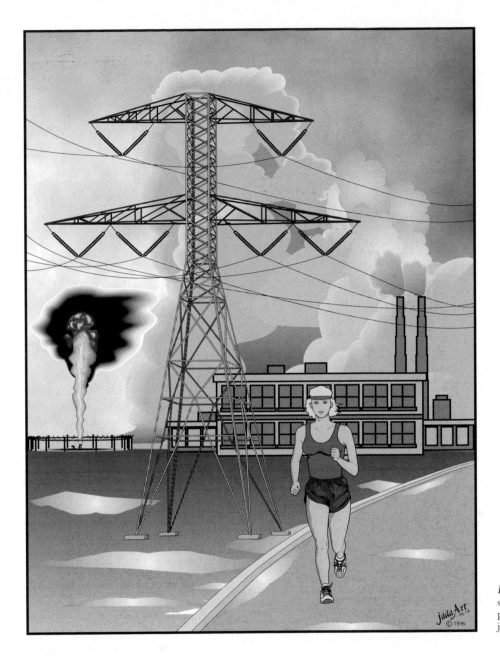

Figure 3 – There seems little sense in a perfect athletic performance in a planetary junk-yard

Protecting the body means not embarking on training schedules and techniques which have adverse health effects. Rigorous performance schedules for gymnastics and women's events may precipitate menstrual dysfunction and eating disorders with both short-term (malnutrition, starvation) and long-term (osteoporosis, hip and vertebral fractures) consequences. The dangers of blood doping and performance enhancement drugs are described in Chapter 4. Athletes using such drugs, especially steroids, are sacrificing their bodies for short-term achievements. The I.O.C. has rightly taken a hard stance on drugs in sport.

Protecting the environment means athletes and their associations insisting upon protection of their environment. If the purpose of sport (exercise) is to enhance our health (physically and intellectually), then it is irrational and dangerous to exercise in a polluted environment (the main determinant of our health status). Athletic events should only be staged in cities and countries with a commitment to safe and clean environments. The alternatives are clear.

The urban athlete inhales above average quantities of air pollutants (when respiratory minute volume increases up to 20 ×) which bypasses the nose (filter) with the open mouth (after R J Shephard, 1984).

There is: drying of the airways, possible cold/dry air induced bronchospasm, respiratory muscle fatigue and the toxic effect of pollutants. Such effects are maximal in marathons and road races (cycle/foot).

Air pollutants are either reducing or oxidant forms of smog. Reducing forms (carbon fuels) consist of smoke particulates, SO_2 or SO_3. These may induce bronchospasm with later respiratory infection and viral myocarditis, especially in children in big cities. Oxidant forms (vehicle exhausts with sunlight) are CO, hydrocarbons, ozone and nitrogen oxides. These agents affect athletic competition. CO may be lethal (cardiovascular death in elderly and possibly in the young athlete in competition). Swimming times are slower when levels exceed 30 ppm (parts per million). Ozone and nitrogen oxides impair the respiratory system. Competitive cyclists on open roads absorb lead emitted from cars which increases with training. Similarly, amateur cyclists suffer airway irritation from ozone.

Team doctors have been required to advise on accommodation in smog ridden cities, identify congested roads for athletes to avoid (80% of CO comes from cars; pollutants concentrate in tunnels). Training has been curtailed when ozone levels are high. Whether adaptation to pollutants occurs and is desirable is debatable.

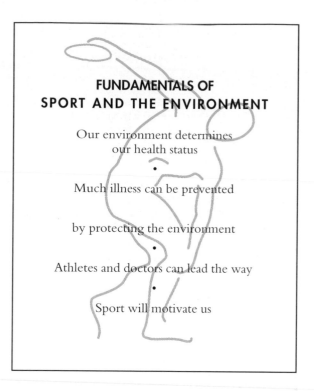

FUNDAMENTALS OF SPORT AND THE ENVIRONMENT

Our environment determines
our health status

•

Much illness can be prevented

by protecting the environment

•

Athletes and doctors can lead the way

•

Sport will motivate us

There must be an awareness of the need for ecological compatibility of athletic performance with the environment in which they are competing. Future Olympic Games such as **the Sydney 2000 Games** are being planned with this in mind. **"Greening-up for the Games"** means these Games are being staged in sympathy with the needs and protection of the environment (Fig. 4). The construction of the Olympic Stadium at Homebush Bay (a 760 hectare site of saltmarsh and wetlands which was previously an industrial dump) has provided the impetus for the biggest and perhaps the "greenest" single urban remediation. This has involved the preservation of a number of valuable animal (the rare green and golden bell frog) and plant species. Engineers have constructed a system of sub-surface drains to collect leechate from contaminated materials to send (isolated from the natural habitats) to treatment areas.

The development of the facilities is being based on the principles adopted at the 1992 United Nations Earth Summit. These 2000 Games are being held with a commitment to energy and water conservation, waste minimisation, air, water and soil quality and protection of cultural and natural environments. In particular, it is intended to use passive solar building design, collect wastewater for recycling and protect natural nearby ecosystems.

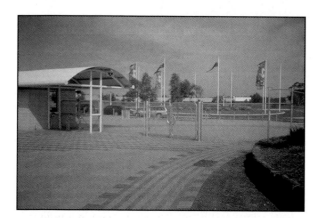

Figure 4 – The Sydney 2000 Olympic site under construction

Precious resources should not be squandered. It is important to avoid constructing huge Olympic monuments to excess and waste with a legacy of poor future usage and a financial burden for coming generations (Montreal 1976) nor to dangerous Political Ideologies (Nazism in Berlin 1936; Communism post-1956, Commercialism in the 1990s). Jack Lovelock (NZ) single-mindedly won the glamour event of the 1500 m in Berlin 1936, blithely unaware of the Nazi funfare about him (Fig. 5).

The Medic-O-Games (Medical Olympics) – Inaugural meeting in Sydney 1998 will provide a forum for medical doctors to discuss the health and environment problems facing us over the next millennium and to participate in Olympic sporting events themselves. It's aim is to harness the Olympic spirit to restore idealism to the practice of medicine. Doctors and sports medicine specialists need to be aware of the impact of an (adverse) environment on health and their athletes. They need to know how to detect and diagnose environmentally related problems, identify environmental hazards and appropriately advise patients/athletes. Physicians in the USA are joining the US Environmental Protection Agency in the desire to preserve the environment and promote global health.

It is a new concept of harnessing the Olympic Spirit which should establish an environmental model for the next century.

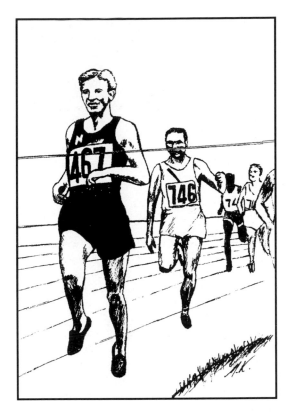

Figure 5 – Jack Lovelock (NZ) winning the 1500 m in Berlin (1936).

4

THE ENVIRONMENT AND SPORT, MEDICAL PROBLEMS, DRUGS IN SPORT

Donald Kuah
Carolyn Broderick
Mark Freeman

THE ENVIRONMENT AND SPORT

Donald Kuah

INTRODUCTION

This chapter will discuss various medical issues involving environmental effects on the sportsperson. Many of these are potentially serious but may often be prevented by adequate preparation, anticipation and education.

TEMPERATURE EXTREMES
(HEAT ILLNESSES, COLD ILLNESSES)

An understanding of thermoregulatory factors is important in discussing this topic. Thermoregulation in the human body results from reflex responses from various temperature receptors in the skin, central vessels, viscera, and anterior hypothalamus, signalling sympathetic shunting of blood and sweat gland stimulation.

The body attempts to maintain its core temperature between the normal range of 36.1 to 37.8 °C by a balance between heat production or gain and heat loss. Heat is produced in the body by metabolic functions and work done by muscles (smooth and skeletal). Heat is also exchanged with the environment by the following avenues (Fig. 1): radiation, evaporation, convection and conduction.

The Wet Bulb Globe Temperature (WBGT) takes into account air temperature, solar and ground radiation, humidity and wind velocity. The American College of Sports Medicine in 1984 recommended that endurance events were unsafe to be held if the WBGT >28 °C

HEAT ILLNESSES

These are a group of clinical presentations due to increased core temperatures which are generally classified into mild, moderate or severe (Fig. 2). There is an increased risk in children and female athletes (where prolonged exercise in the luteal phase).

Mild: This is clinically manifested by one or any combination of heat fatigue, cramps or syncope. Symptoms of weakness, fatigue and muscle cramps often occur during exercise, whereas fainting or

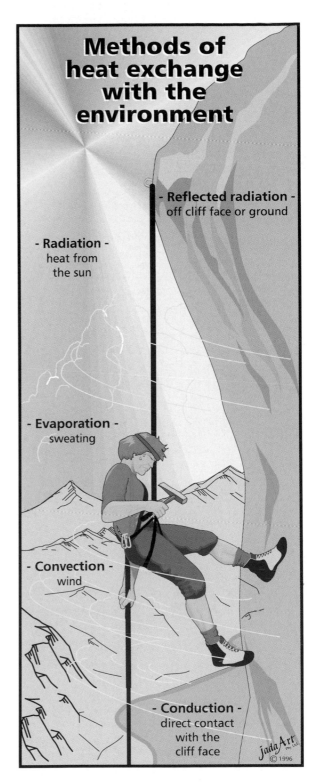

Figure 1 – Methods of heat exchange with environment (Radiation/Evaporation/Convection/Conduction)

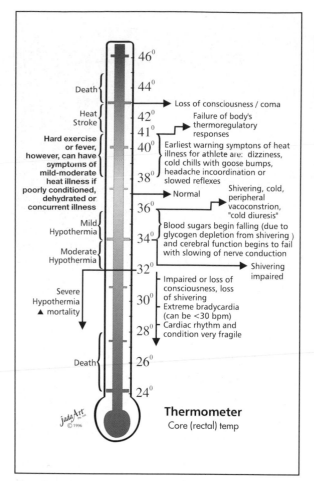

Figure 2 – Approximate core temperatures related to symptoms and sign of heat and cold illness

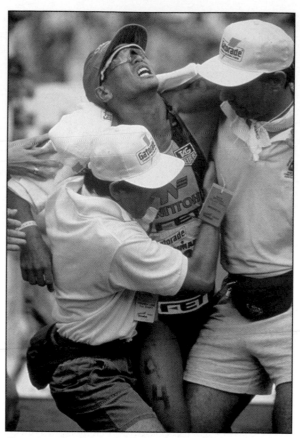

Figure 3 – Syncope at end of a race. Usually postural hypotension but made worse in presence of dehydration and heat illness

dizziness usually occurs at the end of exercise (Fig. 3), when venous blood pools in legs. Signs are of muscle tightness or spasm. Also postural hypotension and tachycardia.

Treatment: Rest, ice and massage cramps. Oral fluids. Lie in cool area and elevate legs if syncope. Remove excess clothing.

Moderate: Commonly described as heat exhaustion. Athlete usually suffers from headache, weakness, exhaustion, nausea, vomiting, ataxia and mild confusion. Examination reveals increased sweating, hypotension (especially postural) and tachycardia. Raised core temperature is present but its significance is doubtful since well marathon runners can have temperatures up to 41 °C. However, rectal temperature should be used to monitor athlete status and to rule out heat stroke.

Treatment: Measures as for mild, as well as ice packs to groin and axillae and possibly intravenous fluids.

Severe: Commonly known as heat stroke (core temp >41°C). Collapse with impaired consciousness owing to exercise. Clinical picture may be masked by having hot, dry skin or cold and sweaty skin (therefore always take rectal temperature).

Treatment: Rapid cooling and intravenous fluids. Transfer to nearest hospital as this is a medical emergency with potentially life threatening multi-organ complications.

PATHOPHYSIOLOGY AND COMPLICATIONS

In severe heat illness, a chain of events commonly occurs:

> Heat injury ➡ gut ischaemia ➡ endotoxins enter portal circulation ➡ hepatic clearance overwhelmed ➡ cytokine release

Dehydration and cytokines both contribute to hypotension and other complications.

Complications of severe heat illness include:

- **Cardiac**   Postural hypotension, myocardial infarction, and cardiac failure.

- **Neurological** Convulsions, cerebro-vascular events and coma.

- **Abdominal**   Gastrointestinal bleeding, liver damage and renal failure.

- **Other**   Rhabdomyolysis or breakdown of skeletal muscle membrane. This results in toxic metabolites such as myoglobin which may lead to renal failure. Present with myoglobinuria (brown urine) and raised serum phosphokinase and potassium. An associated disseminated intravascular coagulation may also develop.

PREVENTION

- Wear appropriate cool, light coloured clothing

- Stay well hydrated before, during and after exercise (Fig. 4).

- Adequate physical fitness preparation for sport/event/conditions. This may include heat acclimatisation. The physiological adjustments in increased blood volume, venous tone and especially sweating, seen during acclimatisation usually require two weeks to take effect (although this is variable).

- Avoid exercise in extreme heat (and humidity). At-risk events and sports should have guidelines under medical advice.

- Avoid exercising with intercurrent illness.

- Adequate planning such as fluids, sunscreen and medical or first aid cover.

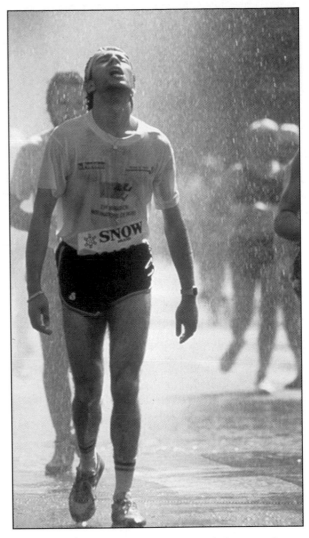

Figure 4 – Cooling and hydration is important during a marathon

- Education of early signs of heat illnesses.

Hyponatraemia -   Can cause collapse associated with exercise in heat and is commonly mistaken for heat stroke. Usually only seen in ultra-endurance events (>34 hours) and is thought to be caused by fluid overload from hypotonic drinks.

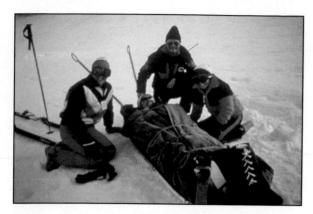

Figure 5 – Injuries in snow or water sports are especially at risk of hypothermia

COLD ILLNESSES

These include various degrees of hypothermia and frostbite. Those involved in snow, adventure, and mountaineering sports are particularly at risk (Fig. 5) as are endurance events held in cold temperatures Hypothermia can be classified into mild, moderate or severe and their clinical features vary accordingly (Fig. 2):

Mild: Core temp (34-36°C). Athlete usually displays cold extremities, shivering, tachycardia, tachypnoea, urinary urgency, and slight incoordination.

Moderate: Core temp (32-34°C). Blood sugars begin to fall and cerebral function begins to fail at 35°C, with unsteadiness, muscle weakness, cramps and decreased coordination. If warmth, shelter and food are found at this stage, recovery is rapid. However, if exposure to the cold continues, a failure of shivering and a loss of vasoconstrictor tone results in an accelerating loss of temperature control. Speech becomes slurred, fatigue, dehydration, amnesia, poor judgement, drowsiness, anxiety and irritability takes place.

Severe: Core temp (<32°C). There is significant mortality with total loss of shivering, inappropriate behaviour, impaired or loss of consciousness, muscle rigidity, hypotension, pulmonary oedema, extreme bradycardia, and cardiac arrhythmias (especially ventricular fibrillation).

Treatment: Measurement of rectal temperature is essential in assessing the severity of hypothermia and in monitoring of status. The general principles of treatment involve basic life-support measures (such as

fluids, nutrition, and cardiac support), minimising further heat loss, re-warming, treatment of other injuries and transportation. It is a flawed presumption that voluntary activity increases body heat. Instead, movement increases peripheral blood flow, pumping air/water through the body to replace the warmer film around the body surface, and increases body surface area exposure to the surrounding elements, resulting in increased heat loss and body heat requirements.

Re-warming may be:

a) **passive** – insulation from wet, wind and cold. Removal of wet clothing and drying the body (even in dry snow!). Allowing the body to gradually re-warm by its **own** metabolic heat.

b) **external active** – hot packs and baths, electric blankets, another body are examples (Fig. 6).

   Caution should be exercised in severe cases where shift of already reduced fluid volume to a warmed periphery may cause hypotension and a cardiac event.

c) **internal active** – warm drinks or food are reasonable simple measures. However, haemodialysis, airway warming or warm intravenous infusion should be left for a hospital setting where close monitoring can occur.

FROSTBITE

Frostbite is a local destruction of superficial tissues caused by cold exposure (commonly toes, fingers, ears). This is classified into (Fig. 7): Frost nip, superficial, deep frostbite.

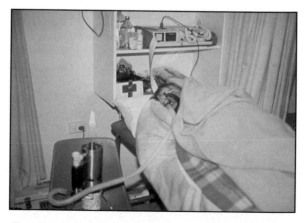

Figure 6 – External active heating is appropriate treatment for mild hypothermia; inhalation re-warming also demostrated

Treatment: Local re-warming, analgesia, protection (with blanket cotton wool) and gentle handling. Avoid rubbing area or applying snow and watch for secondary vascular occlusion by oedema, gangrene and infection (Fig. 9).

COLD URTICARIA

This is a disorder in which patients exposed to cold similarly develop urticarial eruptions which may evolve into angio-oedema. This may be associated, in severe cases, with hypotension and syncope. It is a chiefly mast cell mediated, IgE dependent disorder, although cryoglobulins and cold agglutinins may be recognised in the blood. The urticaria may affect only the exposed limb. Previous asymptomatic exposure to cold stimuli does not exclude cold urticaria.

Treatment is by re-warming, antihistamines and sympatheticomimetic agents if severe (Fig. 10).

ALTITUDE MEDICINE

Various distinct medical problems are encountered in sport at high altitudes. These are made worse with rapid ascent (Fig. 12). Performances at high altitudes are affected positively by reduced wind resistance and gravity, and negatively by the reduced oxygen concentration (Fig. 13). Also, dropping temperatures can have an effect on performances (temperatures reduce by about 2 °C for every additional 300m above sea level).

A resolution was made at the 20th World Congress of Sports Medicine (Melbourne 1974) urging extreme caution at altitudes of more than 2290m (8700ft) and

FROSTBITE TYPES	
• Frost nip	incipient frostbite with sudden blanching of skin and is painless
• Superficial	skin place, waxy and firm but not frozen (Fig. 8)
• Deep frostbite	cold, pale, solid, fragile tissue

Figure 7

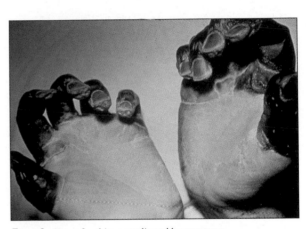

Figure 9 – Deep frostbite complicated by gangrene

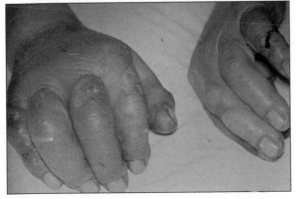

Figure 8 – Superficial frostbite following re-vascularisation of fingers

PREVENTION OF COLD ILLNESSES
• Adequate preparation, including clothing, communication, equipment, weather forecasts (Fig. 11).
• Keep well hydrated and nourished.
• Avoid exercising to exhaustion.
• Appropriate fitness level for proposed activity including cold and altitude acclimatisation if indicated (NB. Cold acclimatisation is less effective than heat acclimatisation).

Figure 10

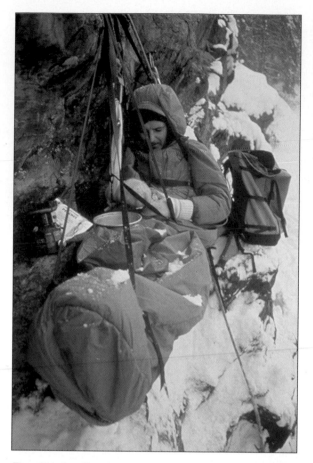

Figure 11 – A well-equipped and prepared mountaineer can combat the elements and prevent hypothermia

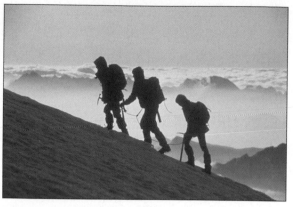

Figure 12 – Mountain climbers are more susceptible to altitude illnesses with rapid ascents. Modern day climbers (unfortunately) are able to be flown to base camps

an absolute prohibition of contests above 3050m (10000ft). Various adaptations occur over varying time frames at altitude, including a reduction in bicarbonate, an increase in haemoglobin levels, a restoration of blood volume and an increase in various tissue enzymes. Illnesses encountered at altitudes include the following:

Mountain sickness

Non-specific symptoms such as headache, dizziness, nausea, vomiting, irritability and insomnia are a result of the hyperventilation and associated acid-base disturbances. This is usually a temporary condition affecting the first 2 or 3 days of a rapid ascent over 2000m. Symptomatic treatment is usually sufficient although in severe cases return to lower altitudes is advisable and the use of acetazolamide may help (beware diuretic effect on plasma volume).

Pulmonary oedema

This is a life threatening condition occurring in the first few days of an ascent and manifests with symptoms of dyspnoea, blood-stained frothy sputum, coughing, and chest discomfort. It is more common in people with intercurrent cardio-respiratory conditions. Treatment includes rest, oxygen, diuretic and return to a lower altitude.

Cerebral oedema

This is a rare condition which may result in headaches, confusion, hallucination, impaired consciousness or coma. It is usually associated with rapid ascents above 4000m. Treatment is again urgent. Return to low altitude, oxygen and intravenous corticosteroids.

Retinal pathology

Small retinal haemorrhages which are mainly benign may occur above altitudes of 4000m. However, visual impairment can occur with central scotomata and impaired colour vision.

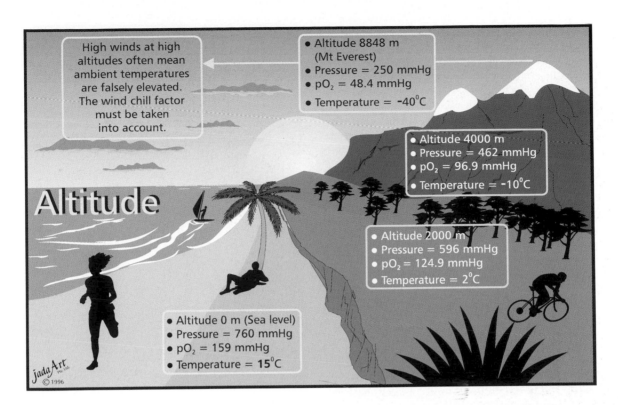

Figure 13 – Oxygen concentrations, atmospheric pressures and ambient temperatures at various altitudes

PREVENTION OF ALTITUDE ILLNESS

- Avoid rapid ascents

- Altitude acclimatisation (Fig. 15). Approximately 3 weeks at a moderate altitude (2500 - 3000m)

- Appropriate medical screening

- Education of participants about early symptoms, signs and management of altitude illnesses

Figure 14 – Prevention is possible and essential

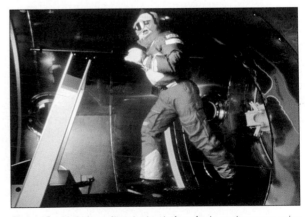

Figure 15 – Altitude acclimatisation in hypobaric environment prior to an attempt on Mount Everest

UNDERWATER MEDICINE

The sport of **scuba** (self contained underwater breathing apparatus) diving has had a rapid growth in popularity over the last 20 years. Whilst the injury rate is surprisingly low, there are a disproportionate number of serious and fatal incidents from diving (Fig. 16). A basic understanding of the physics of the underwater environment is required to consider the medical problems in diving.

PHYSICS

In the ocean, pressure increases by one atmosphere with each 10 metre increase in depth and results in gas filled spaces undergoing their greatest volume changes near the surface. Boyle's law states that at constant temperature, the volume of the gas decreases proportionately to the absolute pressure (Fig. 17). This relates to the various sites of barotrauma that can result from a rapid ascent.

Henry's law states that at a constant temperature, the amount of gas dissolved in a liquid is proportional to the partial pressure of the gas over the liquid. A good model of this law and it's implications to decompression sickness is demonstrated when a carbonated bottle of drink is opened, reducing the pressure and allowing gas previously dissolved in the drink to form gas bubbles.

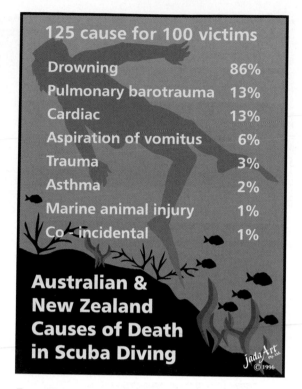

125 cause for 100 victims	
Drowning	86%
Pulmonary barotrauma	13%
Cardiac	13%
Aspiration of vomitus	6%
Trauma	3%
Asthma	2%
Marine animal injury	1%
Co - incidental	1%

Australian & New Zealand Causes of Death in Scuba Diving

Figure 16 – Causes of death in diving accidents. Many of the "drowning" deaths are thought to be due to arterial gas embolism or nitrogen narcosis

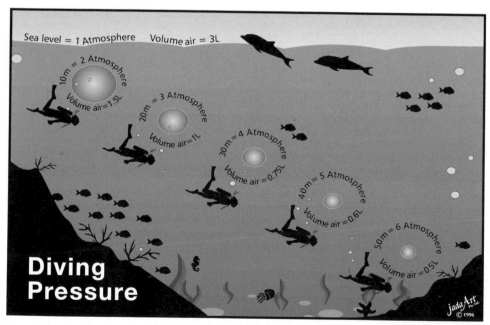

Sea level = 1 Atmosphere   Volume air = 3L

10m = 2 Atmosphere   Volume air = 1.5L

20m = 3 Atmosphere   Volume air = 1L

30m = 4 Atmosphere   Volume air = 0.75L

40m = 5 Atmosphere   Volume air = 0.6L

50m = 6 Atmosphere   Volume air = 0.5L

Diving Pressure

Figure 17

BAROTRAUMA

Barotrauma (BT) can affect any gas filled space in the body and refers to injuries caused by pressure imbalances between gas spaces in the body and adjacent body tissues or fluids.

• Middle Ear BT (or "Squeeze")

This is the commonest form of BT and may be caused by inability to equalise middle ear pressures via the Eustachian tube usually during descent. This results in marked negative pressure in the middle ear, bleeding oedema and possible tympanic membrane rupture. All cases require audiograms - management involves analgesia, decongestants and antibiotics.

• Inner Ear BT

Middle ear BT may occasionally have an effect on the inner ear, causing vertigo and tinnitus. This is usually from rupture of the round window. The patient should be rested sitting up in bed and should avoid increasing intracranial pressure (e.g. coughing). Urgent ENT review is mandatory.

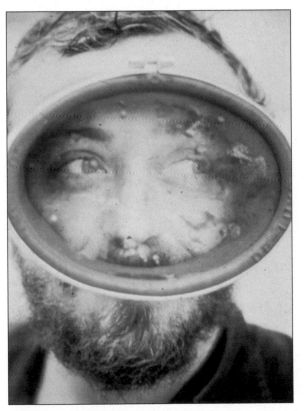

Figure 18 – Sinus barotrauma with blood in the mask

• Sinus BT

This commonly presents as blood in the face mask (Fig. 18) and pain but is usually not serious. Symptomatic relief from a nasal decongestant may be used.

• Pulmonary BT

This is a common cause of diving deaths and is encountered after rapid or uncontrolled ascent (without exhaling) or conditions causing air trapping (e.g. asthma). Various forms include arterial gas embolism (AGE), pneumothorax, surgical emphysema or pulmonary infarcts. The most serious complication is cerebral arterial gas embolism or CAGE, where gas bubbles escape from ruptured alveoli into the circulation and migrate to the brain. CAGE must be suspected in any neurological presentation and is probably the true cause of death in many drownings. Symptoms ranging from headache, confusion through to unconsciousness usually present within 5 min of ascent. Patients should be administered 100% oxygen and be nursed horizontally (to avoid further bubbles migrating to the brain). Stabilisation of pneumothorax if present and urgent recompression are the definitive treatments.

• Face Mask Squeeze

This benign condition results from reducing pressure in the face mask during descent due to failure of the diver to equalise the pressure in the mask. There is oedema of the face, sub-conjunctional haemorrhage or petechiae and occasionally temporary blindness.

DECOMPRESSION SICKNESS (DCS)

DCS (also known as the 'bends' or 'caisson disease') involves a wide variety of multi-organ conditions as a result of previously dissolved nitrogen forming bubbles in the tissues of bloodstream of the body during ascent (this follows Henry's law). The longer and deeper a dive, the more nitrogen that is forced into solution within the body. The symptoms and signs of DCS usually occur within the first 24 hours following ascent. Decompression stops during ascent are designed to allow the diver to expel extra gas from the tissues before bubble formation.

The most common presentation of DCS is persisting lethargy, general malaise and musculoskeletal pain. It is important to note that any or all types of DCS can co-exist (Fig. 19) including:

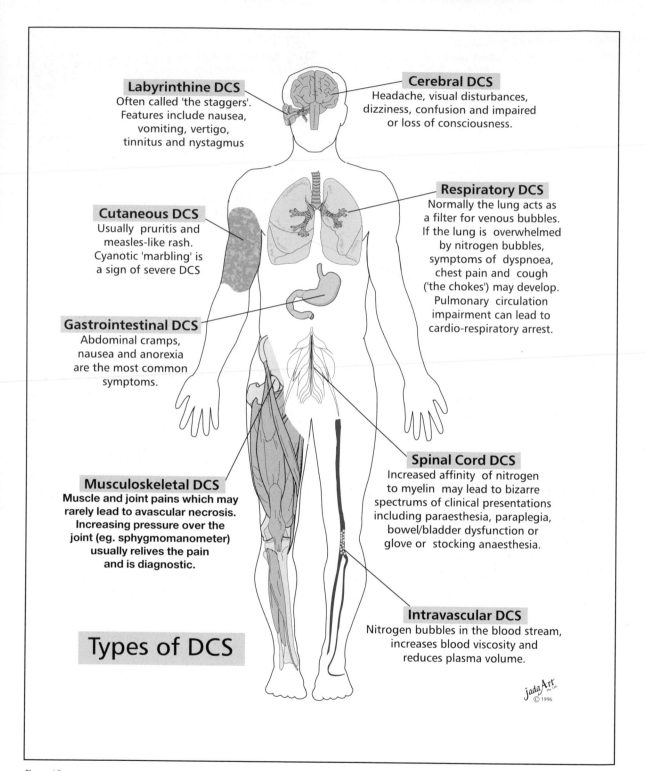

Labyrinthine DCS
Often called 'the staggers'.
Features include nausea,
vomiting, vertigo,
tinnitus and nystagmus

Cerebral DCS
Headache, visual disturbances,
dizziness, confusion and impaired
or loss of consciousness.

Cutaneous DCS
Usually pruritis and
measles-like rash.
Cyanotic 'marbling' is
a sign of severe DCS

Respiratory DCS
Normally the lung acts as
a filter for venous bubbles.
If the lung is overwhelmed
by nitrogen bubbles,
symptoms of dyspnoea,
chest pain and cough
('the chokes') may develop.
Pulmonary circulation
impairment can lead to
cardio-respiratory arrest.

Gastrointestinal DCS
Abdominal cramps,
nausea and anorexia
are the most common
symptoms.

Spinal Cord DCS
Increased affinity of nitrogen
to myelin may lead to bizarre
spectrums of clinical presentations
including paraesthesia, paraplegia,
bowel/bladder dysfunction or
glove or stocking anaesthesia.

Musculoskeletal DCS
Muscle and joint pains which may
rarely lead to avascular necrosis.
Increasing pressure over the
joint (eg. sphygmomanometer)
usually relives the pain
and is diagnostic.

Intravascular DCS
Nitrogen bubbles in the blood stream,
increases blood viscosity and
reduces plasma volume.

Types of DCS

jadaArt
© 1996

Figure 19 – Various clinical presentations of decompression sickness

- Musculoskeletal
- Intravascular
- Neurological – spinal
              – cerebral
- Labyrinthine ("Staggers")
- Respiratory ("Chokes")
- Cutaneous
- Gastrointestinal

Remember that many of these presentations **may be bizarre and life threatening,** but the common link is the history of a recent dive (Fig. 20).

Treatment: Early treatment can reverse even severe symptoms and signs of DCS and involves 100% oxygen, intravenous fluids, and horizontal, appropriate transport of the patient to a hyperbaric recompression chamber (Figs. 21 & 22).

Nitrogen Narcosis

This is often labelled "rapture of the deep" and usually occurs only at depths exceeding 30 metres. The increasing exposure to nitrogen leads to an anaesthetic effect and may mimic alcoholic intoxication. Symptoms may include euphoria, terror, poor judgement, slowed reflexes and reduced mental alertness. Treatment is gradual ascent.

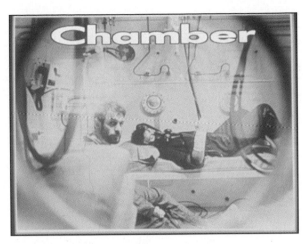

Figure 21 – Patient undergoing recompression in hyperbaric chamber

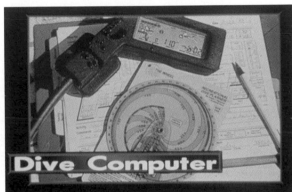

Figure 22 – A dive computer is part of the essential safety equipment in scuba diving

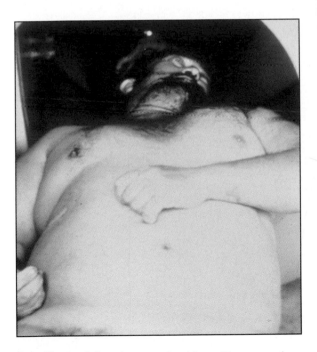

Figure 20 – Death from decompression sickness. Note gross oedema and rash

---

PREVENTION OF DIVING ACCIDENTS

- Adequate medical screening, including spirometry and audiograms.
- Appropriate training and certification.
- Strict adherence to safety procedures.
- Current safety equipment regularly checked (Fig. 22).
- Avoid diving after alcohol /drug use.
- Avoid airplane travel 24 hours after previous dive.
- Awareness and recognition of early symptoms and signs.

Figure 23

MEDICAL PROBLEMS IN SPORT

Carolyn Broderick

INTRODUCTION

While most of the focus in sports medicine is on the assessment and treatment of musculoskeletal injuries, sports people will often present to their medical practitioners with medical complaints, brought on or exacerbated by exercise. Management of a sporting population requires some knowledge of these conditions and their management. It is important to consider pre-existing conditions prior to sport participation (Fig. 24) and to perform a pre-participation assessment (Fig. 25).

Pre-participation examinations are becoming increasingly required at various levels of sporting activity.

PRE-PARTICIPATION SPORTS SPECIFIC EXAMINATION
Developmental Age
• Presence (extent) facial/axillary/pubic hair
Health History
• Chronic illness/hospital care/dental appliances/ past injury/psychological problems/tetanus status
Examination
• Height/weight/BP/P/vision
• ENT/chest/CVS/GI/GU/spine/musculo skeletal assessment
• Urine analysis/Hb/vaccination status
Clearance for
• Collision/contact/endurance/leisure-sports subgroups

Figure 24

PRE-EXISTING CONDITIONS AND SPORT PARTICIPATION		
	Contact Sport*	**Non-Contact Sport****
Carditis	No	No
Hypertension	Yes (after specialist evaluation)	Yes
Acute viral illness		No, until careful individual assessment
Detached retina		Ophthalmic review
Loss of eye		Use eye protection/ ophthalmic review
One kidney present	No	Yes
Epilepsy	Only when well controlled for 12 months	
Diabetes	Only when well controlled	Yes
History of head/neck injuries	No	Yes
Asthma	Yes	Yes
Enlarged spleen	No	Yes
Enlarged liver	No	Yes
Atlanto axial instability	No	Yes (not strenuous)

* contact sports (e.g. boxing, football, ice hockey, skiing, volleyball i.e. contact with another athlete or surface)
** non-contact (e.g. aerobics, track and field, table tennis, archery)

Figure 25

Although reasonable for children/adolescents, older athletes and disabled athletes there is no clear evidence of the effectiveness of screening on the overall incidence of injury. A sports-specific examination would seem reasonable and cost effective (Fig. 25). Following this, exercise stress testing may be indicated (when > 40 years age; 2 or more major risk factors present or confirmed disease), consider disability and pathology then devise an exercise prescription (based on the concept of METS, see Chapter 19).

RESPIRATORY CONDITIONS

EXERCISE-INDUCED ASTHMA

Presentation

The most common respiratory condition seen in the exercising person is exercise-induced asthma (EIA). It is characterised by shortness of breath, cough or wheeze which comes on with, or immediately following, a bout of moderately intense exercise. It is classically worse in cold, dry conditions and the sufferer often gives a family history of asthma or atopy.

Aetiology

It may be caused by drying of the airways (as in cold, dry air) which causes hyperosmolarity of the epithelial fluid. This results in the release of inflammatory mediators such as histamine and leukotrienes which produce bronchospasm. This "airway drying" theory would explain why sports such as cycling, running and cross-country skiing are more likely to produce EIA than those performed in higher humidity such as swimming. It is for this reason that many asthmatics take up swimming and that a not inconsiderable number of current elite swimmers are asthmatics.

Refractory Period

The symptoms of exercise-induced asthma classically come on after about five min of moderate or intense exercise. In sprinters the symptoms are often worse following a race than during it. About 50% of all people who suffer from EIA have a "refractory period" during which a further episode of bronchoconstriction cannot be provoked. This lasts for about one hour. Many athletes make use of this refractory period prior to competition. This is best done by performing a vigorous warm-up 15-20 minutes prior to competition. Bronchoconstriction occurring at this time can be treated and the athlete (if one of the lucky 50%) is then assured of being symptom-free for the following hour.

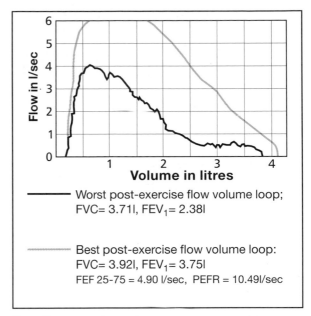

Figure 26 – Graph of flow/volume curve EIA vs Normal (From T.A. Kaplan, *The Physician and Sports Med. 23;8: pp54).*

Diagnosis

Diagnosis is from the history. Physical examination between episodes will usually be unremarkable. Simple confirmatory tests can be done in the office with spirometry equipment (Fig. 26). The subject's FEV1 and peak flow are measured pre- and post-exercise to see if there is any fall. A fall of greater than 15% of FEV1 suggests EIA. This should be reversible with bronchodilators. More detailed investigations should be performed in those whose symptoms are difficult to reproduce or are less classical. A hyperventilation challenge test is a very sensitive indicator of EIA. In this situation large volumes of dry air are inspired (consistent or greater than those volumes inspired during maximal exercise). Changes in FEV1 and response to bronchodilators are recorded. A negative hyperventilation challenge test makes the diagnosis of EIA very unlikely.

Management

Management of EIA in the past has focused on relief of symptoms with the use of bronchodilators. It is not uncommon at half-time in football matches to see many players in the team using puffers. Current treatment protocols however are largely aimed at prevention. These include:

- avoid exercise in cold, dry air where possible (cover face with scarf on long, early morning cycling trips).

- make use of the refractory period.

- use preventative medications (inhaled corticosteroids, sodium cromoglycate and nedocromil sodium to reduce the hyperactivity of the airways. Inhaled beta agonists can also be used prior to exercise).

EXERCISE-INDUCED URTICARIA/ANAPHYLAXIS

This was described in 1979, with the clinical features ranging from skin warmth, flushing and pruritis to urticaria, angio-oedema, laryngeal oedema, bronchospasm and hypotension. To date, there have been no reported deaths associated with exercise-induced anaphylaxis.

CHARACTERISTICS OF EXERCISE-INDUCED URTICARIA/ANAPHYLAXIS

There is a strong correlation between this condition and atopy. It classically occurs with exercise of moderate intensity and females are affected more than males in a ratio of 2:1. In some instances there are family clusters. Jogging is the activity most commonly associated with exercise-induced anaphylaxis. A number of co-precipitating factors have been identified. These include exercise with heat, cold, humidity, following certain foods, alcohol and medications.

Treatment

Treatment of the **acute episode** is the same as that for anaphylaxis of other origins and includes airways maintenance, circulatory support and the use of adrenaline. Prevention of **recurrent episodes** involves avoidance of any known co-precipitating factors or avoidance of vigorous exercise if symptoms warrant. Use of prophylactic non-sedating antihistamines has been successful in preventing symptoms. Cromolyn has also been used with success prior to exercise.

GASTROINTESTINAL CONDITIONS

Gastrointestinal complaints in sport are common, particularly in endurance exercise. The most common gastrointestinal complaints include nausea, vomiting, diarrhoea, cramps and gastrointestinal bleeding. To

understand this it is necessary to review the redistribution of blood flow which occurs with exercise.

SPLANCHNIC BLOOD FLOW DURING EXERCISE

During exercise, blood is shunted from the splanchnic circulation to the exercising muscles. The degree to which this occurs depends on the intensity and duration of the exercise. In severe endurance exercise, blood flow to the abdominal organs can be reduced as much as 80%. Although there is an increase in the oxygen extraction by these organs during this time, it does not compensate for the marked reduction in blood flow. Dehydration will further compromise splanchnic blood flow to the abdominal organs because more efficient oxygen usage in the exercising muscles, and a higher cardiac output, means less shunting of blood from the splanchnic circulation is required. Gut ischaemia is thought to produce some of the gastrointestinal symptoms we associate with endurance exercise.

CAUSES OF GASTROINTESTINAL SYMPTOMS

Certain factors contribute to the high frequency of gastrointestinal symptoms in endurance athletes (Fig. 27).

CAUSES OF GASTROINTESTINAL SYMPTOMS IN ENDURANCE ATHLETES

- Common use of NSAID
- Slow rate of gastric emptying with moderate and severe exercise
- Diet (often very high in fibre)
- pre-competition nerves

Figure 27

Nausea and vomiting occurring during or soon after exercise may be due to gut ischaemia, gastric erosions secondary to use of NSAID, or poor gastric emptying in combination with an inappropriate pre-event meal. High proportions of fat or protein in a meal prior to exercise will reduce the rate of gastric emptying as will high concentration carbohydrate drinks during exercise. If simple measures such as modification of the diet, avoidance of dehydration and use of antacids or

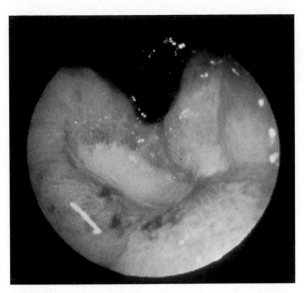

Figure 28 – Gastric erosion seen at endoscopy

H_2 antagonists do not improve these symptoms, further investigations such as an endoscopic examination are necessary (Fig. 28).

Abdominal cramps and diarrhoea are also common complaints. Here again, if simple measures such as ensuring good hydration, reducing the pre-exercise fibre intake and dealing with pre-competition nerves do not improve the symptoms, a more thorough investigation should be undertaken. Athletes are not immune from the gastrointestinal diseases that affect the sedentary population. Inflammatory bowel disease, infectious causes and bowel tumours need to be excluded.

GASTROINTESTINAL BLEEDING

Gastrointestinal bleeding (often occult) is common following events such as an Ironman Triathlon. The site of blood loss is most commonly the stomach and the most likely causes are gut ischaemia and gastric erosions secondary to the use of aspirin or NSAID. The mechanical effect of running on hard surfaces may also contribute to gastric blood loss. It is often difficult to determine how fully to investigate these athletes but if the preventative measures described above and withdrawal of non-steroidal anti-inflammatory medication does not resolve the bleeding, then endoscopic evaluation should be arranged to rule out other pathology.

CARDIAC CONDITIONS

Cardiac symptoms differ in their type and significance depending on the age of the exercising person. Symptoms of ischaemic heart disease such as chest pain and dyspnoea are not uncommon and should be thoroughly investigated in the over-35 athlete. Younger athletes, although less frequent, may also present with cardiac symptoms. The most common complaints in the under 30 age group include palpitations, dizziness and syncope. These may be benign and insignificant or they may be the only warning to suggest a person has a severe congenital cardiac defect. Sudden cardiac death (SCD) during sport, although rare, is particularly tragic. Many of these people have no previous warning signs but some have given a prior history of palpitations or dizziness or syncope. It is for this reason that these symptoms must be taken seriously.

PALPITATIONS

Palpitations are relatively frequent in athletes and resting ECGs commonly demonstrate frequent ectopic beats. These ectopic beats however should become less frequent, rather than more frequent with exercise. Any person who complains of palpitations with exercise should be investigated with an ECG and an exercise stress test. If symptoms cannot be reproduced during a stress test a 24 hour Holter monitor may be able to capture the rhythm. Treatment will depend on the nature of the arrhythmia, the frequency of symptoms and the presence of any underlying heart disease.

DIZZINESS AND SYNCOPE

Dizziness following exercise is not uncommon, especially if the athlete suddenly stops exercise when exercising upright. This causes blood to pool in the lower limbs and the cardiac output suddenly drops. Dizziness or actual syncope may result. It is more pronounced in hot weather when maximal skin vasodilation is present. To avoid this, runners and cyclists are best advised to continue slowly jogging or gently peddling following finishing an exercise bout, to avoid the sudden drop in venous return.

Dizziness or syncope during heavy exercise is a more sinister symptom. Anyone who reports syncope (after excluding dehydration) during exercise should undergo a full cardiac investigation including ECG, CXR (X-ray) and echocardiography to exclude a congenital cardiac defect such as hypertrophic cardiomyopathy (which is the most common cause of sudden cardiac death during exercise in the under 30 age group).

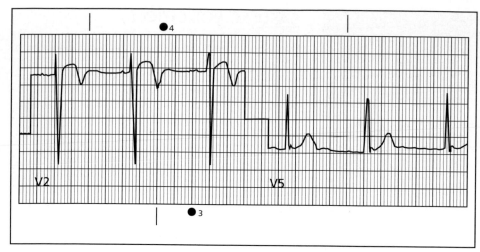

Figure 29 – ECG of athlete's heart characterised by sinus bradycardia, first degree AV block and tall QRS in praecordial leads (Ts may be inverted)

Dizziness or syncope during exercise in the older age group is more likely to represent an arrhythmia secondary to ischaemic heart disease. Also requires a thorough cardiac workup.

THE ATHLETE'S HEART

When interpreting the ECG of a person who has cardiac symptoms with exercise, it is important to be able to differentiate pathological changes from the ECG changes characteristically associated with the normal athlete's heart (Fig. 29). Changes in cardiac dimensions depend on the type of training undertaken. Resistance athletes (eg weight lifters) often demonstrate an increase in ventricular wall thickness whereas endurance athletes commonly display an increase in heart volume.

ECG CHANGES

Features of the ECG of an athlete's heart often include:

- voltage criteria for LVH (left ventricular hypertrophy)

- sinus bradycardia

- frequent premature ventricular contractions at rest

- prolonged PR interval (1st and 2nd degree heart block are common in athletes at rest). This should shorten with exercise.

- wandering atrial pacemaker

- non-specific ST segment and T wave changes.

SUDDEN CARDIAC DEATH

CAUSES

Sudden cardiac death (SCD) during sport is fortunately rare. The cause of SCD differs according to the athlete's age. In the **over 35** age group, coronary artery disease is easily the most common cause. In the younger age group (**less than 35**) congenital cardiac anomalies are the most common cause (hypertrophic cardiomyopathy, Marfan's syndrome and congenital coronary artery anomalies). Of the congenital cardiac abnormalities, hypertrophic cardiomyopathy is the most common cause of death in the younger age group.

HYPERTROPHIC CARDIOMYOPATHY

Pathology

Hypertrophic cardiomyopathy (HCM) is a congenital condition in which there is asymmetric hypertrophy involving the left ventricle and septum. In some people with HCM there is left ventricular outflow obstruction but the cause of death in this group is usually ventricular arrhythmias.

Clinical Features

These athletes will often give a history of dyspnoea, chest pain, palpitations and exertional syncope. There may also be a family history of sudden death with exertion. Physical examination if often unremarkable but may reveal a systolic murmur, louder with standing, in those with outflow obstruction. The ECG is often indistinguishable from that of the athlete's heart.

MARFAN'S SYNDROME	
CLINICAL FEATURES	
System	**Abnormalities**
• Cardiovascular	Weakness in aortic media causing dilation of aortic root and potential of dissecting aneurysm of proximal ascending aorta
• Musculoskeletal	Long fingers, pectus excavatum/pectus cavinatum, high arched palate, ligamentous laxity, increased length of tubular bones (arm span often greater than height)
• Eyes	Lens dislocation/subluxation

Figure 30

Diagnosis

Only about one-quarter of cases of HCM are diagnosed with physical examination, ECG and chest X-ray. The diagnosis is made with echocardiography and this reveals thickening of the septum (>15 mm) with the septum often >1.3 times the thickness of the free left ventricular wall. In patients with outflow obstruction, the echocardiogram will demonstrate systolic anterior motion of the mitral valve.

Treatment

Strenuous exercise should be avoided in all patients with HCM. Beta-blockers and calcium antagonists are often successful in relieving the symptoms of chest pain and palpitations but there is no evidence that they reduce the incidence of sudden death.

MARFAN'S SYNDROME

Marfan's syndrome, an autosomal dominant condition, is another cause of SCD in young athletes. The cause of death is aortic rupture or dissection. It is important when screening athletes pre-season to be on the look out for Marfanoid features because these people are well-suited to sports in which height is an advantage such as basketball, volleyball and high jumping (Fig. 30). Advice regarding exercise in athletes with Marfans syndrome should be individualised according to the presence of aortic changes. An echocardiogram should be performed to determine the presence of aortic root disease.

CORONARY ARTERY DISEASE

Coronary artery disease is the commonest cause of sudden cardiac death in the over 35 age group. Many athletes believe that because they are physically active they are immune from this condition. People in this age group complaining of exercise related dyspnoea, chest pain, palpitations or syncopal episodes should be investigated with an exercise stress test and thallium 201 scanning or coronary angiography if indicated.

HEADACHE

Headache is common amongst the sporting population. The majority of headaches suffered by athletes are of the same aetiology as those suffered by the general population (migraine, cluster headaches, viral illnesses, sinusitis and drug related causes). There are however a number of causes of headache which are more commonly seen in athletes (Fig. 31).

ATHLETES HEADACHE
• Benign exertional headache (especially in weight lifters)
• Post-traumatic headache (boxing and the football codes)
• "Exertional migraine"
• Cervicogenic headache (also seen in the non-sporting population)

Figure 31

THE HISTORY GIVES THE BEST CLUE AS TO THE CAUSE

Benign Exertional Headache

Benign exertional headache occurs following relatively intense exertion, commonly weight lifting and running. The cause of this type of headache is not known but it may be related to a disturbance in cerebrovascular autoregulation. The onset of headache is usually acute and severe but this lasts for only a short time (seconds or minutes) and is followed by a dull ache which may last for many hours. This headache occurs only with exercise and if it is recurrent it should be investigated due to the fact that **ten percent** of all so-called "benign exertional headaches" are associated with some form of intracranial pathology. NSAID have been used with some success in those without any obvious cause of their symptoms.

Post-traumatic Headache

Minor head injuries are common in contact sports (boxing and the football codes). Headache is almost universal following a concussive episode and may last for days or even weeks following a head injury. (Post-traumatic headache may even occur after trivial head traumas such as "heading" the ball in soccer). If headache persists following a minor head injury, a thorough neurological examination and a CT or MRI scan should be performed to rule out the possibility of a sub-dural haematoma or other cerebral bleed. The majority of these sports people, however, have no abnormality on imaging and are diagnosed as having "post-concussion syndrome", a condition in which symptoms such as headache, poor concentration, dizziness and fatigue persist for weeks following an episode of concussion (see Chapter 6).

Exertional Migraine

"Exertional migraine" presents as a classical or common migraine but usually occurs following relatively vigorous, often prolonged activity. It usually, but not always, occurs in subjects with a history of non-exertional migraine. The precipitating factor is thought to be hot weather and dehydration may play a role. The headache, as with classical migraine, is often preceded or accompanied by visual and sensory symptoms, nausea and vomiting. It is classically retro-orbital and comes on at the completion of exercise. Treatment is the same as that for classical migraine (usually pharmacological). Identification and modification of possible causative factors such as drugs (oral contraceptive pill,

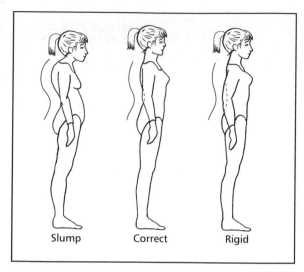

Figure 32 – The characteristic posture of a person with cervical headache vs corrected posture

caffeine, vasodilators, alcohol), exercising in hot weather and inadequate hydration is important in reducing the number of episodes.

Cervical Headache

Cervicogenic headache is common in both the sporting and non-sporting population (Fig. 32). It differs from migraine in its intensity and duration. Cervical headache is classically worse with neck movements and dull in nature. It usually lasts for days without variation in its intensity, unlike migraine which is more short-lived and severe. Features such as visual disturbances and vomiting are not features of cervical headache, although dizziness may be present. Physical examination of any sports person presenting with headache should, as well as including a full neurological examination, include an examination of the cervical spine. Cervical spine examination should involve; assessment of range of motion, palpation for tenderness over the spinous processes, facet joints and cervical musculature, and attempts at provocation of symptoms by palpation or neck movements. Postural factors may contribute to the development of cervical headache with hyperextension of the cervical spine increasing the load on posterior structures such as the facet joints. These factors should be addressed with a neck flexor strengthening programme and emphasis on chin retraction. Mobilisation of the intervertebral joints and soft tissue treatment to the muscles will also improve symptoms.

Athletes are not immune to the neurological diseases which affect the general population. If headaches are persistent, severe, recurrent or associated with systemic or neurological symptoms, investigations should proceed as for the non-athlete.

FATIGUE

CAUSES

The causes of fatigue in an athlete are numerous (Fig. 33).

HISTORY

When assessing such an athlete with fatigue, a thorough history including a diet and training diary are essential. The cause of fatigue is often apparent following the history. The training diary should be examined to assess the rate of progression of exercise duration and intensity and the frequency and duration of recovery periods. Other important details in the history should include:

- Current medications
- Menstrual history
- History of recent overseas travel
- Presence of systemic or localising symptoms
- Social history including work and home situations
- Presence of stressors.

PHYSICAL EXAMINATION

Physical examination of the "tired athlete" is often unrewarding but should include a full cardiovascular, respiratory and gastrointestinal workup. Look specifically for the presence of pallor, lymphadenopathy, hepatosplenomegaly and thyroid enlargement.

INVESTIGATIONS

In many cases, the diagnosis will be apparent from the history and examination, and further investigations will not be required. The type of investigations performed in other cases will depend on the clinical suspicion but the following investigations are often useful in differentiating between the common causes of fatigue.

- Urinalysis
- FBC, ESR, EUCs, liver function tests, fasting plasma glucose
- Serum iron studies, B12, folate
- Thyroid function tests
- Pregnancy test
- Viral serology, including EBV, CMV, toxoplasmosis, Hepatitis A, B and C.

OVERTRAINING SYNDROME

Overtraining is characterised by tiredness, irritability, poor motivation, sleep disturbances, lowered immunity to infection and deteriorating performance. The history will usually suggest the diagnosis but other markers of overtraining include changes on psychological tests, elevation of early morning heart rates, and deterioration in performance tests. A psychological test commonly employed is the Profile of Mood States (POMS) and overtrained athletes record low scores for vigour and high scores for anxiety and depression on this test. While there is no simple blood test that is pathognomonic of overtraining, a number of trends may be observed on blood testing. These include

CAUSES OF FATIGUE IN ATHLETE	
• Overtraining • Viral/post viral illness • Nutritional factors • Anaemia/iron deficiency • Pregnancy	• Medications e.g. beta blockers, sedatives • CFS (chronic fatigue syndrome) • Metabolic/endocrine causes such as diabetes and hypothyroidism • Malignant disease

Figure 33

depression of the serum testosterone:urinary cortisol ratio, decreased plasma glutamine levels, decreased urinary noradrenaline levels, elevation of the white cell count and depression of the serum ferritin level. The presence of definite immunological markers of overtraining may be possible in the future.

Management of Overtraining Syndrome

Management of this condition involves reduction in training volume and intensity. Prevention, however, is the preferred method with training programmes designed cyclically to incorporate adequate recovery periods and light training periods interspersed with the heavy sessions. This allows for consolidation of gains and recovery of muscle tissue. Modification of the training schedule will require close collaboration with coaches and relatives.

VIRAL ILLNESS

The presence of a viral illness is usually apparent from the history and examination. Tiredness may persist for weeks or months following some viral infections (hepatitis, EBV). Premature commencement of training following such an illness may prolong the fatigue. Athletes with hepatomegaly or splenomegaly associated with a viral illness should not play contact sports until these findings have resolved. Athletes with recurrent viral illnesses should have their training programmes assessed to exclude the possibility of overtraining syndrome.

NUTRITIONAL DEFICIENCIES

Inadequate nutrition is a very common cause of fatigue in the sports person. This may be due to one of the following:

- Inadequate caloric intake to match energy expenditure

- Inadequate carbohydrate intake to restore muscle glycogen

- Inadequate iron intake or poor iron absorption.

Caloric Intake

In athletes with suspected dietary related fatigue, a diet diary and training diary should be examined to assess whether the caloric intake is enough to compensate for the energy output. Weight loss in an athlete suggests that the output exceeds the intake.

Carbohydrate Intake

Subjects involved in endurance sports require a high percentage of carbohydrate in their diet (60-70%), as carbohydrate is the main source of energy in this group. Inadequate carbohydrate stores will result in poor performance and early fatigue.

Iron Intake

There are two main types of iron in the diet and their absorption varies considerably. Haem iron is the type found in meat and its absorption is 10-20%. Non-haem iron which is found in green vegetables, legumes and cereals is poorly absorbed with absorption being less than 10%. Vegetarians are therefore at increased risk of iron deficiency. There are a number of foods which, if taken with iron, will reduce its absorption. These include phytates (in cereals) and tannins (in tea). Vitamin C, if taken with iron-containing foods, will enhance its absorption and is beneficial in the treatment of iron deficiency. Female athletes are also at greater risk of iron deficiency as a result of increased loss of iron through the menstrual cycle.

Iron Deficiency

Iron deficiency anaemia has a marked effect on endurance training as a result of the impairment in oxygen transport. Iron deficiency, without the presence of anaemia, has also been known to cause tiredness and poor performance. This may be due to the widespread role of iron in energy metabolism. Iron stores can be estimated by measurement of serum ferritin. A serum ferritin of less than 30 mg/ml in females and 50 mg/ml in males is thought to represent a reduction in iron stores and should be treated with dietary modification or iron supplements. Athletes with persistent iron deficiency, despite an adequate dietary intake, should be investigated for blood loss or malabsorption (Fig. 34).

EXERCISE AND THE IMMUNE SYSTEM

There is conflicting evidence in this area. Athletes in training report increased susceptibility to infection (versus recreational activities). This can disrupt their training schedules. Moderately intense exercise (<60% VO_2max) is immunopotentiating whilst intense exercise (>60% VO_2max) is immunosuppressive. Elite

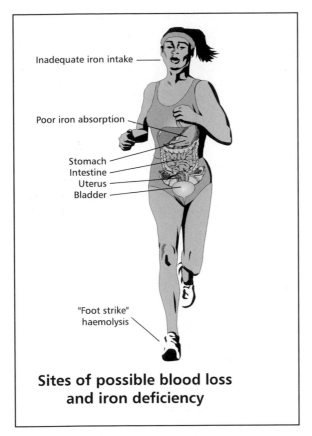

Inadequate iron intake

Poor iron absorption

Stomach
Intestine
Uterus
Bladder

"Foot strike"
haemolysis

**Sites of possible blood loss
and iron deficiency**

Figure 36 – Sites of possible blood loss and deficiency

athletes, in prolonged training, may experience immunosuppression. Of interest, recreational skiers experience a similar range of minor infections as is seen in general practice (such as URTI and gastrointestinal infection). There is a need to set some simple guidelines (Fig. 35).

HIV/AIDS IN SPORT

There is no documentation of transmission in sporting activity. However, travelling athletes need to be aware of possible higher infection rates outside their home countries (will influence medical treatment and sexual contacts).

Training of moderate intensity has not been shown to adversely affect the health of HIV positive athletes.

Hepatitis B and C are much more easily transmitted on the playing field.

Asymptomatic HIV-positive athletes benefit from exercise and competition. However, competition needs to be curtailed when the CD4 count <500 or when AIDS develops.

EPILEPSY AND THE ATHLETE

This is a brief, paroxysmal disturbance of the brain which may be focal (simple/complex/leading to generalised) generalised or unclassified.

Primary generalised may have tonic/clonic seizures; onset in childhood, a normal brain and be inherited (or no cause). Controlled in >75% cases.

Secondary generalised are usually tonic/clonic, akinetic or multi-focal; onset in childhood with diffuse brain damage. Difficult to treat.

There are over 400,000 young epileptics in the USA.

Such patients are not at risk for seizures during exercise, in fact regular exercise may improve control of seizures. These athletes have no higher injury rates than non-epileptics. The most frequent cause of death during a seizure is drowning (in the bath tub).

GUIDELINES FOR TRAINING FOLLOWING MINOR/MAJOR ILLNESS (AFTER BLOOMFIELD, FRICKER AND FITCH , 1995)		
	Minor URTI Headache (mild)	**Major** Fever Severe URTI/GI upset
Action	Only intensity training	No training until no systemic complaints
Return to training	Full training in 1-4 days	Gradual return days to week

Figure 35

It is generally thought that epileptics can play all sports (contact and non-contact) if there has been good seizure control for 12 months.

Epileptics in competition must adhere strictly to their recommended drug medications to prevent break-through seizures. When such seizures occur in competitions exclude head injury, hyperthermia, metabolic/electrolyte problems, fatigue and check serum anticonvulsant drug levels.

DIABETES MELLITUS

Diabetics are able to exercise (though usually reluctant) and will benefit from it. Insulin-dependent diabetics achieve better glucose control (increased insulin sensitivity and glucose utilisation) and it may lessen long-term diabetic complications (decreased cardiovascular risk factors, improved serum lipids). Non-insulin diabetics may avoid the diagnosis in the first place and not require the use of medication (tablets or insulin) (decreases insulin resistance and improves glucose utilisation). In particular, exercise keeps the weight down for this second group.

The complications of diabetes may indicate the safer type of sporting activity (neuropathic or vascular foot, no impact sports; proliferative retinopathy, no weight-lifting which may raise the BP and no scuba diving). It is best to keep activity at a moderate level (50 to 70% VO$_2$ max, 30 min, 3 times/week). In general, young diabetics in good control with no complications need have no restrictions. Brittle diabetics can exercise but under close supervision with frequent blood glucose tests (high or low blood glucose levels in exercise are dangerous). Never exercise alone and always carry glucose tablets.

It is important to establish a careful insulin regimen with monitoring (keep blood glucose >100 mg/dl, and <250 mg/dl; correct Ketonuria). Measure blood glucose before and after exercise (**less than 130 mg/dl** use 2 carbohydrates exchanges for 30-45 min of light-to-moderate exercise, <60% VO$_2$ max; 3 exchanges for heavy exercise; **level 130-180 mg/dl** one carbohydrate load for 30-45 min moderate and 2 for heavy exercise; when **level 180-240 mg/dl** no carbohydrate load; **when >240 mg/dl** no exercise). When exercising over several hours, reduce insulin 20 to 50% and use carbohydrate exchange every 30-45 min.

Post-exercise hypoglycaemia does occur and so exercise is best done in the morning (avoid nocturnal hypoglycaemia). Diabetics using the above approach have completed marathons and climbed mountains.

DRUGS IN SPORT

Mark Freeman

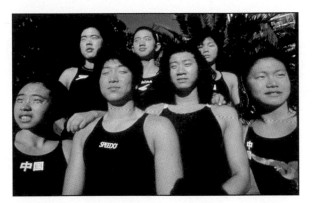

Figure 36 – The Chinese Swimmming Team disqualified in 1994 for breach of drug sporting regulations

Various performance-enhancing techniques, legal and illegal, are employed by athletes seeking to gain an advantage over their rivals (Figs. 36 & 37). Since Canadian sprinter Ben Johnson's dramatic 1988 Seoul Olympic 100 m disqualification for testing positive to the anabolic steroid stanozolol, the widespread abuse of drugs in sport has become patently clear. There was a concern that up to 75% of the track and field athletes at the Atlanta Olympics (1996) were using performance enhancement drugs. The International Olympic Committee and many individual sport's governing bodies now continually seek to improve their testing methods to try to keep elite athletes "clean". The IOC's hypersensitive High Resolution Mass Spectrometer (HRMS) has detected traces of urine steroid allegedly taken more than 3 months previously. Conversely, athletes seek to remain a step ahead of the detection systems and turn to newer drugs with shorter elimination times so they can continue taking performanceenhancement drugs closer to their competition dates. Testing difficulties obviously exist for the increasingly popular naturally-occurring substances such as erythropoietin, blood, Insulin-like growth factor-1 (IGF-1) and human growth hormone, which can all give a competitive edge. Use of performance-enhancing drugs is not limited to the elite, with gyms around the world being a focus of supply to the non-elite athlete. The major classes of drugs and doping methods in sport are described below.

• Stimulants

Cocaine, amphetamines, crack, caffeine, beta-agonists, phenylpropanolamine, ephedrines.

These are used at competition time (sprinters and weight lifters) to hasten reflexes, improve confidence and diminish an athlete's sense of fatigue. Away from major events, their appetite-suppressant effect can be used to help lose weight (gymnasts, figure skaters, weight class sports). Performance enhancement is questionable with adverse effects including anxiety and psychosis, and in the case of cocaine and crack, dependence.

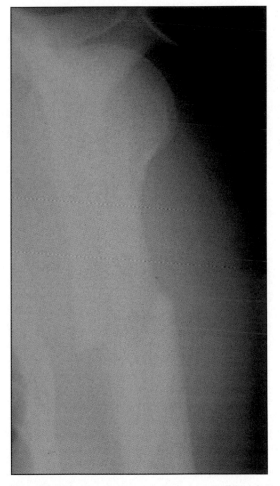

Figure 37 – Pathological fracture of humerus in weightlifter on anabolic steroids

This group of IOC-banned substances includes those commonly ingested inadvertently such as caffeine, the ephedrines (in decongestants) and beta-agonists (asthmatic medications). The IOC has approved some beta-agonists for asthmatics as "allowed" medications. The beta-agonist clenbuterol has been specifically banned due to its ergogenic effects. Clenbuterol has a significant lipolytic effect and stimulates fast-twitch muscle hypertrophy secondary to increased muscle protein aggregation. Clenbuterol is difficult to detect more than 48 hours after use, and is often used with undetectable growth hormone as an alternative to anabolic steroids which athletes fear being tested and caught for.

• Blood Doping and Erythropoietin

A higher level of red blood cells in the circulation increases the oxygen-carrying capacity of the blood and enhances an athlete's endurance. These methods are favoured by cyclists, cross-country skiers, orienteers, triathletes and marathoners. Improvements in endurance capacity, VO$_2$max, and race times are undeniable but the exact relationship to the increased haemoglobin level is uncertain.

Blood doping entails reinfusion of 275-500 ml of an athlete's own previously stored, or type-matched, packed red cells with saline 1-7 days before competition. Up to 12% increases in haemoglobin levels have been detected after reinfusion. Levels remain high for 4-6 weeks, tapering back to normal levels in 3-4 months. Some risks associated with non-medical transfusion include allergic skin rash, acute haemolytic reaction of mismatched donor blood, transmission of viral hepatitis or AIDS.

Recombinant human erythropoietin (rEPO) was developed to treat anaemia and is almost indistinguishable from the natural kidney hormone. Infusions or subcutaneous injections stimulate erythropoiesis in a sustained manner, giving an athlete elevated red blood cell concentrations for extended periods after the blood concentration has diminished to undetectable levels. The blood profile post-rEPO can approximate that due to high-altitude training. Very serious side-effects follow from excessive use of rEPO since elevated haemoconcentration and blood viscosity can lead to young athletes, especially whilst resting or sleeping, have been attributed to erythropoietin use.

Urinalysis cannot detect either of these methods so blood sampling of athletes may become necessary to detect use of rEPO.

• Anabolic-Androgenic Steroids and Hormones (stanozolol, methanedienone, hCG, growth hormone, IGF-1)

Anabolic steroids are synthetic analogues of the natural male hormone testosterone. The chemical modifications are aimed firstly at increasing the efficacy of the drug by reducing liver metabolism and secondly at maximising the desired anabolic (muscle-building) effects and minimising the unwanted androgenic (masculinising) effects of the drug.

Potential benefits of anabolic steroids include increased muscle bulk and an enhanced ability to perform high-intensity training. Anecdotal evidence suggests that most strength gains occur when hard training is undertaken concurrently with the steroid "cycle". The "cycling" regimen consists of alternative 6-12 week cycles on/off the drug(s) at 5-100x physiologic male testosterone levels up to 3 times/year and normally away from competition times. "Stacking" of 1-2 oral and 1-2 transdermally injected anabolic steroids at the one time is perceived by some bodybuilders and athletes to give increased benefit. Human chorionic gonadotrophin (hCG) is sometimes taken concurrently by males to minimise the unwanted side-effects of testicular atrophy and gynaecomastia (breast development).

These drugs are widely used by non-elite athletes, often adolescents concerned with the development of a muscular physique. The side-effects are numerous, including the very serious hypertrophic cardiomyopathy and sudden death. More common are increased aggressiveness, acne, facial hair, accelerated baldness, menstrual irregularities, gynaecomastia, testicular atrophy and mandible enlargement. Sperm production remains faulty for up to 2 years.

Advances in testing for steroids (the IOC's HRMS) mean that some athletes are now using tablets and absorbable gel steroids instead of the injectable forms. These preparations are very quickly metabolised and excreted, allowing the athlete to continue taking them up to 2 weeks prior to a competition. Random out-of-competition drug-testing in most IOC-sports is now the biggest deterrent to elite athletes taking banned drugs.

Growth hormone is produced naturally in the human pituitary gland and controls our growth from infancy. The synthetic version is identical to the natural version and hence undetectable. HGH has an overall anabolic effect similar to anabolic steroids, but without many of the side-effects. It stimulates muscle protein and nucleic acid synthesis, increases lipolysis. The adverse effects include diabetes, gigantism in prepubescents and acromegaly in adults.

IGF-1 is another natural hormone which promotes growth of all cells. It can increase natural strength by 5-15% and as such is far more potent than growth hormone. It is extremely expensive but of considerable attraction to the power athletes. Side-effects are similarly more potent than for growth hormone and include swelling of the brain, hypertrophic cardiomyopathy, sudden death and diabetic coma.

• Other Drugs

The narcotic analgesics (morphine, pethidine, buprenorphine) are IOC-banned substances since they may give an increased pain threshold, feelings of invincibility and euphoria, and a diminished recognition of injury. Of this group, however, Codeine is now IOC-approved as a pain-killer for athletes.

Beta-blockers (Sotalol, Atenolol) are IOC-banned substances because they decrease tremor and improve steadiness, giving possible benefit to archers, shooters and biathletes.

Corticosteroids, apart from topical preparations and some inhalation treatments, are IOC-banned. The non-specific systemic energising effects of these include a feeling of well-being which may translate into sporting improvement in a way similar to the stimulatory effect of amphetamines, but with more of a psychological component. Non-steroidal anti-inflammatory drugs are recommended by the IOC for treatment of sports-related injuries.

Probenicid and related masking agents alter the integrity and validity of urine samples. They are IOC-banned since they are used by some athletes in conjunction with anabolic steroids to reduce urine steroid concentration.

Diuretics are IOC-banned because of the possibility of weight-category sports people abusing their acute weight-losing effects to satisfy a weight limit. Diuretics also dilute urine, making detection of other substances more difficult.

Phosphate loading works by elevating the level of 2,3-DPG, which shifts the oxygen-dissociation curve to the right and allows increased oxygen unloading at the tissues. Benefits are unclear.

Bicarbonate loading works by neutralising muscle lactic acid build-up. It is used by middle-distance runners, who take 300 mg/kg common baking soda 30 min before their event. Small decreases in running times have been noted.

CONCLUSION, THE TEAM DOCTOR

Sports medicine involves the management of medical problems in athletes as well as the diagnosis and treatment of musculoskeletal conditions. Although moderate, regular physical activity has health promoting effects, athletes are not immune to the general illnesses which affect the non-sporting population. The common medical presentations of the sporting population have been outlined in this chapter. Early recognition and treatment of these conditions will usually enable a prompt return to their chosen sport.

The team doctor has an important role to play in treating the illness and injuries of athletes (referring on when indicated); make decisions regarding athletes eligibility to join the team and to return to play after injury. The responsibilities are firstly to the athlete (as patient), the team, family and administrators. It should not be a position of burden but of pleasure in being able to practice a broad spectrum of medicine covering internal medicine, orthopaedics, gynaecology, pharmacology and exercise physiology. Always preserve the athlete's (patient's) confidentiality and practice to the best Hippocratic ideals.

Most teams find the combination of primary care doctor and orthopaedic surgeon ideal (most injuries are musculoskeletal). However sports medicine physicians are able to provide this comprehensive care.

It is best to adopt a team approach (the athlete, doctor, coach and the trainer).

Administration is important to ensure proper facilities for treatment, transport and the safety of athletes (smog-free and terrorist-safe transport routes to facilities) and public relations.

5

THE FALLEN ATHLETE
The Acute Management of the Sick and Injured Athlete

Stuart Stapleton

INTRODUCTION

Sport and recreational injuries are not uncommon. Such injuries account for up to 20% of total injury costs, with the cost in Australia alone (in 1990) being nearly $1 billion. The number that are life-threatening is probably low. The risk of these injuries or illness amongst athletes depends upon factors, such as the type and level of sport (amateur versus professional), and the athlete's previous illness or injury and level of fitness. It is important to have a simple approach to use in any case of potential life-threatening injury (Fig. 1) or illness.

SICK AND INJURED ATHLETES

Resuscitating patients falls into two basic groups - **non-trauma** related or **trauma related** (Fig. 2). Various treatment algorithms have been designed for each group (Australian Resuscitation Council, American Heart Association, Early Management of Severe Trauma, Advanced Trauma Life Support). For athletes requiring resuscitation it is essential to determine from **the onset of first aid, if there has been any trauma** present. If there is uncertainty about the presence or absence of trauma, **assume trauma is involved and treat accordingly** (Fig. 3).

BASIC DIFFERENCES BETWEEN NON-TRAUMA RELATED AND TRAUMA RELATED ILLNESS IN ATHLETES		
	Non-trauma Related	**Trauma Related**

Examples	Dehydration
	   Exertional heat
	   illness (heat stroke)
	
	Cardiac disease (e.g.
	   angina,
	   heart attack,
	   or arrhythmia)
	Exercise induced
	   acute asthma
	Epilepsy
	Diabetic
	   hypoglycaemia
		Contact sports
		   – spear tackle
		     (rugby)
		   – boxing
		Motor sports
		Water sports
		   – near-drowning
		   – diving into
		     shallow water
		Falls
		   – rock climbing

Airway Management	Standard Basic Life Support (see below)	Must protect the neck and prevent head movement

Circulation Management	Standard Basic Life Support (see below)	Require early intravenous therapy
		Obvious external bleeding must be stopped
		   – pressure
		   – bandage
		Do not use tourniquets

Figure 2

ON FIELD APPROACH TO INJURY		
Injuries can be:		**Action**
1. Minor	– cuts/abrasions/sprains/cramps	Return to game
2. Moderate	– sprains (swelling, pain, ▼ ROM)	Treat on site/later refer

3. Severe	– severe pain, swelling, deformity	Expert medical care
		   (severe sprains , fractures,
		   dislocations)

4. Life threatening	– stroke, head/neck injury, heart attack	Resuscitate

Use:
  A airway
  B breathing
  C circulation

History:
Brief talk to athlete or witness/details of accident/extent pain/assess severity.

Examine:
Check for: swelling/deformity/tenderness/ROM and classify (as above).

Treat.

Figure 1

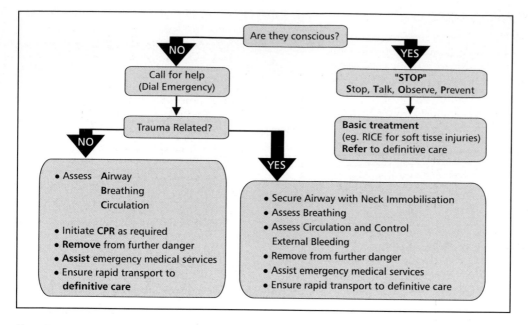

Figure 3 – Initial assessment of the sick or injured athlete

CARE OF THE COLLAPSED OR SERIOUSLY ILL ATHLETE

The basic principles of the resuscitation of collapsed or seriously ill patients are outlined (Fig. 4).

The steps in this Chain of Survival are:

1. **Early Access** to emergency medical services. This "call for help" allows the rapid delivery of care in the field by ambulance services to commence early stabilisation and delivery of the patient to a hospital for definitive care.

2. **Early commencing of bystander CPR (car-diopulmonary resuscitation)**, when required. This will buy time for the arrival of ambulance personnel, particularly in the setting of cardiac arrest, where early defibrillation is the most important factor determining survival.

3. **Early Defibrillation** is the most important factor in determining survival in cardiac arrest due to either ventricular fibrillation or pulseless ventricular tachycardia.

4. **Early Advanced Care** implies the rapid delivery of the seriously ill patient to hospital. In the non-trauma related illness this allows the early administration of advanced medical care.

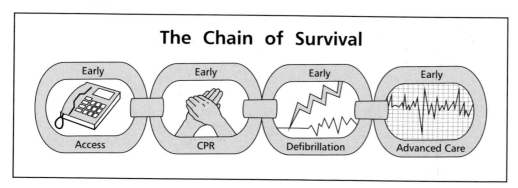

Figure 4 – The Chain of Survival (adapted from the American Heart Association Guidelines for Cardiopulmonary Resuscitation and Emergency Cardiac Care)

EARLY ACCESS TO EMERGENCY MEDICAL SERVICES

Emergency medical services are able to achieve **two major goals:** the early resuscitation and stabilisation of the seriously ill patient, and the rapid delivery of the patient to definitive care. This is best achieved when bystanders call for help as the initial step in the caring for the seriously ill patient. If two or more bystanders are present, one person should dial the Emergency telephone number, while the other commence CPR. When doing this it is important to relate clear information regarding the location of the patient, and any other information requested by the operator.

For the infant or child, in arrest, the most likely cause is an airway problem. In this setting it is best to commence CPR, then call for help.

"Call for help" also implies gaining assistance at the scene, before the ambulance arrives. Even for people experienced in resuscitation, CPR is always easier with two or more people lending help. Don't hesitate to seek help.

COMMENCING EARLY CPR

The window of opportunity for survival from cardiac arrest is small. As such, the aim of bystander CPR is to increase the time before death occurs, allowing emergency medical services the opportunity to deliver early defibrillation, and other advanced care techniques.

After assessing the person's responsiveness, the steps in bystander CPR or basic life support for the collapsed patient are as follows (Fig. 5):

1. Secure the airway

   To do this requires two actions, firstly **clearing the airway,** and **then opening the airway**. Clearing the airway removes any foreign bodies from the airway including dentures, broken teeth, food, vomit or blood. It is achieved by the finger sweep, although care must be taken not to dislodge any loose teeth, especially in young children. When available a suction device should be used. After clearing the airway, it may need to be opened by a combination of extending the head, chin lift and jaw thrust (Fig. 6). Various devices such as oropharyngeal airways or Geudel's airway (Fig. 7) should be used if available.

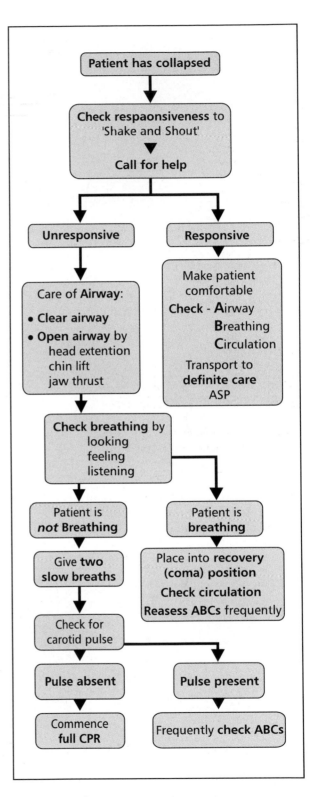

Figure 5 – Basic Life Support

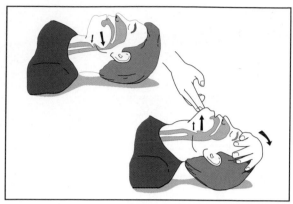

Figure 6 – Opening the airway. Note how each of the manoeuvres results in moving the tongue from the back of the pharynx. Remember in the injured patient not to use the head extension, as this may damage the cervical spine.

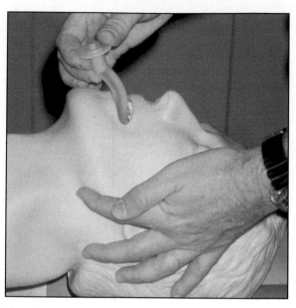

Figure 7 – An oropharyngeal (Geudel's) airway. When inserting the airway take care not to dislodge teeth as the airway is rotated into position. This is especially important in young children with primary dentition.

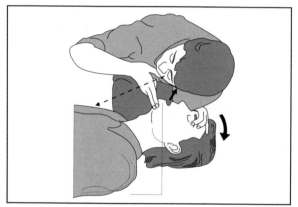

Figure 8 – Assessing the adequacy of breathing. By adopting this position it is easy to look for the chest moving, feel for the chest moving, and listen for the movement of air, while keeping the airway open.

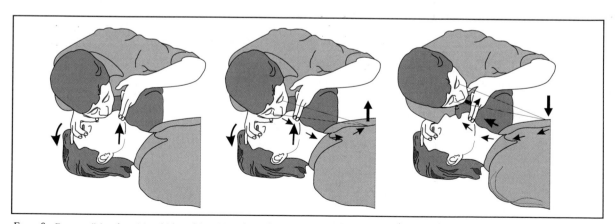

Figure 9 – Rescue (Mouth to Mouth) breathing. Note how the rescuer is able to assess the adequacy of rescue breathing by watching the chest move, while maintaining an open airway.

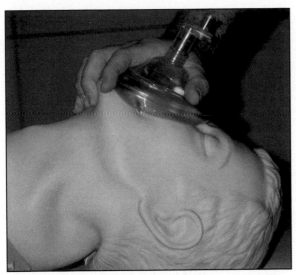

Figure 10 – Mouth to mask ventilation. Such devices are portable and reduce the risk to the rescuer due to vomiting and infectious diseases. They should only be used by people adequately trained in their use

2. Assess and ensure breathing (rescue breathing or expired air resuscitation)

To assess the presence or absence of breathing one must look for movement of the chest with inhalation and exhalation, feel for chest movement and listen for the movement of air. This can be easily achieved by using the technique shown in Figure 8.

If there is no evidence of breathing, rescue breathing should be commenced immediately. This is commenced with two slow breaths, by the mouth-to mouth technique, ensuring that the chest rises (Fig. 9). If a mouth to mask device is available (Fig. 10), this may be used, reducing any risk of infection.

The rates and ratios of external cardiac compression and rescue breathing are shown in Figure 11.

3. Assess and maintain circulation

(external cardiac compression)

To assess the circulation the rescuer feels for the carotid pulse, in the neck at the angle of the jaw. **If the pulse is present,** but the patient is not breathing spontaneously, continue rescue breathing at a rate of 15 breaths per minute, until either help arrives or spontaneous breathing commences.

If there is no detectable carotid pulse, commence external cardiac compression (ECC) immediately. The hands are placed on the lower third of the sternum, with the arms locked at the elbows and the rescuer kneeling over the patient (Fig. 12). Compressions are approximately 5 cm deep in the adult, at a rate of between 80 to 100 compressions per minute. This is tiring work, if continued for a prolonged period, so don't hesitate in getting help from other bystanders, changing every few minutes.

To determine the adequacy of ECC, the carotid pulse should be felt for, and after every 2 min of full CPR, a check should be made for the return of spontaneous breathing and circulation. Full CPR should be continued until either help arrives, or there is return of a spontaneous circulation.

4. Stabilisation and Transport

When the patient begins to maintain their own airway and breathing, and has return of a spontaneous circulation, they should be placed in the coma position until help arrives (Fig. 13). Airway patency, adequacy of breathing and circulation, should be frequently reassessed, and any deterioration should be acted upon immediately. Once available, the patient should be transported to hospital, as soon as possible.

RATIOS OF BREATH TO CHEST COMPRESSIONS FOR CARDIOPULMONARY RESUSCITATION			
	Ventilation	**Chest Compressions**	**Ratio** (Breaths to compressions)
One Rescuer	15 breaths/min	80 to 100/min	15 to 2
Two Rescuers	15 breaths/min	80 to 100 /min	5 to 1

Figure 11

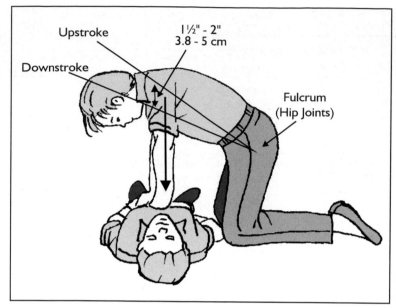

Figure 12 – Technique of CPR. Hands over lower ⅓ of sternum, elbows locked, rescuer kneeling over patient.

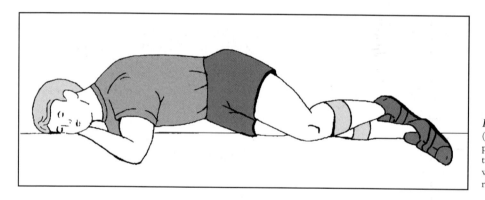

Figure 13 – The Recovery (coma) Position. Placing the patient in this position allows the patient to keep their airway open, and reduces the risk of aspiration of vomit

THE APPROACH TO THE SEVERELY INJURED ATHLETE		
At the scene, it is important to prevent further injury by removing the patient from any danger. It is essential to care for the patient's **neck** whilst doing so.		
Primary Survey	Airway and cervical spine immobilisation	Immobilise head and neck with in-line stabilisation Clear airway Open airway - remember **not** to extend the neck
	Assess and ensure adequate **breathing** (ventilation)	Commence rescue breathing
	Control bleeding and maintain **circulation**	Apply pressure to external bleeding Commence external chest compression, if no pulse
	Assess **disability** (neurologic function)	If unconscious, assume major head injury and transport to hospital ASAP If unable to move arms or legs, assume spinal cord injury, and prevent further injury by not moving until help arrives
	Control **environment**, and be able to clearly explain the **events** causing **injury**	Remove from danger Prevent excessive cooling if injured Be clear about the mechanism of injury (events), as this is important in looking for injuries later
Resuscitation phase	Any immediately life-threatening problem found in the primary survey is addressed	
Secondary Survey	Usually done in hospital Head to toe, front to back examination looking for injuries Usually includes X-ray and blood tests	System by system examination Thorough history: **Allergies** **Medications**, last tetanus **Previous** illness/surgery **Last** ate **Event** - what happened
Stabilisation and Transport	Re-assess ABC, before moving Splint any limb injuries	Transport to hospital as soon as possible

Figure 14 – Approach to the severely injured athlete

THE SERIOUSLY INJURED ATHLETE

The approach to the seriously injured athlete is similar to that of the seriously ill athlete, with a couple of points of note. The system taught in Advanced Trauma Life Support and the Early Management of Severe Trauma courses, is an easy-to-remember system for dealing with such cases (see Fig. 14).

Remember the following points:

1. **Remove from danger**, in order to prevent further injury. While doing so it is essential to protect the patient's neck, to prevent any trauma to the cervical spine and spinal cord. Figure 15 shows how this may be achieved.

2. **Airway management including care of the cervical spine.** In the non-injured patient, one of the first airway opening manoeuvres is to extend the neck. This should not done in the injured patient, especially if unconscious, as it may damage the cervical spine. All airway manoeuvres must be accompanied by in-line cervical immobilisation. When available, the neck should be immobilised with a rigid cervical collar (see Fig. 16).

3. In controlling the circulation, **control blood loss**. This can be achieved over the site of any external bleeding by pressure (Fig. 17). Limb tourniquets should not used, as they may cause arterial or nerve damage. Any long bone fractures, especially fractures of the femur, should be splinted to reduce blood loss and help control pain (Fig. 18).

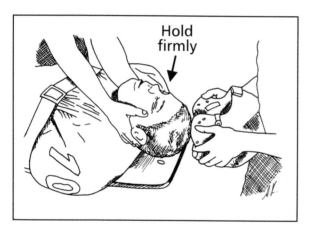

Figure 15 – Moving the patient with a possible neck injury. It is important to prevent any movement of the head or the neck as when removing football helmets

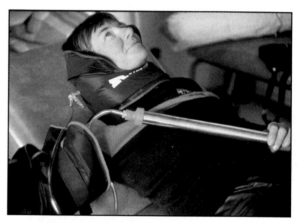

Figure 16 – A rigid cervical collar on a skier

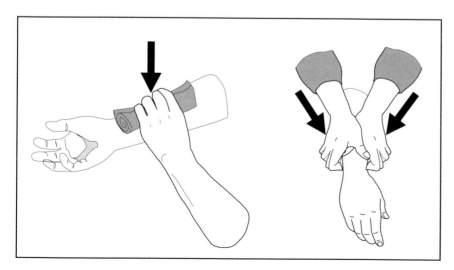

Figure 17 – Controlling external haemorrhage with local pressure is essential in managing the circulation of trauma-related injuries

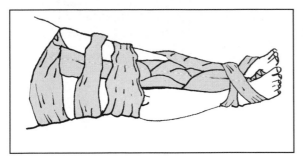

Figure 18 – Splinting a fractured shaft or femur will help to control pain as well as reduce blood loss into the fracture site

4. In the unconscious, injured athlete **always consider severe head injury**. These patient need rapid stabilisation and transfer to a hospital to allow a further assessment for potentially life-threatening intracranial bleeding, which will require urgent operation (Fig. 19).

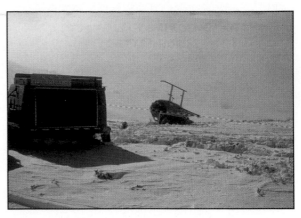

Figure 19 – Over-snow ambulance at rescue after helicopter crash on ski fields

Part II

Regional

6

HEAD

Jeffrey Compton
Michael Foster

INTRODUCTION

Head injuries occur in all sports (Fig. 1) and are more common in contact sports, particularly where the aim of the sport is to inflict injury to the head (boxing, kick boxing) (Fig. 2). Whilst most head injuries are minor there is the potential for every injury to lead to permanent disability or even death. The accurate assessment of the nature of the head injury and subsequent treatment can mean the difference between life, death or a lifetime of disability (Fig. 3).

The brain's susceptibility to injury is a function of its **softness**. It is basically a soft fluid structure enclosed within a very rigid box. The fact that the head is supported on a **relatively long neck** also

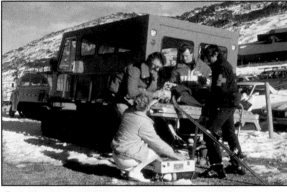

Figure 3 – Accurate early assessment and treatment of head injury can mean the difference between life and death or a lifetime disability

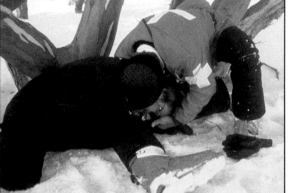

Figure 1 – Skier pinned under tree with acute cerebral contusion (died 4 hours later)

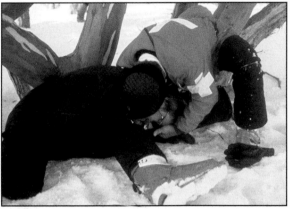

Figure 2 – A direct blow to the head in boxing (coup) with contre-coup can result in serious or fatal injury (40% of all boxing injuries are head injuries). Repeated punches may result in "Dementia Pugilistica".

INJURY TO BRAIN
• Directly (to brain and neural pathways)
• Indirectly (from bleeding arteries/veins)
• Structures adjacent (cranial nerves, meninges)

Figure 4 – Mechanism of Injury to brain

allows injuring forces to be magnified. Injury can occur to the brain and neural pathways directly or the brain can be injured as a result of bleeding from arteries or veins in relation to it. Injury can also occur to structures attached or adjacent to the brain (the cranial nerves or brain linings) (Fig. 4).

ASSESSMENT

Assessment of the severity of head injury is vital in allowing an accurate plan for the management of the injury and indicating what investigations and treatments are required.

The history of the injury itself can suggest its severity as well as allowing an assessment to be made of whether the patient's clinical condition is improving or deteriorating. It is important to remember that **not all cases of reduced conscious state in sport** are due to head injury, hence the importance of history taking in distinguishing head injury from other causes such as spontaneous intracranial haemorrhage or metabolic causes of unconsciousness (Fig. 5). It is

CAUSES OF REDUCED CONSCIOUS STATE

- Head injury
- Spontaneous intracerebral haemorrhage
- Metabolic (diabetic/uraemic/hepatic/hypothermia)
- Drugs (alcohol/narcotics/barbiturates/CO)
- Epilepsy
- Infection (meningitis)
- Psychiatric (hysteria, catatonia)

Figure 5 – Causes of reduced conscious state

important to collect information from **witnesses** to the event. In particular, it is important to record the **mechanism of injury**, the **extent of the reduction in conscious state** and the **length of any period of unconsciousness.**

Even untrained witnesses are able to confirm whether the patient was talking or opening his eyes or obeying commands. They are also able to attest to the victim's level of orientation or confusion. Witnesses are also able to give information in relation to the **absence of jerking** movements, **changes in pattern of respiration** or **skin colour** or **loss of continence** which may suggest **seizure** activity.

Injuries are classified as focal or diffuse (Figs. 6 & 7). The most common head injury in sport (concussion) is further sub-classified to guide practitioners (Fig. 8).

Types of Intracranial Haematomas

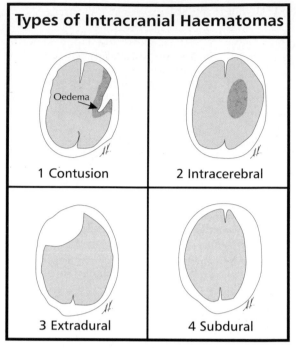

1 Contusion   2 Intracerebral

3 Extradural   4 Subdural

Figure 7 – Focal head injuries may be contusion, intracerebral haematoma, extradural haematoma or subdural haematoma

ON-FIELD MANAGEMENT (FIRST AID)

First aid treatment for head injuries is of importance as even a minor head injury has potential to be made significantly worse by coincident hypoxia, prolonged seizure activity, aspiration or other complications. In the acute injury state maintenance of an adequate

CLASSIFICATION OF HEAD INJURIES

Focal	–	**cerebral contusion** (ill defined area damage/translational force/contre-coup injury)
	–	**intracerebral haematoma** (deep/force over small area)
	–	**extradural haematoma** (middle meningeal artery/temporal skull fracture/ high mortality/ classic presentation *(LOC ➡ lucid ➡ LOC ➡ coma in only 10-30%)
	–	**subdural haematoma** (bridging veins torn/acute or subacute/70% mortality)
Diffuse	–	concussion (most common, see guidelines return to sport)
	–	diffuse axonal (severe brain dysfunction)
★ LOC – loss of consciousnes		

Figure 6 – Classification of head injuries

GRADING OF CONCUSSION	
I (mild)	Confusion/no LOC or amnesia Lucid in 5-15 min
II (moderate)	No LOC but confusion and retrograde amnesia (for few min)
III (severe)	LOC, confusion and amnesia (retrograde and post-traumatic).

Figure 8 – Grading of concussion

GUIDELINES TO RETURN TO SPORT AFTER CONCUSSION			
	1st episode	**2nd episode**	**3rd episode**
I	When asymptomatic > 20 min	When asymptomatic > 1 week	When asymptomatic > 3 months
II	When asymptomatic > 1 week	When asymptomatic > 1 month	When Next season if asymptomatic
III	When asymptomatic	off for season > 2 weeks	off for season

Figure 8 – Guidelines to return to sport after concussion

airway is of critical importance. The patient should be rolled into the coma position so that the airway is not obstructed by the tongue. Likewise the airway should be cleared of any vomited material or foreign bodies (e.g. mouth guards). It is important to be aware of the possibility of coincident spine injury and the patient should be rolled and positioned so that the spine is not bent or twisted during the process.

If the patient suffers seizure activity then the airway is further at risk. Most seizures are of short duration and self terminating. No effort should be made to lever the jaws apart. This can result in damage to the patient's teeth or the bystander's fingers.

If the patient remains unconscious for more than a few minutes an ambulance should be summoned and the patient transferred to the nearest appropriate hospital for further management.

MEDICAL MANAGEMENT

Most head injuries are minor and will require no medical treatment. If the patient has not lost consciousness then it is probably safe for them to return to competition once any symptoms have resolved. They should not compete if they suffer with dizziness, headache, are poorly orientated or have any neurological symptoms. There are now uniform guidelines in this area (Figs. 9 & 10).

If the sportsman has lost consciousness then they should not be allowed to compete in a situation where further head injury is possible for a period of one week or until any symptoms have resolved. The patient should be seen by a medical practitioner so that any evidence of post concussion symptoms can be assessed and appropriate investigation and treatment undertaken.

TAKE-AWAY HEAD INJURY GUIDE (TO GO WITH PATIENT AND CARER)
1. No play for 24 hours.
2. Liquid diet 8-24 hours.
3. Ice to head (15 min of every 60 min)
4. Panadol (tylenol) only.
5. Awaken patient 2 hourly x 24 hours.
6. Report any of following to Doctor: Nausea/vomiting/visual problem/ear ringing/confusion/disorientation/lack co-ordination/ drowsiness/worse headache/persistent headache (<48 hours)/unequal or slowly reacting pupils/convulsions/tremors.
7. Follow-up with usual doctor.

Figure 10 – Take away head injury guide

If the patient has been rendered unconscious for longer than **5 min** then hospital admission, observation and, if necessary, further investigation and treatment are required.

HOSPITAL MANAGEMENT

Upon hospital admission the patient should have their level of consciousness formally assessed and assessment made for the presence of any other injuries. The most

GLASGOW COMA SCORE		
Best Open	Spontaneously	4
	To speech	3
	To pain	2
	None	1
Best Verbal Response Sound	Orientated	5
	Confused	4
	Inappropriate Words	3
	Incomprehensible	2
	None	1
Best Motor Response	Obey commands	6
	Localises pain	5
	Flexion to pain	4
	Abnormal flexion	3
	None	2
		1

Figure 11 – Glasgow Coma Score is used to assess the severity of head injury.

widely accepted schema for assessment of the level of consciousness is the Glasgow Coma Scale (Fig. 11). The coma scale has been shown to be a reliable indicator of severity of injury and gives good information in terms of the likelihood of significant intracranial pathology being present and the patient's prognosis.

If the Glasgow Coma Score (the sum of numeric values assigned to levels on the coma scale) is **greater than 8** then the patient should be admitted for neurological observation. If their coma score fails to **return to 15** within 12 hours or if it deteriorates then have a CT scan performed. The patient should be observed until their coma score has returned to 15 and once the coma score has been at 15 for a period of time they should be discharged into the charge of a responsible adult with warnings given to **return to the hospital** should the level of consciousness deteriorate, should headache recur or persist, or should the patient develop any neurological symptoms.

If the Glasgow Coma Score is 8 or less there is a high chance that significant intracranial pathology is present. Immediate steps should be taken to stabilise the patient's condition and to reduce the chance of further brain injury. The patient should be anaesthetised, intubated and slightly hyper-ventilated (pCO_2 25-30 mmHg). A brain shrinking agent such as Mannitol

(one gram per kilogram body weight 20%) should be administered and an indwelling catheter inserted. The patient should have an emergency CT scan.

The pathology present can vary from **extradural haematoma** with blood clot forming between the skull and the dural lining of the brain compressing the underlying brain. These haematomas give a classic lentiform appearance on CT scanning (Fig. 12). **Subdural haematomas** lie between the dura and the brain (Fig. 13) and can arise from either tearing of dural vascular structures or disruption of the underlying brain tissue with haemorrhage in the sub-dural space. The so-called **diffuse axonal injury** is also relatively common in patients with a grossly depressed level of consciousness. **Small petechial haemorrhages** can be seen on CT scanning throughout the brain substance.

Surgical treatment is dependant on the pathology that has been displayed. Significant sized haematomas (generally speaking more than 25 cc or with more than 5 mm shift of the midline structures) should be treated by evacuation. In most cases these require craniotomy, removal of the blood clot and haemostasis. In life-threatening situations when neurosurgical treatment is not immediately available as an emergency measure a burr hole can be cut over the haematoma and evacuation begun.

Control of the intracranial pressure after surgery is also of importance, and efforts should be made to keep the intracranial pressure less than 25 mm of mercury. Treating physicians should also be vigilant of the complications in relation to such severe head injuries (electrolyte imbalance, seizure activity, sepsis, recurrent haematoma).

REHABILITATION

All patients who have lost consciousness for more **than 5 minutes or have persisting symptoms** should be assessed by a medical practitioner for, just as soft tissue and musculo skeletal injuries can require rehabilitation, so can neurological injuries.

Symptoms such as headaches, poor memory, poor concentration, personality change such as irritability or unusual placidity, dizziness or double vision and poor mental and physical stamina are common following significant head injuries. Such symptoms can be devastating for work and family situations and intervention from rehabilitation providers can be beneficial

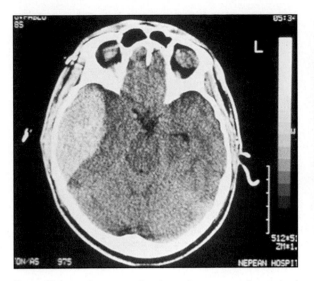

Figure 12 – Axial CT scan showing a large temporal extradural haematoma. The freshly spilt blood is high density (white) on the CT and has the classical lens shape of an extradural haemorrhage

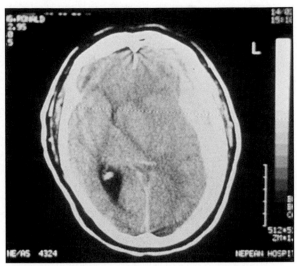

Figure 13 – Axial CT of a subdural haematoma. Compared with Figure 12, the haematoma is more extensive and crescentric in shape, characteristic of subdural bleeding. There is massive midline shift with severe shift of the ventricle evident

in both allowing full recovery from such symptoms and for the provision of aids and coping strategies to minimise their impact.

PROGNOSIS FOR POST-CONCUSSION SYNDROME

SYMPTOMS ARE VARIABLE BUT USUALLY RESOLVE

The prognosis for patients who have been afflicted with severe head injuries is likewise variable. Whilst complete recovery is possible, the progress is often slow and fluctuating. A program of physiotherapy, occupational therapy, speech therapy and psychological intervention supervised by a trained rehabilitation specialist is generally speaking of benefit but even so, some patients will remain significantly disabled (sometimes to the point of requiring institutional care).

PREVENTION OF HEAD INJURIES

- Wear helmets in contact sports (football, cricket, boxing)

- Use mouth guards

- Improved strength of neck extensor muscles may reduce incidence of head injuries

- Monitor necessary games regulation/rules to change dangerous play (scrumming in rugby, speartackling made illegal)

- Supervise children's games and encourage to wear helmets, (Figs 14 & 15)

SECOND-IMPACT SYNDROME

(AFTER HUGHSTON)

A syndrome of rapid brain swelling (may be fatal) from a second minor head injury whilst athlete is still suffering from the initial injury. It is characterised by the rapid development of diffuse brain swelling following a second impact to the head. Within seconds to minutes of this second impact, the initially but stunned athlete collapses. It is because of this syndrome that there are guidelines for the return to play of athletes with head injuries.

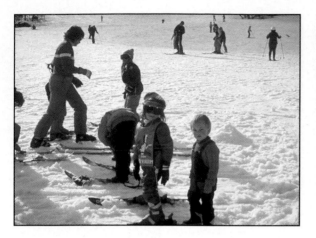

Figure 14 – Children should ideally wear helmets when snow skiing for although the incidence of intracranial injury is low, a helmet with visor will also protect the facial skeleton (Fig. 15)

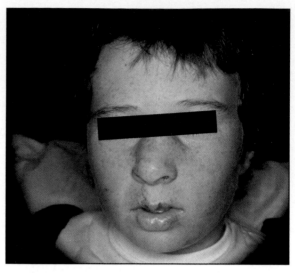

Figure 15 – 6-year-old skier with a broken nose

DEMENTIA PUGILISTICA

The "Punch Drunk" syndrome was first described amongst boxers in 1928. It results from repeated punches to the head (chronic closed head trauma). Its severity correlates with neuro anatomical changes (hydrocephalus, scarring) and presents with cerebellar (Parkinsonian) features, dysarthria, personality changes and deteriorating mental capacity. Modification of activities, head protection, changes to the boxing code and supportive care are required.

7

FACIAL SKELETON

Lydia Lim

FRACTURES OF THE MANDIBLE

Mandibular fractures are the most common maxillo-facial injury from sporting accidents. Common fracture patterns are: condyle, body, angle, symphysis, ramus (rare) and coronoid process (rare). (Fig.1)

CONDYLAR FRACTURES

Condylar fractures are the most common site of mandibular fracture. Most fractures are "sub-condylar" (fracturing through the weak area at the neck of the condyle). This fortunate anatomical design prevents the head of the condyle from being forced through the thin plate of bone lining the glenoid fossa into the middle cranial fossa.

The diagnosis is often missed. The Orthopantomogram (OPG) and PA Mandible X-rays should always be carefully studied by outlining the contour of the condyles bilaterally (Fig. 2).

There is pain and tenderness from the temporo-mandibular joint, pre-auricular swelling, limitation in oral opening, alteration in occlusion with gagging of occlusion on the posterior molars, and deviation in mandibular movements on opening towards the side of fracture.

These fractures may be undisplaced, displaced (antero-medial from pull of the lateral pterygoid muscle, condyle remains within glenoid fossa) or dislocated (Fig. 3).

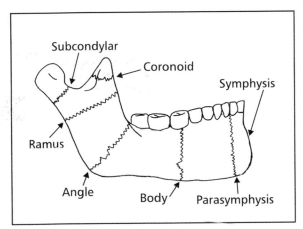

Figure 1 – Fracture patterns in mandibular fracture

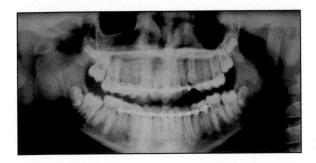

Figure 2 – OPG of subcondylar fracture

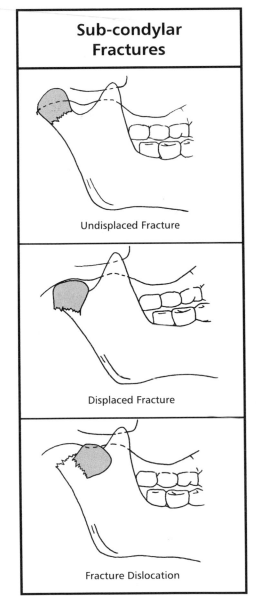

Figure 3 –Types of subcondylar fracture

The management of **children** with condylar fractures is nonsurgical (remodelling occurs with complete regeneration of normal condylar anatomy post-injury). Jaw exercise to attain normal occlusion is sufficient. If the occlusion is not consistently attainable then a short period of intermaxillary fixation (2 weeks) followed by a period of guiding elastics may be required.

In children, an **intracapsular** pattern of fracture is common. Accurate diagnosis with early jaw function is essential to prevent ankylosis and future growth asymmetry problems.

The treatment of adults with sub-condylar fractures remains controversial (open versus closed reduction). I believe that open reduction is indicated for gross fracture dislocations and when the occlusion is not able to be attained by closed reduction. In most cases, the occlusion is minimally altered and the patient is able to attain their correct occlusion with minimal effort. Simple jaw exercises to achieve a repeatable occlusion may be all that is required. If the correct occlusion is not readily achieved by the patient then a closed reduction is indicated. Arch bars are placed and the patient is placed into intermaxillary fixation (for 2 weeks). Intermaxillary fixation is then released and guiding elastics used for the next two to four weeks (Fig. 4).

In body and angle fractures, there may also be altered sensation of the lower lip. A mandibular fracture is diagnosed by (a change in occlusion) asking the patient if their bite feels different and checking the occlusion by manually directing the chin point upwards (note if the teeth interdigitate well into occlusion). A **change in occlusion** means a displaced mandibular fracture. A displaced fractured mandible

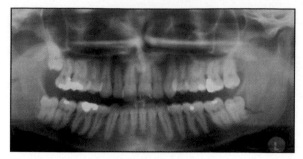

Figure 5 – Angle fracture (involving impacted third molar tooth

(except for condylar fractures) is always open and requires early antibiotic therapy with adequate stabilisation of the fracture.

Altered sensation to the lower lip (injury to the inferior alveolar nerve) is often present with fractures at the angle and body of the mandible.

X-rays required are the OPG and PA Mandible X-rays.

Angle fractures often occur through or adjacent to an impacted third molar tooth ("wisdom tooth") (a line of weakness) and may be associated with a concomitant body fracture or sub-condylar fracture on the contralateral side. A bilateral angle fracture is less common and presents as an anterior open-bite occlusion (where the teeth do not meet anteriorly) (Fig 5).

Fractures of the **body of the mandible** are commonly located by the canine tooth ("parasymphyseal" fractures). Displaced parasymphyseal fractures can be extremely mobile and painful (Fig. 6). There may be loose teeth present on either side of the fracture. Stabilisation of the fracture with a simple wire passed

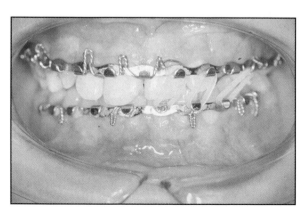

Figure 4 – Subcondylar fracture treated by arch bars and guiding elastics

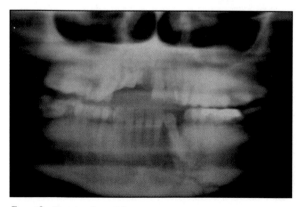

Figure 6 – Parasymphyseal fracture

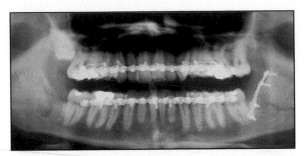

Figure 7 – Internal fixation of mandibular fracture (with mini plates)

inter-dentally and on either side of the fracture can improve patient comfort prior to definitive surgery.

A displaced fracture resulting in altered occlusion requires open reduction and fixation (rigid fixation using titanium mini-plates to avoid inter-maxillary fixation for the traditional 6 week period) (Fig. 7).

Post-operative care includes antibiotics (penicillin), soft diet, and strict oral hygiene. Contact sports are banned for a minimum of 6 weeks.

An undisplaced fracture may not require any surgical treatment but antibiotics, soft diet with regular review.

FRACTURES OF THE MAXILLA

Much less common than mandibular fractures (classified according to the **"Le Fort"** patterns of fracture (Rene Le Fort (Paris, 1900) from cadaver experiments). In all Le Fort fractures the middle third of the facial skeleton is displaced downwards and backwards resulting in an elogated lower third of the face with the mandible "gagging" open with an anterior open bite occlusion and a retropositioning of the upper incisor teeth behind the lower incisors (Fig. 8).

Le Fort Pattern of Maxillary Fractures

Le Fort I Fracture

This is a horizontal fracture affecting only the tooth bearing portion of the maxilla. Produces a mobile maxilla (displaced downwards and backwards). Treatment is an open reduction and internal fixation of (mini-plates at the pyriform and zygomatic buttresses).

Type 1

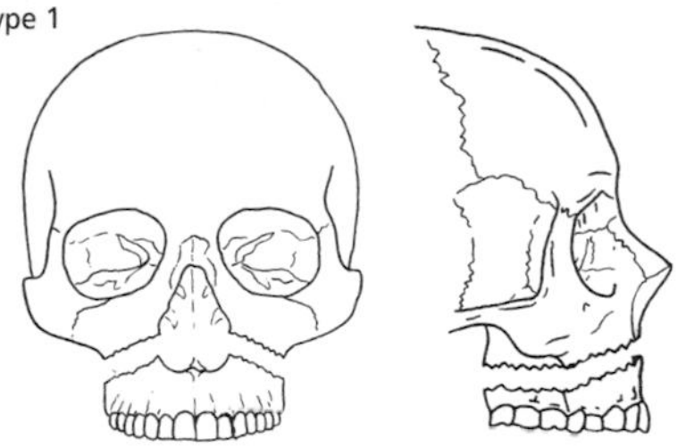

Le Fort II Fracture

The "pyramidal" fracture (involves the nasal bones, the floor of the orbit, the maxillary sinus, the pterygoid plates).

Type 2

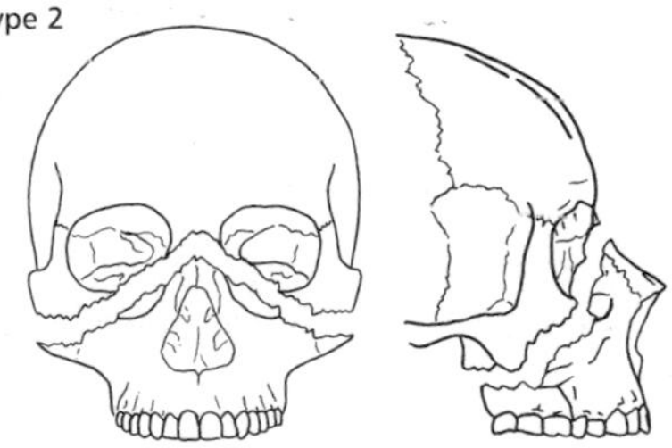

Le Fort III Fracture

From a severe blow to the face with separation of the facial skeleton from the base of the skull ("cranio-facial dysjunction").

Type 3

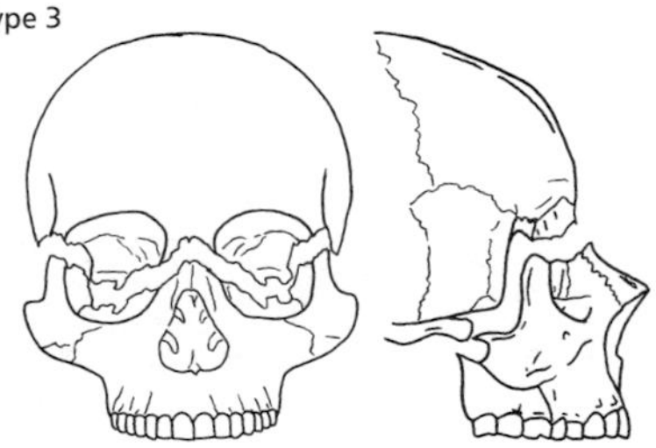

Figure 8 – Le Fort classification of maxillary fractures

Signs and symptoms of Le Fort II and III Fractures are bilateral cicumorbital and subconjunctival ecchymosis (**"racoon eyes"**) and Facial oedema (**"balloon face"**); downward and backward displacement of the middle third of the face (**"dished face"**), **mobility** of the middle third of the face; paraesthesia (infra-orbital nerve distribution); CSF **rhinorrhoea** (ethmoid dural tear) and **diplopia** and **enophthalmos** (when orbital floor comminuted).

Fractures of the middle third of the face cause **serious airway problems** which can be **life threatening**. The middle third of the face is displaced downward and backward, the soft palate impacts against the posterior pharynx and the base of the tongue along with massive bleeding form the fracture site. Treat by disimpacting the maxilla (manually pull the maxilla forwards and upwards). This clears the posterior airway obstruction and reduces the fracture so resulting in decreased bleeding. The conscious patient should be nursed in a sitting position with regular oral suction at hand. Sometimes endotracheal intubation is necessary.

Surgical treatment depends upon the severity and involves a combination of open and closed reduction techniques.

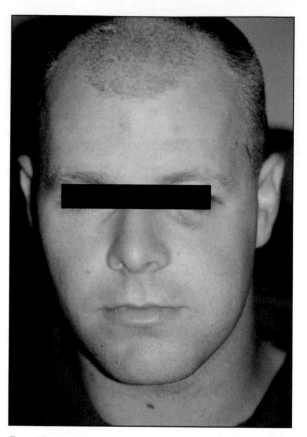

Figure 10 – A patient with a zygomatic complex fracture (footballer)

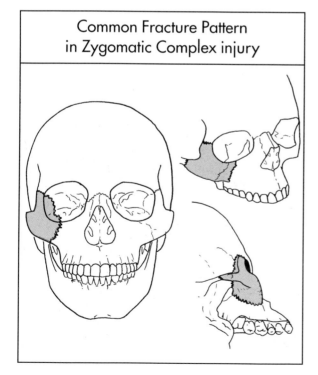

Figure 9 – Common fracture pattern in zygomatic complex injury

FRACTURES OF THE ZYGOMA

Common facial injuries in sporting accidents because of the zygoma's prominent position. The zygoma is a four sided anatomical pyramid (not a tripod structure) (Fig. 9).

The **first priority** in examining a zygomatic complex fracture is to assess the **globe** and **exclude ocular damage.** (Ocular injuries occur in 5%).

Signs and symptoms of these fractures include: periorbital ecchymosis and oedema, flattening of the zygomatic prominence, indentation, deformity (palpable step defect) of the infra-orbital margin, ecchymosis and tenderness to palpation at the maxillary buttress, subconjunctival ecchymosis, diplopia, limited oral opening, and mandibular lateral extrusion towards the side of fracture, paraesthesia of infra-orbital nerve distribution, epistaxis, air emphysema and enophthalmos (rare) (Fig. 10).

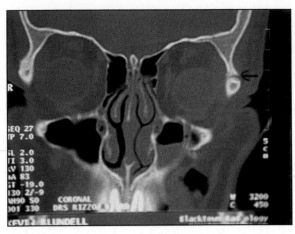

Figure 11 – CT of a zygomatic fracture

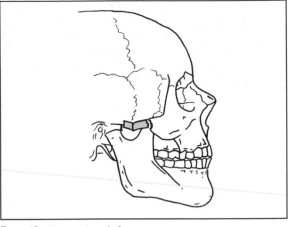

Figure 12 – Zygomatic arch feature

X-rays to be taken include: occipitomental views, submentovertex and CT scan (coronal) (Fig. 11).

For minimally displaced cases, a simple elevation of the zygoma (via a Gillies' temporal approach) is all that is required.

More often an open reduction with internal fixation is required (rigid fixation rather than traditional wire fixation). The frontozygomatic suture represents the thickest bony buttress of the zygoma and fixation by a plate in this region has been shown to be effective. Two point fixation is often necessary in severely displaced fractures and with plates placed at a combination of either the frontozygomatic suture, infra-orbital rim or maxillary buttress.

The orbital floor may need to be explored and fixed if diplopia is present.

A fracture of the **zygomatic arch alone** without involvement of the body of the zygoma may require elevation (Fig. 12).

ORBITAL BLOW-OUT FRACTURE

A fracture of the orbital floor, without a fracture of the orbital rim, caused by a blow to the orbit resulting in a sudden rise in intraocular pressure (thin orbital floor). This mechanism acts like a safety valve and spares the globe. Often described as a "trap-door" fracture because the fracture gives way in the infra-orbital canal appearing like a trap-door.

Paraesthesia of the infra-orbital nerve is common. The orbital contents may herniate through the fracture into the maxillary sinus or become entrapped in the fracture site (gives diplopia or enophthalmos).

Signs and symptoms include paraesthesia of infra-orbital nerve, diplopia, and enophthalmos.

X-rays include the occipitomental views and a coronal CT scan (Fig. 13).

Treatment is controversial. Surgery necessary for enophthalmos, diplopia (persisting after 10 to 14 days) and in the presence of large blow-out defect (greater than 1.5 cm) with orbital content herniation.

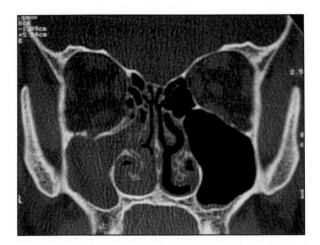

Figure 12 – A coronal CT scan of a blow-out fracture of the orbital floor

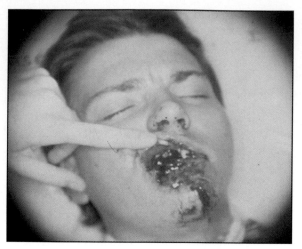

Figure 14 – Male skier with extensive facial lacerations and avulsed teeth from collision with rocks

Small blow out fractures without diplopia need no surgery. Antibiotics (cephalosporin) needed and avoid nose–blowing (to prevent periorbital emphysema).

NASAL FRACTURES

Can be either low or high velocity type fractures. Most from sport are low velocity and can be treated by closed reduction.

Signs and symptoms include nasal swelling, epitaxis, nasal deviation and deformity, mobility and crepitus, septal deviation, and obstruction to breathing.

Radiographs include nasal bone views.

Often the nose has previously been broken. Treated by closed reduction with internal packing.

TEMPOROMANDIBULAR JOINT INJURY (TMJ)

A blow to the TMJ area may cause haemarthrosis, capsulitis, discal damage or subluxation/dislocation. Check for limited mouth opening with pain or deviation, mal occlusion, clicking or difficulty closing the mouth.

Treatment includes initial ace bandages, soft diet, moist heat, NSAID (7-10 days) or surgery (arthroplasty). A dislocation is reduced by grasping each side of the jaw with thumb (inside mouth away from teeth) and pushing down and posteriorly. Post surgery avoid contact sports for 2 to 3 months and use mouth guard.

DENTAL INJURY

Teeth may be impacted, displaced, avulsed or broken (Fig. 14). Exclude associated facial injuries and organise careful dental assessment including X-rays (CXR to find inhaled tooth).

TREATMENT
• Replace avulsed tooth (into clean socket)
• Light bite
• Antibiotic cover
• Suture lacerations
• Exclude alveolar fractures
• Light diet (2 to 3 weeks)
• Use mouthguard

8

EYE

Eugene Hollenbach
I-Van Ho

INTRODUCTION

Sporting injuries to the face are very common, especially to the eyes, ears, nose and teeth. The eye may be injured even though it is protected by the reflex lid closure and the bony orbit. High risk sports include basketball (fingers and elbows), racquet sports (badminton and squash) and high-velocity contact sports (martial arts and football). Effective daily performance relies heavily upon adequate visual acuity, so it is important to perform routine visual acuity assessments in pre-competition examinations.

Many ocular injuries are preventable.
Remember:

1. **Protective** eyewear is important, e.g. polycarbonate spectacles or goggles in high risk environments (high risk sports, working with corrosive substances). Contact lenses offer **no protection** at all!

2. **First Aid** in common ocular injuries **is copious washing** with bland water for chemical injuries/splashes to the eye; **gentle handling** with **no compression** or forced opening of the eye in suspected penetrating injuries.

3. In the event of an **eye injury**, early medical evaluation and ophthalmic review.

Contact sports should be strongly discouraged and use of protective eyewear enforced in the presence of **only one good eye** (e.g. in severe amblyopia (lazy eye), ocular trauma, infections), history of **retinal detachments** or presence of **retinal tears**; diabetic retinopathy; Marfan's syndrome; haemocystinuria; severe myopia (as the elongated globe is at risk for retinal injuries) and recent eye surgery.

History and examination is essential (Fig. 1). Include a check list for eye injuries (Fig. 2).

Thorough examination of the anterior segment requires slit-lamp biomicroscopy with fluorescein stains to show corneal defects (bright green under normal light and bright yellow under blue light). Local anaesthetic (amethocaine 0.5%) may be helpful if pain restricts adequate examination but should never be used to relieve pain for the extension of sporting play. Short-acting mydriatics (0.5% tropicamide) may be used to visualise the fundus.

Note the danger signs of potentially serious eye injury (Fig. 3). Have available the essentials of emergency kit for eyes (Fig. 4).

HISTORY AND EXAMINATION	
Management of eye trauma involves consideration of injuries to both of the globe and the adnexae (lids, lacrimal apparatus and orbit).	
History	*Check for:* 1. Symptoms experienced – pain, blurred vision, diplopia, decreased visual acuity, diminished visual fields, photophobia, floaters or flashes, epiphora (watery eye), altered facial sensations. 2. Possible intraocular foreign body – velocity of injury or particles, type of particles involved – sand, iron; blunt injury vs projectiles 3. Possible injuries sustained and if fellow eye is also affected 4. General medical and ophthalmic history 5. Type of chemical and time of injury
Examination	*Good ophthalmic examination requires:* 1. Adequate illumination 2. Adequate magnification with hand-held monocular or binocular loupe, ophthalmoscope, slit-lamp biomicroscopy 3. Local anaesthetic drops and short acting mydriatics, and fluorescien 4. Eyelid speculum

Figure 1 – History and examination of the injured eye

CHECK LIST FOR EYE INJURIES	
Visual acuity	• Estimate with a Sellen chart or simple reading of differing newpaper font sizes/ sign-boards/counting fingers and perception of a light at various distances. • Pinhole vision • Always done on each eye seprately, **before** installation of eye-drops (mydriatics) and with the best corrected vision (wearing glasses if necessary). The exception is chemical injuries (e.g. line markings) where washing of the eye takes precedence over examination.
Eyelids and lacrimal system	• Eversion of eyelids is necessary for a complete eye examination. Instruct patient to look down with their chin elevated). • Inspect for sub-tarsal foreign bodies and signs of trauma. • Lacerations of the upper eyelids may affect the levator muscle whilst lacerations of the medial eyelids or canthus commonly involve the lacrimal system. Lacerations may involve the orbit itself. Simple bruising may mask an underlying **lacrimal system damage!**
Cornea, conjunctiva and sclera	• Examination using a magnifying lens or a loupe. • Look for surface irregularities, perforations, subconjuctival haemorrhages, iris prolapse, foreign bodies etc. with flourescein.
Pupil	• Note -size, shape, irregularity, iridodonesis (tremulousness of the iris due to lack of support (eg. lens subluxation), abnormal light reflexes, aniscoria (unequal pupil size). • Swinging torch sign indicates retinal or optic nerve damage (relative afferent pupillary defect). A positive RAPD involves pupillary dilation when a light is swung from the normal to abnormal eye.
Anterior chamber fundus	• Any haziness or blood should be noted, and depth of anterior chamber (versus other eye). • Fundus examination may be difficult to interpret in small pupils or hazy media but any definite abnormalities must be noted. • Using an ophthalmoscope – look for the red reflex and any changes in this reflex e.g.. opacities, grey colour (in retinal detachment).
Fellow eye	• Always remember that the patient has two eyes.
Face	• Exophthalmos, enophthalmos. • Look for signs or orbital fracture, nerve palsies, altered facial sensation.
	• Ensure that there are no other more urgent injuries sustained.

Figure 2 – Check list for eye injuries

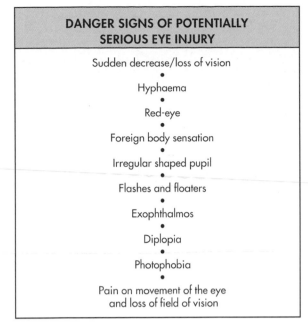

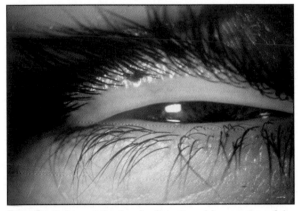

DANGER SIGNS OF POTENTIALLY SERIOUS EYE INJURY
Sudden decrease/loss of vision
•
Hyphaema
•
Red-eye
•
Foreign body sensation
•
Irregular shaped pupil
•
Flashes and floaters
•
Exophthalmos
•
Diplopia
•
Photophobia
•
Pain on movement of the eye and loss of field of vision

Figure 3 – Danger signs of potentially serious eye injury

ESSENTIALS OF EMERGENCY KIT FOR EYE INJURIES
Visual acuity card, pin hole
Penlight
Flourescein
Eye-wash (plastic squeeze bottle)
Eye shield (plastic/metal)
Topical anaesthesia (amethocaine)
Antibiotic and short-acting mydriatics
Tape
Plastic sandwich bags
Eye speculum
Ophthalmoscope

Figure 4 – The essentials of an emergency kit for eye injuries

NON-PENETRATING INJURIES

MECHANICAL

Conjunctival Lacerations

The conjunctiva may be torn in sporting injuries to the eye but is seldom serious and seldom requires suturing. It is important to exclude lacerations to the orbit itself (i.e. scleral penetration). **Never apply ointment** to the eye if penetrating lacerations are suspected. Refer to ophthalmologist.

Conjunctival Foreign Body

Commonly occurs when dirt or sand is thrust into the eye in the course of being tackled in contact sports with facial contact with the ground. It is usually very painful and obvious, provided the eyelids are everted during examination. If high velocity injury, consider intra–ocular penetration.

Treatment:

• Wash with sterile saline or water, or use a sterile cotton bud to remove.

• Evert eyelids to ensure removal of all foreign bodies (Fig. 5).

Figure 5 – **Subtarsal foreign bodies.** Found by eversion of the eyelids

• Refer to ophthalmologist if removal of foreign body is not successful.

Conjunctival or Eyelid Oedema

• Eyelid oedema: apply crushed ice in a plastic sandwich bag taped to the eye.

• Conjunctival oedema (severe chemosis): tape all edges of a plastic sheet around the eye to create a "moist chamber" to prevent drying of the conjunctiva.

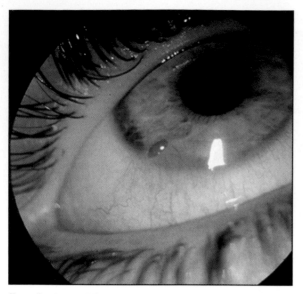

Figure 6 – **Corneal foreign body from insect**. Examine with the slit-lamp

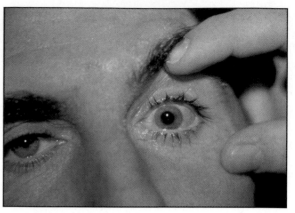

Figure 7 – **Heterochromia** the difference in iris colour is due to iron deposition in this man's left eye after along standing hyphaema. The Fe comes from the haemoglobin! (Pupils are dilated with mydriasis).

Corneal Foreign Body

Usually arises from the same mechanism as with conjunctival foreign body. Metallic foreign bodies tend to stick and leave a rust ring upon removal (Fig. 6).

Treatment:

- Anaesthetise and stain the eye with Fluorescein/ Amethocaine to assist with examination and procedure.

- Stabilise the patient's head, eyes (ask patient to look at a point) and open eyelids.

- Remove by gentle leverage with a sterile 24-gauge needle under magnification and bright illumination; ideally using a slit-lamp.

- All corneal foreign bodies overlying the pupil must be referred to the ophthalmologist for removal.

- If rust-ring remains: chloramphenicol and mydriatic drops or ointments, pad eye, review in 24 hours when the rust-ring often separates easily (Fig. 7).

Small rust rings not in the visual axis should be left alone but those that are within the visual axis should be referred to an ophthalmologist.

The following are common injuries seen after a blunt ocular injury:

CORNEAL ABRASIONS

Corneal abrasions commonly follow a fingernail scratch to the eye or foreign bodies in the eye, and present with pain, photophobia and epiphora. Fluorescein dye will delineate the extent and region of abrasions.

Treatment:

- Chloramphenicol ointment, cyclopentulate 1% (dilates pupil and the accompanying decrease in ciliary spasm increases comfort) and pad firmly.

- Review 24 hourly, and continue padding, until fluorescein stained abrasions not visible.

- Look for: sub-tarsal foreign bodies, corneal lacerations, signs of infection.

- Padded eyes should not be disturbed for swifter healing, but the eyes should be re-examined 24 hourly for presence of infection.

- Contact lenses must not be worn until complete healing and local anaesthetic should never be used as long-term analgesics as it disrupts the corneal healing process.

- Tetanus prophylaxis must be considered for all corneal injuries.

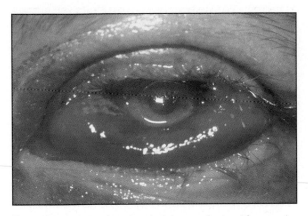

Figure 8 – Severe subconjunctival haemorrhage with extensive protrusion of the conjuctiva. Investigate further for other ocular damage (refer) such as orbital fracture

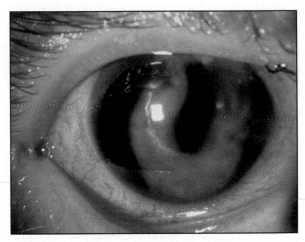

Figure 9 – Severe (non–penetrating) blunt trauma to the eye with hyphaema, oval shaped/irregular pupil and 360° iris detachment. These injuries are emergencies and must be referred to the ophthalmologist

CORNEAL LACERATIONS

A laceration is an extension of an abrasion and must always be treated with great care. Refer to ophthalmologist.

Treatment:

- Assume penetrating injury !

- Do not increase intraocular pressure: by forcing eyelids open, squeezing eye closed, pressure on eye, physical activity. Increased intraocular pressure in the presence of a penetrating injury may lead to decompression and loss of the globe.

- Lightly pad and transfer to hospital with ophthalmological department.

- No topical preparation if perforation suspected.

- X-ray or ultrasound to exclude intraocular foreign bodies.

SUBCONJUNCTIVAL HAEMORRHAGE (SCH)

Common injury arising from a blow to the eye, weight lifting or scuba diving where there is a change in intravascular pressure (Fig. 8). It can also occur in very trivial injuries or spontaneously (usually in the elderly).

Treatment:

- No treatment as it is usually settles in 1-3 weeks.

- **Beware**

    - hypertension: must investigate further.

- no posterior limit to SCH: possible orbital or cranial injury that must be excluded by careful examination and radiological investigations.

- frequent SCH: possible blood dyscrasias need to excluded.

- SCH may conceal a scleral rupture; indicated by a collapsed appearance of the eye.

HYPHAEMA

Haemorrhage into the anterior chamber by small iris vessels. This is an **extremely common sports** related injury usually following blunt trauma (hit by a squash ball, shuttlecock). A serious condition **in children** due to a high incidence of a more severe secondary haemorrhage, usually leading to a severe form of glaucoma (Fig. 9).

Symptoms: blurred vision, red eye, pain, photophobia, drowsiness (due to concussion or hyphaema).

Signs: hazy anterior chamber that settles within a few hours to form a fluid level when sitting upright, slowly reactive and irregular pupil (traumatic mydriasis), associated orbit, ciliary body, retinal damage are common.

Treatment:

- Ocular emergency due to high rate of rebleed.

- Pad both eyes, sedation, absolute bed-rest with head elevated, no strenuous exercise.

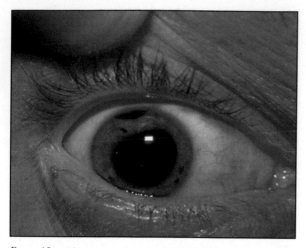

Figure 10 – Blunt trauma causing **iridodialysis** of the superior iris (11 o'clock) and **traumatic mydriasis**. Not uncommonly encountered and easily missed if not looked for.

- Hospitalise and obtain an ophthalmological consult.

- Ophthalmic follow-up to detect/manage complications: (rebleed, secondary glaucoma, cataracts, corneal staining).

- Cyclopegics may be considered for relief of ciliary spasms to increase comfort.

- Topical steroids.

TRAUMATIC MYDRIASIS/IRITIS

Common in blunt injuries due to damaged iris sphincter and is often associated with accommodative paresis. May recover spontaneously. Traumatic iritis may also lead to a miosis (Fig. 10).

Symptoms: blurred vision, photophobia, pain.

Signs: irregular and minimally reactive pupils in traumatic mydriasis.

Treatment: exclude other ocular injuries; ophthalmic review.

IRIDODIALYSIS

Avulsion of a portion of the iris root in severe blunt trauma. A 360° iris root avulsion may occur in very severe injuries. It is always associated with a hyphaema and is managed as such. Retinal dialysis must be excluded.

LENS INJURY

Traumatic lens subluxation or dislocation may be present and results in iridodonesis or phacodonesis. Vitreous humour may also appear in the anterior chamber of the eye.

Cataract formation is more common with penetrating injuries and is usually not seen until days or weeks later. The pattern of the cataract is typical of trauma with the anterior and posterior layer of the lens affected. Lens injury requires urgent hospitalisation and ophthalmological consult.

Posterior segment involvement in ocular trauma

Not uncommon such as choroidal ruptures and haemorrhage; retinal oedema (especially in the macular region), tears, haemorrhage and leading to detachments and optic nerve damage; potentially resulting in visual loss. Thus, if visualisation of fundus is difficult (vitreous haemorrhage) or posterior segment is suspected, urgent hospitalisation and ophthalmological consult is required.

RETINAL INJURIES

Haemorrhage and oedema usually affect the macular region and may not necessarily be associated with anterior segment injuries. Peripheral oedema may be asymptomatic and resolve in several weeks without any permanent sequelae.

Symptoms: blurred vision, sudden shower of floaters.

Signs: haemorrhage may be seen on or within the retina or in the vitreous, whitish elevation of the retina in oedema (best appreciated using a slit-lamp or indirect ophthalmoscope), decreased pupillary reflex.

Retinal detachments/dialysis commonly follow severe blunt injuries with the temporal quadrant most often affected (Fig. 11). It is usually secondary to retinal tears or dialysis. Supero-temporal detachments affects the macula earliest as gravity assists in the process of detachment. Retinal detachment, especially with macular involvement, leads to visual loss thus it is an ocular emergency. Most detachments are now treated with lasers.

Symptoms: flashes, floaters (new dark ones, sudden showers), dark curtain coming down over vision.

Signs: early detached retina appears elevated and once detached, becomes grey in appearance with the vessels

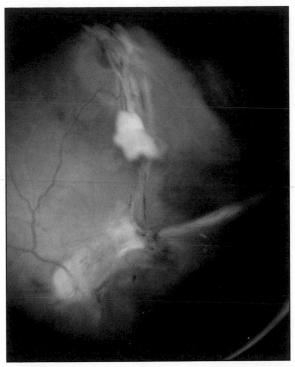

Figure 11 – Fundoscopy shows a Fractional Retinal detachment from a penetrating eye injury

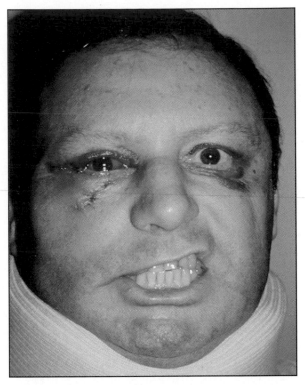

Figure 12 – **Head and Ocular Trauma (R)**. The important features here are SCH, lacerations on the lower eyelid and obvious VIIn palsy. This demonstrates the importance of never limiting an ophthalmic examination to the ocular structures only!

being black, red–reflex becomes grey, decreased pupillary reflex.

Choroidal rupture follows severe blunt trauma and is usually associated with a retinal haemorrhage. Examination shows a whitish retinal area circumscribing the optic disc. Prolonged rest is needed for recovery.

Optic nerve may be injured from direct injury but more commonly follows blunt head injury with no ocular damage, producing permanent blindness. Fracture of the optic canal is not commonly found. The visual loss is most likely a result of tearing of the nutrient vessels to the nerve by the shearing stress. Examination may reveal abnormal pupillary light reflex and a pale, swollen disc.

ORBITAL INJURY

May or may not be associated with fracture of orbital bones. Retrobulbar haemorrhage and oedema may lead to exophthalmos and limitations of eye movements with diplopia, even in the absence of blow-out fractures (Fig. 12).

Blow-out fracture (Figs. 13 & 14) occurs in severe blunt injuries that suddenly increases the intraorbital pressure markedly. Punching, kicking or being hit in the eye with a **squash ball** commonly results in a blow-out fracture. The strong orbital margins usually remain intact whilst the thin orbital floor, offering little resistance, may fracture. Intraorbital contents may herniate through the fracture site and consequently become trapped within. Orbital floor and the medial wall are the most common fracture site.

Clinical features include:

- Periocular signs: ecchymosis, oedema, subcutaneous emphysema.

- Enophthalmos: usually with a downwards displacement as the intraorbital contents herniate through the fractured floor. A narrowed palpebral fissure and deep superior sulcus may be seen.

- Intra-orbital nerve anaesthesia (orbital floor fractures): lower lid, cheek, side of nose, upper lip, upper teeth and gums.

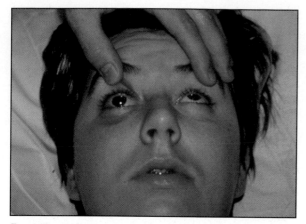

Figure 13 – (R) Orbital floor fracture. Note periocular ecchymoses, restricted elevation of the (R) eye. Orbital floor fractures are common in blunt injuries and require full ophthalmic examination and X-ray

- Supra-orbital paraethesia from fracture of orbital roof.

- Diplopia: inferior rectus and orbital fat is commonly trapped in the fracture side, limiting vertical movements. Limitation of movement may also be due to oedema, haemorrhage, muscular damage.

- Ocular damage: must be assessed.

Medial wall fracture usually occurs with floor fracture and the following must be considered:

- Nasolacrimal duct involved leading to occlusion and epiphora and commonly a secondary dacrocystitis.

- Subcutaneous emphysema is more common and is usually the initial presentation. This is accentuated by the patient blowing their nose, which should be discouraged as it may blow infected sinus contents intra-orbitally.

- Medial rectus entrapment

- X-rays may demonstrate a maxillary sinus clouding, herniated contents into maxillary sinus, air in the orbit, fracture (very rarely seen). CT scan offers better resolution and should be used in doubtful cases.

Treatment:

- Antibiotics to prevent orbital cellulitis, especially if maxillary sinus involved.

- Light padding of the eye and instruct patient not to blow their nose.

- Ophthalmological consult.

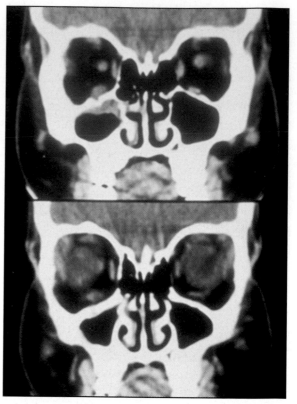

Figure 14 – CT scan (coronal). Shows obvious fracture in the (R) orbital flow with herniation of intra-ocular tissue (fat or inferior rectus muscle)

Treatment is usually **conservative**, as some fractures will unite, otherwise surgery.

CHEMICAL

Alkali and Acid Burns

Alkali and acid injuries to the eye are ocular emergencies. Line markings on sporting fields contain **lime** and may result in a chemical injury to the eyes (Figs. 15 & 16).

Management:

- First aid involves instillation of topical anaesthetics and oral analgesics, washing copiously with water or sterile saline; eyelids must be everted to ensure all chemical/particles are removed (especially in lime injury).

- Neutralising chemicals.

- Immediate hospitalisation and ophthalmic consult.

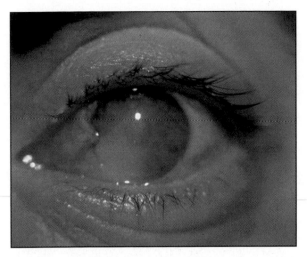

Figure 15 – **Alkali burn of eye.** Subtle, easily missed, devastating. Note the scleral whitening and corneal cloudiness due to the alkali infiltration into the deeper corneal layers. **Ocular emergency!**

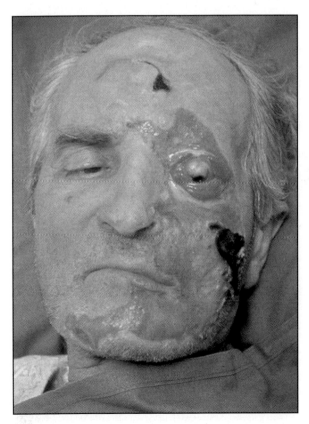

Figure 16 – **Acid Burn** to face and eye (not as severe as alkali, which penetrates the eye) from accident. Note the extensive facial burns and the destroyed globe. Left eye cannot be saved (needs a prosthetic eye). Must take good care of his only remaining (R) eye.

The immediate injury often appears deceptively mild but can lead to severe damage, especially with alkali burns as it **penetrates deeply** into the eye, producing gross corneal and conjunctival scarring, iritis, uveitis, lens changes, secondary glaucoma, ophthisis bulbi.

Radiant Burns

Ultraviolet light causes epithelial damage to the conjunctiva or corneal surface. This is common in water or snow sports; where there is ample surface reflection of the UV-light.

Symptoms: excruciating pain, blepharospasm, epiphora, photophobia, developing a few hours later.

Signs: multiple small epithelial defects over corneal surface visualised with fluorescein stain.

Management:

- Mild cases - soothing drops (e.g. liquifilm and albalon)

- Severe cases - hydrocortisone ointment, firm padding, systemic analgesics.

These cases usually settle with minimal sequelae.

Heat burns by fire usually have accompanying facial burns and requires hospitalisation and specialist attention.

PENETRATING INJURIES

Penetrating injuries may always be suspected or excluded in all ocular injuries. The signs are hyphaema, subconjunctival haemorrhage, asymmetrical depth of anterior chamber and difference in intraocular pressures. If the history is suggestive, then assume a penetrating injury (Figs. 17 &18).

Teardrop shaped pupil strongly suggests a corneal perforation and iris prolapse, with the apex pointing to the perforation. Beware that subconjunctival haemorrhages may conceal a scleral perforation.

Treatment:

- Do not manipulate the eye, forcefully open the eye for detailed examination or attempt removal of an obvious penetrating foreign body (e.g. nail in the eye) as this may cause further damage.

- No drops, light pad only.

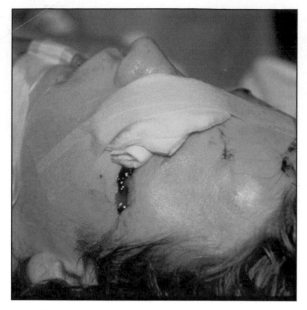

Figure 17 – **Penetrating injury of the eye.** This lady was brought into casualty with a firm, triple layered eye pad for ocular trauma suspected penetration

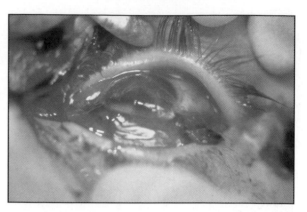

Figure 18 – Note the damage done to the eye if intra-ocular pressure in increased in the presence of ocular perforation. **Never firmly pad or manipulate a suspected penetrating injury of the eye**

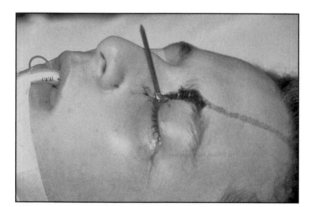

Figure 19 – Nail in eye from nail-gun. CT to determine whether intra-orbital or intra-ocular. **Do not remove nail** (leave to eye surgeon)

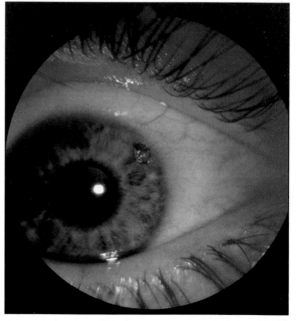

Figure 20 – **More subtle penetrating injury.** There is an obvious corneal lesion, (near the limbus), with a reactive ciliary injection. Note from inspecting the pupil carefully there is a small intraocular foreign body. (The corneal lesion is the perforation site)

- Light padding and urgent transfer to hospital, ophthalmological consult.

- X-ray or CT done to exclude intra-ocular foreign body.

If there is no intra-ocular foreign body, meticulous repair with microsurgical techniques. However, the prognosis is much worse if the lens is damaged, or if ocular contents extruded.

Remember:

Intra-ocular foreign bodies occur after high-velocity projectile injuries (Figs. 19 & 20). Visual loss may result from: direct damage to ocular structures, infection or retained foreign particles (especially copper or iron). The penalty for leaving copper or iron particles is loss of the eye due to dispersion of the particles, occurring up to years later. Non-reactive particles such as glass or plastic are best left alone unless they can be removed without much harm to the eye.

(Slides courtesy of Dr Michael Hargraves, Eye Surgeon, Sydney).

PREVENTION OF EYE INJURIES

Identify

- High risk sports
  - squash (small ball fits inside the orbit)
  - cricket (large ball outside orbit)
  - UV radiation from skiing
  - boxing, wrestling, martial arts

- High risk athletes
  - Functional one-eyed athlete (only **low contact sports** with eye protection)

Wear

- Use **eye protection** (polycarbonate 3 mm centre thickness, 2 mm for low contact; with sturdy frame and posterior rim or moulded temple; anti-fog treatment; have properly fitted).

After injury

- Return to sport when eye comfortable with good vision and "valsalva manoeuvre" is safe.

Figure 21- Prevention of eye injuries

9

SPINE

Ian Farey
Can Huynh

INTRODUCTION

During the past 20 years, there has been a significant increase in participation in competitive and recreational sporting activities. This has led to an increased incidence of injury. Fortunately, injuries to the spine occur infrequently. Less than 10% of reported sports-related musculoskeletal injuries involve the spine. However, these injuries are potentially devastating to the sportsperson (Fig. 1). Football, water sports (particularly diving), and trampolining are the commonest causes of sporting-related spinal injuries (Fig. 2).

Correct evaluation and diagnosis is the key to appropriate treatment and prevention of potentially devastating consequences of spinal column injuries

EVALUATION

The evaluation of an injured spine in a sportsperson requires that a detailed history and physical examination be performed (Fig. 3).

CLINICAL EXAMINATION

The spine should be examined posteriorly, to evaluate the posture and structural deformities. Cutaneous lesions such as midline dimple or neurofibroma should be noted as they may be associated with underlying spinal abnormality. Palpation will determine local tenderness and is helpful in the assessment of muscle spasm and spinal alignment. The range of motion of the spine and its rhythm and any pain reduction should be noted. In the lumbar spine, the neural tension signs (straight leg raising test, Lasegue test, crossed straight leg raising test and femoral nerve stretch test) should be elicited. In the cervical spine, extension combined with rotation may precipitate

radicular pain or symptoms in patients with cervical disc protrusion or spondylosis. Complete neurological examination is mandatory as is assessment of gait. In suspected lumbar spinal injuries, examination of the abdomen and hips is essential, as symptoms arising from these regions can be misinterpreted as arising from the lumbar spine.

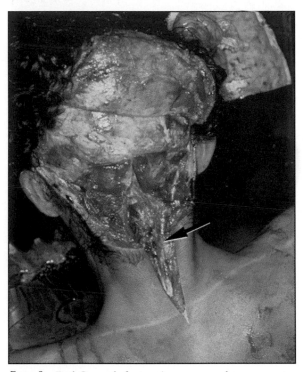

Figure 2 – Fatal C_2 crush fracture in a young male cross-country skier from an uncontrolled slide down a slippery slope

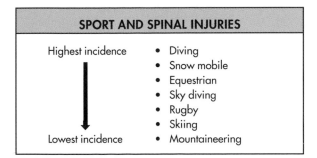

Figure 1 – Relative risks of sporting spinal injury

SPORT AND SPINAL INJURIES	
Highest incidence	• Diving
	• Snow mobile
↓	• Equestrian
	• Sky diving
	• Rugby
	• Skiing
Lowest incidence	• Mountaineering

HISTORY
• Mechanism of injury
• Pain profile
- site
- character and severity of pain
- frequency
- radiation
- exacerbating/relieving factors
- symptoms of nerve root/ spinal cord compression
- recent alteration in activity level, training technique or equipment
- systemic symptoms
- disability

Figure 3 – Approach to the athlete with a suspected neck injury on the field

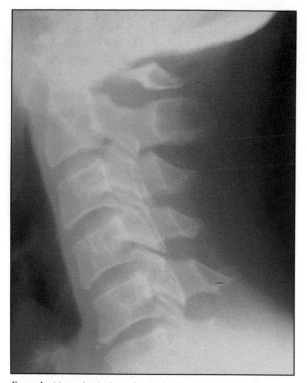

Figure 4 – Normal spinal canal/vertebral body ratio is 1:1

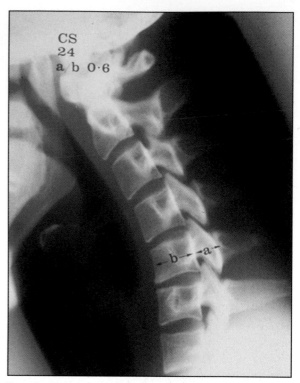

Figure 5 – Congenital canal narrowing where ratio a/b is 0.6

RADIOLOGICAL INVESTIGATION

Major advances have occurred in the radiological evaluation of spinal disorders with imaging modalities such as computed tomography and magnetic resonance imaging. To gain maximum information, the imaging techniques must be used appropriately.

PLAIN RADIOGRAPHS

A very useful tool in the initial imaging of spinal trauma. Assessment of vertebral alignment, fractures and ligamentous injury. Adequate cervical spine radiographs must include C1-T1. Spinal canal narrowing and congenital fusions can be assessed.

CONGENITAL CERVICAL SPINAL CANAL STENOSIS

Athletes with congenital canal narrowing are more susceptible to spinal cord injury, even in the presence of minor disc protrusion or subluxation. Assessment of canal dimensions with Torg's canal to vertebral body width ratio eliminates magnification effect. The normal ratio is 1:1. A spinal canal is narrow if this ratio is less than 0.8 at C3-C6 (Figs. 4 & 5).

COMPUTED TOMOGRAPHY

Provides useful assessment of fractures/dislocations including number, size and position of bony fragments. Aids in surgical planning. Spinal canal contents are poorly visualised. CT rarely depicts disc protrusion in the cervical spine. CT/myelography may be used to visualise compressive lesions when MRI is unavailable.

MRI

MRI with its multi-planar capabilities and superb soft tissue contrast is the modality of choice to investigate suspected spinal cord, disc or ligamentous injuries. Assessment with MRI for disc protrusion is essential in bilateral facet joint dislocations to prevent possible cord compression by disc material prolapsed behind the vertebral body following reduction of the dislocation.

BONE SCAN

This investigation may be useful in cases of unexplained pain - occult fracture, infection, tumour. However, bone scanning lacks specificity.

INJURY CLASSIFICATION

The majority of sports-related injuries to the spine occur in the cervical region. Injuries may be classified as follows:

1. Soft tissue injuries
   - sprains
   - ligamentous injuries with instability
   - intervertebral disc lesions
   - spinal cord injury without fracture/dislocation
   - stinger/burner syndrome.
2. Fracture/dislocations.

SOFT TISSUE INJURIES

CERVICAL SPINE

Acute Sprain Syndrome

This injury is frequently seen in contact sports. It is usually caused by lesser axial loading, flexion or rotation injury. Pain localised to spine and associated

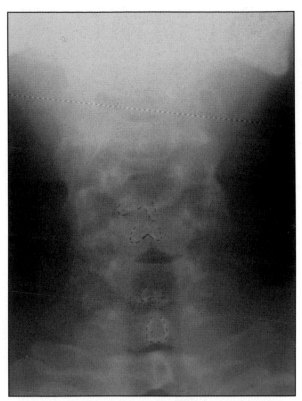

Figure 7 – Increased interspinous distance on X-ray

limitation of spinal motion. Neurological and radiological examination is normal. The exact nature of the injury is usually not determined but minor injury to the disc, ligaments or facet joints may have occurred.

Treatment may include immobilisation, analgesia, anti-inflammatory medication and physiotherapy. Lateral flexion and extension radiographs are indicated after acute symptoms have subsided to exclude instability.

LIGAMENTOUS INJURIES

Mechanism

Ligamentous disruption is usually caused by flexion, often combined with rotational injury. Disruption of the interspinous ligaments, facet joint capsules, posterior longitudinal ligament and posterior aspect of the intervertebral disc can occur (Figs. 6 & 7).

Clinical Assessment

Local tenderness is present with associated restricted motion. Neurological deficit may occur. Ligamentous

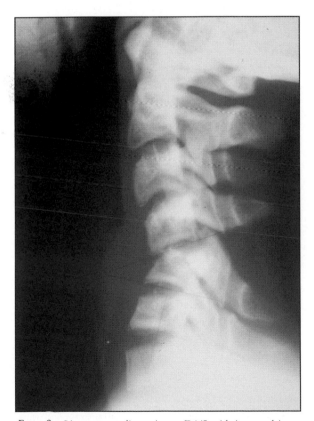

Figure 6 – Ligamentous distruption at D4/5 with increased interspinous distance, angulation and overriding of facets

RADIOLOGICAL SIGNS OF LIGAMENTOUS INJURY
• Widening of interspinous interval (Fig. 7) • Reversal of cervical lordosis • Posterior disc space widening • Subluxation of facet joints or loss of parallelism of joints (Fig. 6) • Anterior vertebral subluxation • Ligament disruption/oedema (MRI)

Figure 8 – Radiological signs of ligamentous injury

CRITERIA FOR INSTABILITY
Upper Cervical Spine • Atlanto-dens interval greater than 3 mm (adult), greater than 4 mm (child) **Sub-Axial Cervical Spine** • Greater than 3.5 mm subluxation (Fig. 10) • Greater than 11° angulation (Fig. 11)

Figure 9 – Criteria for instability

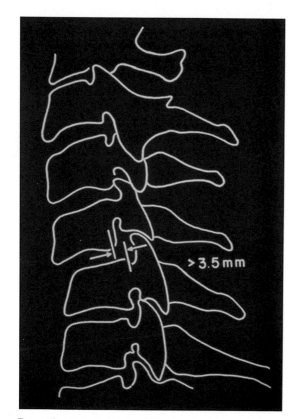

Figure 10 – Criteria for instability in subaxial cervical spine (>3.5 mm subluxation).

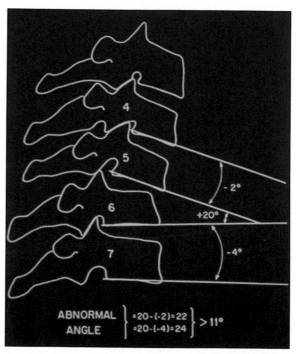

Figure 11 – Criteria for instability in subaxial cervical spine (>11° angulation).

injuries are diagnosed by mal-alignment of osseous structures on radiographs (Fig. 8).

Pseudo subluxation may occur in children, especially at C2/3, C3/4. This is a normal variant in the flexed cervical spine of children.

Flexion extension radiographs are indicated when ligamentous injury is suspected. Ligament disruptions may lead to instability (Fig. 9).

Management

- Unstable injury. Segmental posterior stabilisation and fusion

- Stable injury - brace immobilisation, analgesia, isometric exercises.

INTERVERTEBRAL DISC LESIONS

These are most commonly seen in the lumbar spine (L4/5, L5/S1). Sports-specific lumbar injuries are seen (Fig. 12). The pathomechanics have been described (Fig. 13). A significant incidence occurs in the cervical spine. They rarely occur in the thoracic spine. Disc lesions usually result from flexion/rotation or weight-lifting injury but hyperextension may produce mid cervical disc herniations (C3/4)

General Clinical Features

Intervertebral disc lesions produce axial pain and restricted spinal motion. They also produce symptoms of radicular compression (pain in a dermatomal distribution), weakness, paraesthesia and numbness. Neurological deficit is secondary to nerve root or spinal cord compression (cervical/thoracic may occur) (Fig. 14).

TREATMENT

Non-operative Treatment

Restricted activity, analgesia, anti-inflammatory medication, physiotherapy and orthotic use indicated. Isometric exercises should not be commenced until pain has settled.

Operative Treatment

Indications for discectomy

Absolute:

- Major neurological deficit
  Spinal cord compression
  Cauda equina syndrome (Fig. 15)

| SPORTS-SPECIFIC LUMBAR INJURIES ||
Sport	Injury
Gymnastics	Spondylolysis (hyper extension)
Ballet	Lumbar strain (arabesque position); spondylolysis
Water sports	Diving (back arching), lumbar strain (butterfly stroke) round back (breast stroke)
Weight lifting	Compressive injuries
Football	Transverse process fractures, disc injury, renal contusion (from helmet)
Running	Back pain
Golf	Back pain, disc disease
Tennis	Back pain

Figure 12 – Sports-specific lumbar injuries

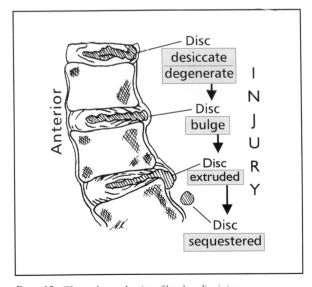

Figure 13 – The pathomechanics of lumbar disc injury

NEUROLOGICAL ASSESSMENT				
Upper Extremity Neurology				
Disc	Root	Motor	Reflex	Sensation
C4/5	C5	Deltoid Biceps	Biceps	Lateral Arm
C5/6	C6	Biceps Wrist Extension	Brachioradialis Thumb/Index	Lateral Forearm Fingers
C6/7	C7	Triceps Wrist Flexion	Triceps	Middle Finger
C7/Tl	C8	Finger Flexion Intrinsics		Ring, Little Finger Medial Forearm
Tl/2	Tl	Intrinsics		Medial Arm
Lower Extremity Neurology				
Disc	Root	Motor	Reflex	Sensation
L3/4	L4	Tibialis Anterior Quadriceps	Knee	Medial Leg and Foot
L4/5	L5	Top Extensors EHL, EDL		Lateral Calf and Dorsum of Foot
L5/Sl	Sl	Eversion	Ankle	Posterior Calf and Lateral Foot

Figure 14 – Neurological assessment of upper and lower extremities

CAUDA EQUINA (SURGICAL EMERGENCY)
• Paralysis of bowel and bladder (urinary retention, bowel incontinence)   • Paralysis lower limb (foot drop)   • Saddle anaesthesia   • Buttock pain

Figure 19 – Cauda Equina Surgical Emergency

Foot drop

• Progressive neurological deficit.

Relative

• Persistent Radicular Pain Unresponsive to Non-Operative Treatment

• Frequent episodes radicular pain.

SURGICAL PROCEDURES

Cervical spine

• Anterior discectomy and fusion

• Foraminotomy (lateral disc protrusion).

Athletes may return to body contact sports following successful single level cervical fusion.

Thoracic Spine

Trans thoracic disc excision — open
                                   — thorascopic

Laminectomy is associated with a significant incidence of paraplegia.

Lumbar Spine

• Partial disc excision — micro discectomy
                        — laminectomy

Recurrent disc protrusion may occur.

STINGER/BURNER SYNDROME

The Stinger/Burner syndrome is a traction injury to the brachial plexus, most commonly an upper trunk lesion.

This injury is common in the rugby codes and also in American football (Fig. 16). Tackling is the usual precipitating event. The injury occurs when the shoulder of a player makes contact with another object. The shoulder is driven caudally and the neck is forced into contra-lateral flexion (Fig. 17).

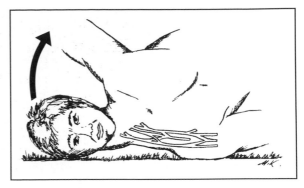

Figure 17 – Mechanism of injury is when the shoulder is driven caudally and the neck is forced into contralteral flexion

Sharp, burning pain radiates from the supraclavicular fossa down the upper limb. Paraesthesia and numbness also occur in a circumferential non-dermatomal distribution. The symptoms usually resolve in a few minutes. Often motor examination is normal. However, weakness may develop in the following hours or days. Weakness, when present, is in the C5, C6 distribution (deltoid, biceps and infraspinatus muscles) (Fig. 18). Significant neck restriction of motion is not a feature. Its presence indicates disc herniation or fracture and requires careful evaluation. Figure 19 outlines the management.

TRANSIENT QUADRIPLEGIA

An acute transient neurological episode of cervical cord origin with sensory changes which may be associated with motor paresis involving both arms, legs or all four limbs after forced hyperextension, axial loading or flexion or the spine. Symptoms and neurological findings are always bilateral.

The patient may also experience Lhermitteís symptoms. Compression of the spinal cord may occur from a hyperextension pincer mechanism in the presence of a congenitally narrow canal. Direct pressure on the spinal cord may occur secondary to disc protrusion or osteophyte impaction following injury.

Fracture or dislocation is not seen on the plain X-ray, but ligamentous instability, congenital fusion or intervertebral disc may be apparent in the presence of congenital spinal canal narrowing. Recovery of neurological function occurs. Patients may return to sport if there is no evidence of instability or degenerative disc disease.

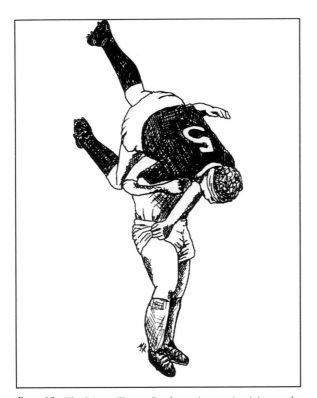

Figure 16 – The Stinger/Burner Syndrome is a traction injury to the brachial plexus not uncommon in rugby codes

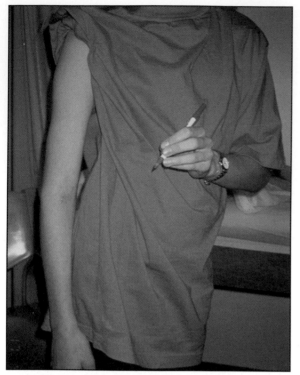

Figure 18 – Transient C5-6 brachial plexus traction injury from trampoline (resolved in 3 months)

MANAGEMENT OF STINGER/BURNER SYNDROME

- Clinical examination
- Monitor neurological status
- Investigate
  Neck pain- radiographs/MRI
  Persistent pain/weakness:
     EMG/radiographs/MRI
- Return to sport
  Normal motor function
- Prevention
  Neck/shoulder strengthening
  High shoulder pads/neck rolls

Figure 19 – Management of Stinger/Burner syndrome.

SPEAR TACKLER'S SPINE

This occurs in an individual who employs the head and neck as the initial point of impact whilst tackling an opponent (Fig. 20). Axial loading of the spine occurs and the patient is at high risk of developing quadriplegia. Radiological findings include congenital narrowing of the spinal canal, reversal of cervical lordosis and slight torticollis. Patient with this spinal configuration should not play contact sport.

FRACTURES AND DISLOCATIONS

Significant spinal column injury must be suspected in any sportsperson who complains of axial pain, restricted motion, paresis, paraesthesia or electric shock-like sensations in the extremities. Any individual who has lost consciousness must be assumed to have a spinal

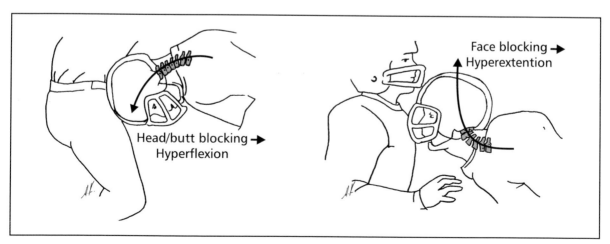

Figure 20 – Head or face blocking in tackling an opponent may result in spear tackler's spine

NEUROLOGICAL DEFICIT

- **Root Injury**
  Dermatomal sensory loss
  Motor and reflex loss appropriate to nerve root

- **Spinal Cord Injury**
  Complete
  No function below level of injury incomplete

- **Central Cord**
  Upper greater than lower extremity involvement
  Motor/sensory loss common. Fair prognosis

- **Anterior Cord**
  Predominant motor loss
  Posterior column motion intact
  Poor prognosis

- **Brown Sequard**
  Ipsilateral motor and position sense loss/
  contralateral pain and temperature loss
  Good prognosis

- **Posterior Cord**
  Rare - loss of position sense
  Poor prognosis

Figure 21 – Neurological deficit can be at both the nerve or spinal cord level

injury until proven otherwise. Only a small proportion of the total number of sports-related spinal injuries result in neurological injury. Neurological injury can occur at both the nerve root or spinal cord level (Fig. 21).

SIGNS OF SPINAL CORD INJURY

The signs of spinal cord injury include:

- Bradycardia
- Hypotension
- Diaphragmatic breathing
- Neurological deficit.

Examination for sacral sensory sparing must be performed as this may be the only indication that an incomplete neurological deficit is present.

Complete spinal cord injury cannot be diagnosed until spinal shock (total loss of motor sensory and reflex function, including absent bulbo cavernosus

reflex) has passed. Spinal shock has resolved when the **bulbo cavernosus reflex** returns (anal sphincter contracts after squeezing the glans penis or by tugging on the urinary catheter).

MANAGEMENT OF SUSPECTED SPINAL COLUMN INJURY

Incorrect management of an unstable injury without neurological deficit can produce neurological deficit. **Prevention of further injury** is the single most important objective of management.

1. At the Scene

- Immobilise head and neck by holding them in neutral position.
- Check breathing and pulse – jaw thrust method to be used for airway clearance.
  Remove mouth guard if present. See Chapter 5, Fig. 5.
- Check consciousness
  - if awake, question regarding pain and symptoms of neurological impairment
- Check neurological status
- Place patient on spinal board or Jordan frame. The body must be kept in line with the head and spine during positioning
- Head immobilisation
- Safe transport.

2. At the hospital

- Resuscitate
- Complete physical examination
- Radiological investigation
- Re-align and stabilise spine
  - traction
  - surgical stabilisation and fusion as indicated
  - orthosis
- Respiratory, pressure area and urinary tract care
- DVT prophylaxis
- Rehabilitation.

High dose steroid treatment if started within the first 8 hours may be effective in improving the prognosis following cord injury (Methylprednisolone, 30 mg/kg, then 4.5mg/kg/hour × 23 hours).

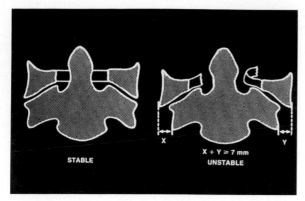

Figure 22 – Criteria for defining unstable Jefferson's fracture (C1)

SPECIFIC FRACTURES AND DISLOCATIONS OF THE CERVICAL SPINE

UPPER CERVICAL SPINE

Jefferson's fracture C1

Fracture of C1 ring, secondary to axial compression (e.g. diving) 75% associated with other cervical vertebrae which require careful evaluation. Unstable fractures have lateral mass spread greater than 7 mm (as seen on open mouth view; Fig. 22) rupture of the transverse ligament on the atlas occurs in this setting. CT scan important for diagnosis.

Treatment:

- for stable use SOMI brace;

- for unstable use Halo brace 3 months; and

- occipito cervical fusion for persistent instability.

Rupture Transverse Ligament of Atlas

Occurs following flexion injury and produces C1/2 instability (ADI greater than 3mm in flexion).

Treatment:
Is surgical with C1/2 fusion.

Odontoid Fractures

Fractures of the odontoid are classified according to the site of fracture (Fig. 23). Pain is experienced in the occipital and sub-occipital regions. Patients may support their chin in their hands to prevent instability. Neurological deficit may present early (cord contusion) or late (instability visualised on AP tomogram). Non-union is prone to occur in Type II injuries (Fig. 24).

Treatment:

- Type I (stable): Soft collar

- Type II (unstable): Halo brace or internal fixation

- Type III (generally stable): SOMI brace.

OS Odontoideum

Result of non-union of odontoid or congenital anomaly. (Fig. 25). Significant instability. Contra-indication to body contact sports.

Treatment: is surgical with C1/2 fusion

Hangman's Fracture (Traumatic Spondylolisthesis)

There is hyperextension causing fracture through the pedicles of C2.

Treatment: is a halo-vest until united (10 weeks). Neurological injury is uncommon.

MID AND LOWER CERVICAL SPINE

Compression Fractures

Wedging of anterior vertebral margin, secondary to flexion injury.

Treatment: SOMI brace immobilisation. If associated with posterior instability - require fusion (greater than 50% of anterior vertebral height and associated posterior ligament injury).

Unilateral Facet Fracture/Dislocation

Flexion rotation injury. Less than 33% subluxation on lateral X-ray (Figs. 26 & 27). Neurological deficit is usually root lesion or Brown-Sequard syndrome.

Bilateral Facet Fracture/Dislocation

Flexion distraction injury with greater than 50% subluxation on lateral X-ray (Fig. 28). Spinal cord injury is commonly associated with this injury.

Treatment: Require reduction, posterior stabilisation and fusion. Pre-operative evaluation with CT scan is required. MRI is required to exclude disc protrusion behind superior vertebral body in all cases of bi-facetal injury to prevent compression of spinal cord by disc material following reduction of dislocation as profound neurological deficit may result.

Types of Odontoid Fractures

Type 1	Type 2	Type 3

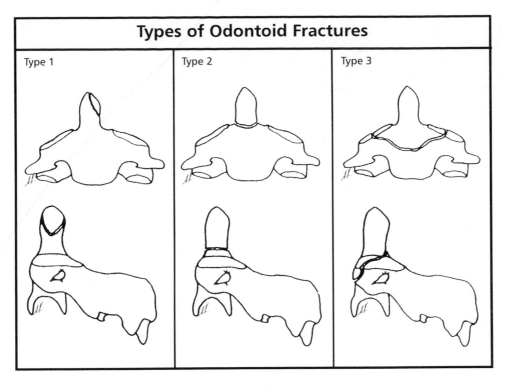

Figure 23 – Three types of odontoid fracture (Anderson, D'Alonzo Classification)

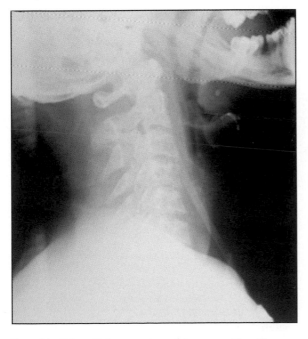

Figure 24 – Odontoid fracture at base of the process (Type II)

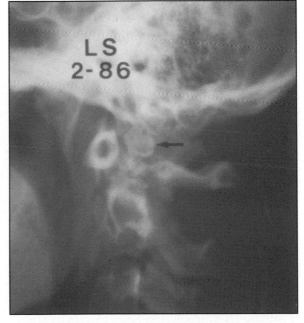

Figure 25 – OS odontoideum

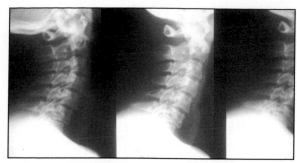

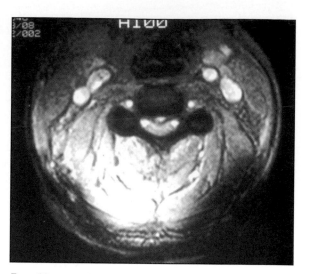

Figure 26 – Unilateral facet dislocation at C6/7

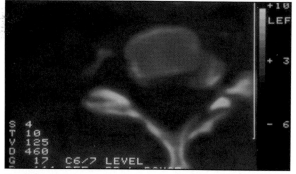

Figure 27 – CT scan showing unilateral facet dislocation with rotation

Figure 29 – Neurological deficit without fracture. MRI shows large disc protrusion and spinal canal compression

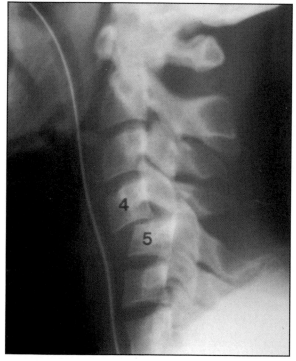

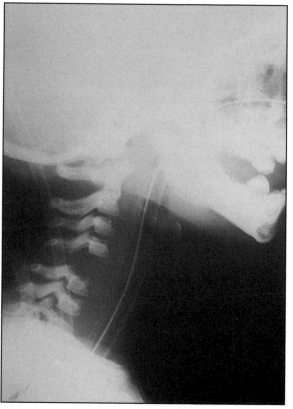

Figure 28 – Bilateral facet dislocation at C4/5

Figure 30 – A 2-year-old with a fatal C4-5 dislocation of the cervical spine (high quadriplegia; no spontaneous respiration; child died within the week)

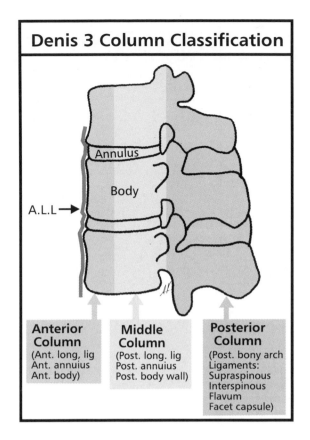

Denis 3 Column Classification

Annulus

Body

A.L.L →

Anterior Column
(Ant. long, lig
Ant. annuius
Ant. body)

Middle Column
(Post. long. lig
Post. annuius
Post. body wall)

Posterior Column
(Post. bony arch
Ligaments:
Supraspinous
Interspinous
Flavum
Facet capsule)

Figure 31 – The three column concept of the spine (Denis) allows stability to be assessed

Burst Fracture

Axial compression injury with fracture fragments displaced into spinal canal. High incidence of spinal cord injury. Non-operative treatment may produce kyphosis and late neurological deficit – generally require anterior vertebrectomy and fusion.

Clay Shoveller's Fracture

Avulsion injury of spinous process (C7, C6 or TI). Stable requires soft collar immobilisation for comfort. Flexion extension radiographs required to exclude instability.

Neurological Deficit Without Fracture

Occurs in patients with congenital narrowing of spinal canal and central disc protrusion, hyper extension injury or following spontaneous reduction of dislocation. MRI mandatory for evaluation (Fig. 29).

Children's spine injuries (Fig. 30) are rare and when

they do occur are at the C1-2 level. It is often a soft-tissue injury with subluxation. Vertebral growth plates may be damaged with later spinal deformity. Spinal cord injury can occur with a normal X-ray (SCIWORA).

Thoraco-Lumbar Spine

The thoracic spine is least susceptible to injury. The rib cage coupled with relative sagittal orientation of the facet joint protects the thoracic spine against injury. However, the thoraco-lumbar junction is the fulcrum between the mobile lumbar spine and relatively immobile thoracic spine and is very susceptible to injury.

The spinal cord usually ends at the Ll/2 interspace. Structural damage in the thoracic spine tends to be associated with neurological deficit. Only 3% of patients with lumbar spine dislocations have neurological deficit. These tend to be at root level and are less debilitating. However, clinical instability of lumbar fractures is common. The lumbar spine supports high physiological loads. Late deformity, pain and occasionally neurological deficit may develop following lumbar fractures. The three column concept of the spine allows stability to be assessed (Fig. 31). Instability is present when 2 or 3 columns are disrupted.

Initial assessment and management is as for cervical spine injuries (Fig. 32).

Specific Thoracic and Lumbar Spine Injuries (outlined in Fig. 33).

Treatment of specific injuries is outlined in Figure 34.

GENERAL TREATMENT THORACO-LUMBAR SPINE FRACTURES AND DISLOCATIONS

- In general for **stable** fractures (well aligned, less than 30° kyphosis and no neurological deficit) is rest, followed by bracing.

- **Unstable** injuries or those with neurological deficit usually require surgery to stabilise the fracture dislocation to preserve or improve neurological function and to prevent late pain, instability and neurological deficit.

Figure 32 – General treatment of thoraco-lumbar spine fractures and dislocations

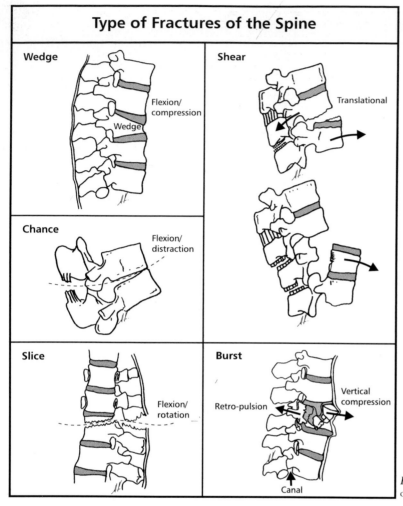

Type of Fractures of the Spine

Wedge

Flexion/compression

Wedge

Shear

Translational

Chance

Flexion/distraction

Slice

Flexion/rotation

Burst

Retro-pulsion

Vertical compression

Canal

Figure 33 – Classification of fractures of the spine

SPONDYLOLYSIS/SPONDYLOLISTHESIS

SPONDYLOLYSIS

Spondylolysis is a stress fracture which develops in the pars interarticularis. It commonly develops in sporting activities which require repetitive hyperextension and rotation. Fast bowlers in cricket, pitchers in baseball, gymnasts, tennis players and weightlifters are prone to this injury. Gymnasts typically develop stress fractures in the upper lumbar spine and these fractures may be present at multiple levels.

Clinically, the patient develops aching low back pain, initially unilateral and then bilateral which increases with extension/rotation of the spine. Nerve root tension signs and neurological deficit are not present but pain can be precipitated by the one-legged extension test and there may be local tenderness.

The stress fracture can be visualised on an oblique X-ray (Fig. 35) but frequently X-rays are normal. A CT scan with reverse angle gantry scan can visualise the defect (Fig. 36). Bone scan (SPECT) may be necessary to diagnose an acute lesion. Chronic lesions will be cold on the bone scan.

Treatment:

Acute - cast immobilisation for two months. There is a significant incidence of fibrous union.

Chronic - symptomatic treatment including restriction of sport, alteration of technique. Flexibility — lumbar and abdominal site exercises.

SPONDYLOLISTHESIS

Anterior displacement of one vertebral body on another (Fig. 37).

SPECIFIC THORACIC AND LUMBAR SPINE INJURIES			
Injury	**Mechanism/Type**	**Treatment**	**Comment**
Compression (wedge)	Flexion	Bed rest/orthosis (Less than 50% loss of vertebral height) associated posterior instability	Neurological deficit uncommon. Stabilisation and fusion if
Chance fracture	Flexion, distraction bony and ligamentous involvement	Bed rest, hyperextension, orthosis or stabilisation and fusion	Neurological deficit uncommon. Duodenal or pancreatic injury common
Shear fracture and slice dislocations	Flexion/rotation	Spinal stabilisation and fusion deficit common	Very unstable - neurological deficit common
Burst	Axial compression	Controversial - <ul><li>neurological deficit surgical decompression and fusion</li><li>no neurological deficit</li><li>bed rest, orthosis unless kyphosis greater than 30° and canal intrusion greater than 50%</li></ul>	Neurological deficit common

Figure 34 – Treatment of specific thoracic and lumbar injuries

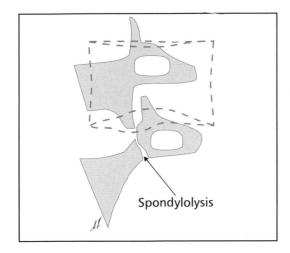

Figure 35 – An oblique view of the lumbar spine may reveal the stress fracture of spondylosis (defect in the neck of the "scottie dog")

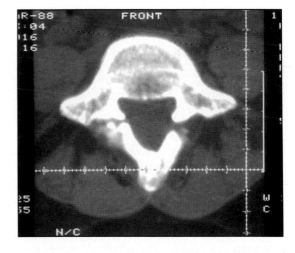

Figure 36 – CAT scan of pars interarticularis defect of lumbar spine

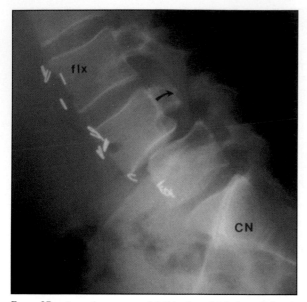

Figure 37 – A grade two spondylolithesis at L4-5 (pars defect is arrowed)

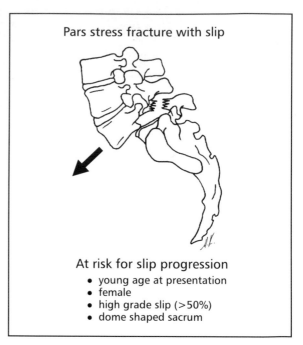

Figure 38 – The risk factors for slip progression in spondylolisthesis

Classification:

    Congenital

    Isthmic (pain interarticularis defect)

    Degenerative

    Traumatic

    Pathological

    Post-surgical.

6% of the population have this condition. The commonest variety is secondary to pars interarticularis defect at L5 producing L5/S1 spondylolisthesis. The degree of spondylolisthesis is graded according to the amount of anterior displacement. Grade I represents 25% forward displacement with grade IV representing 100% displacement.

Spondyloptosis occurs when the superior vertebra is displaced anterior to the inferior vertebral body.

Spondylolisthesis can present as an incidental finding on X-ray. Patients may also experience low back pain and/or radicular pain (L5/S1 spondylolisthesis: L5 radicular pain). Neurological deficit is uncommon. Clinical examination may reveal local tenderness, palpable step at the site of the spondylolisthesis, pain with extension of the spine, heart shaped buttocks in

significant spondylolisthesis (grade III, grade IV) and hamstring tightness.

Sporting activities may precipitate symptoms. The risk factors for slip progression have been described (Fig. 38).

Treatment: Physiotherapy, anti-inflammatory medication, technique modification and trunk exercises may lead to subsidence of symptoms. X-ray guided local anaesthetic and Cortisone injections to the pars interarticularis defect can also be effective. Spinal fusion (in situ) is indicated for persistent pain or painless progression of spondylolisthesis (children). Nerve root decompression is necessary in adults with persistent radicular pain.

VERTEBRAL APOPHYSITIS

Nerve root tension Back pain may be related to apophysitis (Fig. 39). Mechanical pain which is worse with activity and relieved by rest is the presenting feature. Radiographic evidence of changes of apophyseal irregularity at one or more levels without vertebral wedging distinguish this condition from Scheuermann's Disease. The symptoms are produced

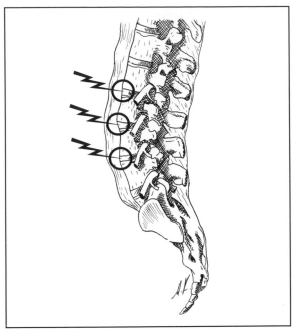

Figure 39 – Vertebral apophysitis is a mechanical cause of back pain in athletes from excessive stress across the spinal apophyses during growth spurts

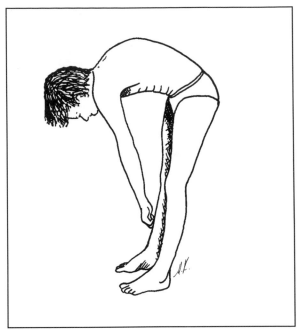

Figure 40 – The risk factors for slip progression in spondylolisthesis

by excessive stress during growth spurts. Treatment includes restriction of activity and strengthening exercises.

CONGENITAL/DEVELOPMENTAL DISORDERS

SCHEURMANN'S DISEASE

Scheurmann's disease produces kyphosis around the time of puberty. Thoracic and low back pain is the presenting feature. The condition is associated with an increased incidence of spondylolisthesis and lumbar disc protrusion.

Clinically, the patient may have increased thoracic kyphosis and lumbar hyper-lordosis (Fig. 40). Spinal motion may be painful.

X-ray criteria for the diagnosis include vertebral end plate irregularity, Schmorlís nodes representing intra-vertebral disc herniation and wedging of 5° anteriorly of at least 3 adjacent vertebral bodies.

Symptoms are commonly precipitated by activities which include rowing and butterfly swimming.

Treatment consists of local modality physiotherapy, strengthening exercises and postural modification. Spinal fusion is occasionally indicated.

KLIPPEL-FEIL ANOMALY

A congenital condition associated with multiple fusions of the cervical vertebrae. Sprengel's shoulder may be associated. Patients with this anomaly should not play body contact sport as there is a significant incidence of cervical spinal canal narrowing and risk of quadriplegia.

CRITERIA FOR RETURN TO SPORT AFTER CERVICAL SPINE INJURY

Cervical spine conditions requiring decision as to whether participation in contact sports is advisable fall into two categories:

1. Congenital or developmental (see above)

2. Post-traumatic (see over page).

The degree of risk of sustaining a spinal cord injury on resumption of body contact sports is variable:

Minimal Risk

Spinous process fracture

Healed lamina fracture

Healed disc protrusion.

Moderate Risk

Facet fracture

Healed odontoid fracture

Acute lateral disc herniation

Cervical radiculopathy, secondary to foraminal osteophyte.

Extreme Risk

C 1/2 instability

Previous upper cervical fusion

Ligamentous instability

Large central disc protrusion with canal narrowing

Multi-level fusion.

Patients in the extreme risk category should not play body contact sport and patients in the moderate risk group should be strongly advised to discontinue.

PREVENTION OF CERVICAL SPINE INJURIES

The incidence of spinal injury can be reduced (as in Schoolboy Rugby Union) by the following:

• Rule modification

• Correct use of protective equipment and play techniques

• Education of athletes, team members and coaching staff

• Avoidance of use of head as initial point of contact in collision situations.

10

SHOULDER

Des Bokor

INTRODUCTION

With its extreme mobility and structural insecurity, the shoulder is probably the most vulnerable joint in the body. The shoulder joint and the muscular supports around it are required to circumscribe large arcs of motion, with high speed and force, to enable the athlete to achieve peak performance. It is not surprising then that the joint is prone to such a variety of injuries with significant stresses being placed on the bones, chondral surfaces and the soft tissues. Between 8 - 13 % of injuries sustained by athletes involve the shoulder (Fig. 1).

ANATOMY AND BIOMECHANICS

The shoulder function is a compilation of coordinated motion between four separate joints. The glenohumeral joint is the main one. The others are the acromio-clavicular, sternoclavicular joints and scapulo-thoracic. Disorders in any of these may be reflected as dysfunction of the glenohumeral joint.

The glenohumeral joint (GHJ) is a ball and socket joint. The humeral head constitutes about one third of a sphere, and the articular surface has a medial angulation of 45 degrees to the shaft and retroversion of about 30 degrees to the transverse axis of the elbow. The glenoid fossa is pear shaped. It's radius of curvature is half that of the humeral head and so the area of bony contact is minimal. The addition of the glenoid labrum increases the depth of the fossa and improves the surface area of contact between the humeral head and the total glenoid cavity. Ligamentous stability is conferred by the superior, middle, and inferior gleno-

humeral ligaments and the capsule. Further stability comes from negative intra-articular joint pressures, the rotator cuff muscles and the coracohumeral ligament (Fig. 2).

The acromioclavicular joint (ACJ) is a diarthrodial joint linking the arm to the axial skeleton. Its bony configuration confers minimal stability to the joint. Within the joint there is a variable fibrocartilaginous disc/meniscus. The capsule with the superior acromioclavicular ligaments stabilise the joint at physiological loads. Further stability is from the coracoclavicular ligaments, the conoid and trapezoid (Fig. 3).

The sternoclavicular joint (SCJ) comprises two incongruent articular surfaces with an intervening fibrocartilaginous disc separating it into two independent joints. It is stabilised by the interclavicular, anterior and posterior sternoclavicular ligaments as well as the costoclavicular ligament (rhomboid ligaments). The joint allows for three planes of motion. The fulcrum of movement is the rhomboid ligament, not the SCJ articulation.

Despite the low weight of the arm, (5% of body weight, i.e. 3.5kg in a 70 kg man) high torque forces

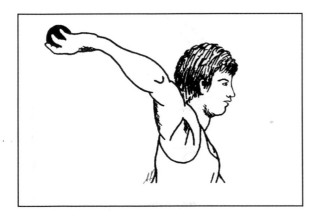

Figure 1 – Action picture of athlete using upper arm in baseball

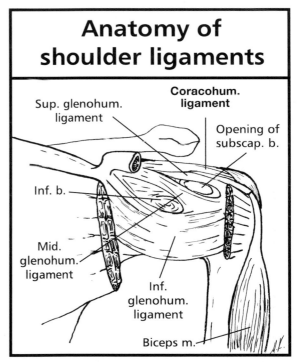

Figure 2 – Anatomy of shoulder ligaments

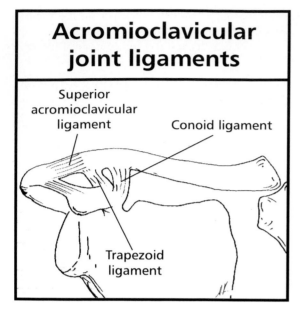

Figure 3 – The acromioclavicular ligaments which stabilise this joint

are generated by the long lever of the arm. The rotator cuff and other shoulder muscles are used to generate movement as well as glenohumeral control. While the shoulder is susceptible to injury from direct forces onto the joint, it is in throwing that all the muscles of the trunk and upper limb work in a synchronised balanced manner to propel an object forward.

Throwing can be divided into: cocking (or wind-up), acceleration and follow-through phases. Imbalance, fatigue, or damage to any structures or muscles may result in pain, tendinitis and/or instability (Fig. 4).

INSTABILITY

Shoulder instability occurs commonly in many sports. Whereas in the past only complete dislocation was recognised, these days a wide spectrum of symptoms occur with a varying degree of slipping of the shoulder. It is common to refer to partial dislocation of the shoulder as subluxation. Many may feel that this is a lesser injury to the glenohumeral joint, however, significant and severe injuries can occur with patients who may have only subluxed their joints. It is better to simply refer to the injuries as **"instability events"** and regard all as potentially damaging to the joint. In the majority of cases (95%) shoulder instability is in the anterior or antero-inferior direction. Other, less common, directions include posterior and multidirectional.

ANTERIOR INSTABILITY

Anterior instability is most likely to occur when the arm is positioned in abduction / external rotation and an anterior load placed on the shoulder joint, as might

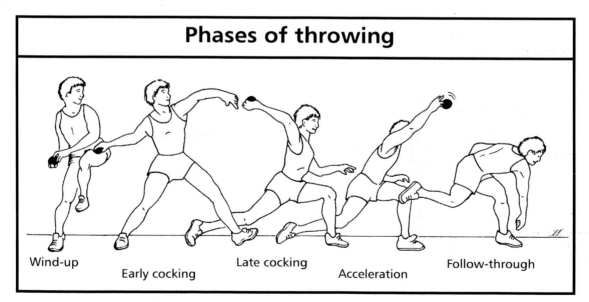

Figure 4 – The phases of throwing

HIERARCHY OF SHOULDER SUPPORT MECHANISMS	
Minimal Loads	Joint Concavity
	Finite Joint Volume
	Adhesion/Cohesion
	Joint Forces
Moderate Loads	Active Co-ordinated
	Cuff Contraction
Massive Loads	Capsulo-ligamentous
	structures
	Bony Supports

Figure 5 – The hierarchy of shoulder support mechanisms

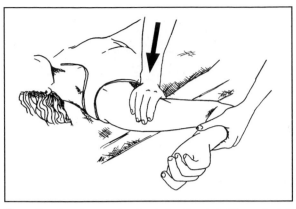

Figure 7 – Anterior apprehension/relocation test. The patient is supine. There may be **apprehension** when the arm is in abduction/external rotation. With downward pressure on the anterior aspect of the arm, the patient feels security (relocation test) and loses any apprehension

occur in a fall on the outstretched hand or tackling a player with the arm out from the side (rugby). In other situations, the instability may occur without an obvious traumatic event. In upper limb, overhead sports (baseball or tennis), gradual stretch of the anterior capsule may occur and give symptoms of the shoulder slipping. There is a hierarchy of support mechanisms controlling glenohumeral stability which, depending on the severity of the force, determine the nature of the damage which might occur (Fig. 5).

The symptoms of instability include: frank dislocation; slipping; pain with the arm in abduction/external rotation; apprehension using the **arm** overhead or a "dead arm" feeling with a tackle or overhead action. **The clinical examination should** include looking at range of motion, strength, increased antero-posterior translation of the humeral head (Fig. 6), apprehension and relocation signs (Fig. 7), coincident tendinitis or labral tears and also signs of ligament laxity.

The natural history of the acute first time anterior shoulder instability is now more clearly described. The chance of **a younger patient** (less than 22 years of age) having a further instability event within 2 years is 62%. Many feel that if these patients participate in contact sports the likelihood of repeat instability is over 90%. **Older patients** have a lesser chance of further instability (in 30-40 year old patients the risk is 25%). Over a 10 year period there is a 12% chance of an instability occurring in the opposite shoulder.

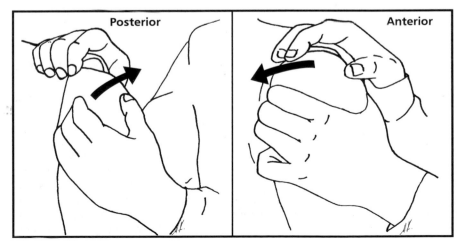

Figure 6 – Clinical demonstration of anterior and posterior glenhumeral translation

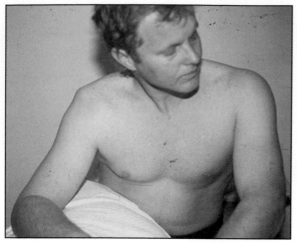

Figure 8 – Typical posture of anterior shoulder dislocation (patient anxious; arm is forward, abducted, internally rotated)

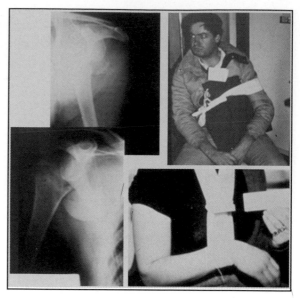

Figure 9 – X-ray anterior shoulder dislocation. Skier with shoulder dislocation; fracture of neck of humerus (apparent after reduction) brachial palsy from dislocation

Most significantly, however, over 10 years there is a 20% incidence of arthritic change on radiograph occurring in the shoulder (9% moderate or severe). This arthropathy is not influenced by the number of dislocations or whether surgery has been performed.

ACUTE DISLOCATION

All patients should be assessed for any associated nerve or vascular injury (Fig. 8). Appropriate X-rays of the shoulder are essential (Fig. 9). Closed reduction can be achieved in the emergency room using either Pethidine/Diazepam/Nitrous oxide or with an intra-articular injection of lignocaine 1%. General anaesthesia may be required where the patient is having excessive muscle spasm. (see Fig. 10 – *Techniques for Closed Reduction of the Dislocated Shoulder*). The arm should be placed in a sling and physiotherapy organised after a 1-3 week period of rest. In younger patients where there is a high risk of recurrence and/or special sporting requirements, an acute arthroscopic assessment and repair may be offered.

RECURRENT DISLOCATION

Where **recurrent** instability becomes a problem, the options of treatment include: modification or avoidance of the precipitating event; a physiotherapy rehabilitation programme to strengthen the shoulder; or surgical reconstruction of the shoulder. A variety of surgical techniques can be used and are divided into those which correct the pathology and those which tighten or use bone blocks to prevent dislocation. Correction of the pathology of instability includes repairing the avulsed inferior gleno-humeral ligament (Bankart Lesion) and correcting any associated capsular redundancy (capsular shift). This is the preferred option in surgical management of the unstable shoulder. The success rate for surgery is approximately 95%. Those procedures which correct the pathology (i.e. anatomical reconstructions) are most likely to restore almost full range of motion. This is important for those athletes involved in upper limb sports requiring a throwing action, e.g. baseball. Many of the non-anatomical reconstructions restrict external rotation and prevent these athletes from being able to perform their sports. (See Fig. 13 - *Types of Surgical Shoulder Reconstructions*)

MULTIDIRECTIONAL INSTABILITY (MDI)

All shoulders demonstrate a variable degree of laxity which is normal. In some patients marked laxity may contribute to symptoms. These may be insidious in onset or be related to a traumatic event. It is important to differentiate laxity from instability. **Laxity** is simply a physical finding, whereas instability is the combination of symptoms and signs. To make the diagnosis of MDI, there is usually instability in at least two directions, inferior plus either/or both anterior and posterior. Patients often have pain and weakness

TECHNIQUES FOR CLOSED REDUCTION OF THE DISLOCATED SHOULDER	
Scapular Rotation Manoeuvre	Patient lies prone on table with injured arm hanging off the edge of the table. The scapula is manipulated to open the front aspect of the joint allowing congruence of the humeral head and glenoid to be restored (inferior tip scapula pushed towards the spine). Elegant and effective (Fig. 11)
Longitudinal Traction Technique	Patient lies supine and the affected arm is slightly abducted. Traction is applied to the arm with the foot (minus shoe) in the axilla or sheet around chest applying counter traction. Simple and effective (Fig. 12).
Stimson's Technique	The patient lies prone. Weight is applied to the arm with the affected shoulder hanging off the edge of a table.
Kocher Manoeuvre	The patient is supine. A sheet is applied around the patients chest. Traction is placed on the arm in slight abduction while the arm is externally rotated, adducted and then internally rotated. Old technique. Painful. May fracture or displace the neck of the humerus.
Forward Elevation Manoeuvre	The patient lies supine. The arm is gently elevated in the plane of the scapula up to about 160 degrees. Traction is a applied in elevation with outward pressure on the humeral head.

Figure 10 – Techniques for shoulder reduction

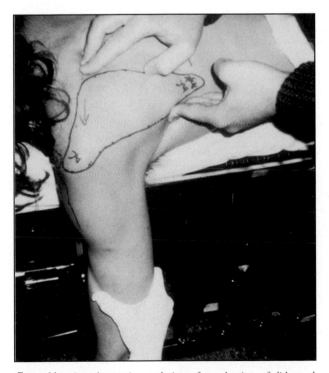

Figure 11 – Scapula rotation technique for reduction of dislocated shoulder. Patient lies prone, arm over side bed and inferior tip of scapula is pushed towards the spine (photograph courtesy of Dr J French, Sydney)

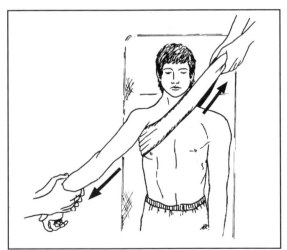

Figure 12 – Longitudinal traction technique for shoulder reduction. Patient supine, affected arm is abducted and traction applied (sheet here used for counter traction)

TYPES OF SHOULDER RECONSTRUCTIONS	
Anatomical Reconstructions	
Bankart Repair	The anterior detached capsule and labrum reattached.
Capsuloraphy	Stretched or redundant capsule is tightened by placation.
Inferior Capsular Shift	Similar to capsuloraphy but mobilisation of the capsule extends inferiorly to take up redundant inferior pouch. Done in patients with very lax shoulders.
Anatomical Reconstructions	
Putti-Plan	The anterior capsule and subscapularis muscles are divided, overlapped and tightened. Similar to converting a single-breasted coat to a double-breasted coat. This decreases external rotation of the arm.
Bristows Procedure	The coracoid process is detached from the scapula and screwed onto the antero-inferior glenoid neck to give extra support to the shoulder.
Magnusen-Stack Procedure	The subscapularis, capsule and a portion of the lesser tuberosity is detached and fixed more laterally on the humeral head. This tightens the anterior shoulder structures, decreasing external rotation.

Figure 13 – Types of surgical shoulder reconstructions – anatomical and non-anatomical

associated with a shoulder that subluxes inferiorly as *well* as anteriorly and posteriorly.

Care is needed in the evaluation of these patients. A small subgroup of MDI patients demonstrate a habitual/voluntary aspect to their problem. This group of patients should be evaluated by appropriate counsellors for associated psychological problems and potential secondary gains. Surgical procedures are likely to fail in this group.

Treatment for these patients focuses around rehabilitation. This includes strengthening of the rotator cuff and scapula stabilisers, proprioceptive/biofeedback techniques and modification of activities. The majority of patients will respond to physiotherapy. If necessary, surgery may be needed and should include an inferior capsular shift with closure of the rotator capsular interval and tightening of the superior glenohumeral ligament. The results of surgery are not as good as in unidirectional anterior reconstructions, however they are still of the order of 80-90%.

POSTERIOR INSTABILITY

Posterior dislocation is uncommon and constitutes about 4% of dislocations. It may occur with a fall, but is more commonly associated with violent muscle contractions such as might occur in an electrocution or grand mal convulsion. The diagnosis is often delayed or missed. The patients may have pain and cannot externally rotate the arm past neutral (Fig. 14). The anteroposterior X-ray may look normal (Fig. 15) however the axillary view is diagnostic (Fig. 16). If there is any doubt then a CT scan should be performed (Fig. 17).

Posterior subluxation can occur in athletes involved in sports such as baseball and should be suspected where the patient experiences symptoms with the arm in front of the trunk. In these situations, it can often be associated with multidirectional instability of the shoulder. Clinical examination may show increased posterior glide, and reproduction of symptoms on posterior load of the shoulder in 90 degrees forward flexion (Fig. 18). The X-rays are often normal.

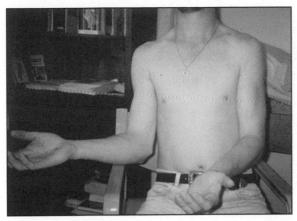

Figure 14 – Left posterior shoulder dislocation. The arm is typically locked in internal rotation

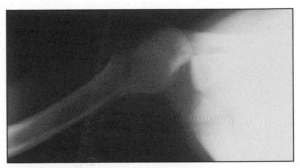

Figure 16 – The axillary x-ray view is diagnostic for posterior shoulder dislocation

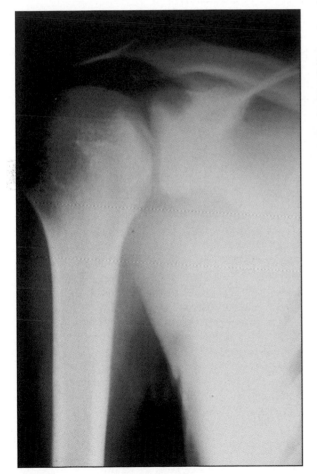

Figure 15 – Posterior shoulder dislocation. The X-ray may look normal but note the tell-tale symmetrical appearance of the humeral head ("ice-cream cone" or "light-bulb" shape). Do not dismiss X-ray as normal until carefully correlated with clinical examination

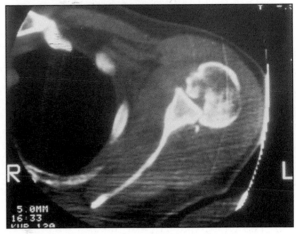

Figure 17 – The CAT scan confirms a posterior dislocation (here locked posteriorly)

Where the shoulder is a **"locked posterior dislocation"**, early recognition and reduction is essential. If the dislocation is longer standing or a large portion of the humeral head is damaged then open reduction with surgical reconstruction of the humeral head defect by autograft, allograft or tuberosity transfer is preferred. Where chondral damage has occurred, total shoulder replacement may be necessary.

In patients with posterior **subluxations and associated multidirectional laxity**, an intensive physiotherapy rehabilitation programme is recommended. Most patients will respond to conservative treatment. If instability continues then surgical reconstruction should be considered. This may be performed from an anterior or posterior approach. The anterior surgery consists of an inferior capsular shift and tightening of the superior glenohumeral ligament. The posterior

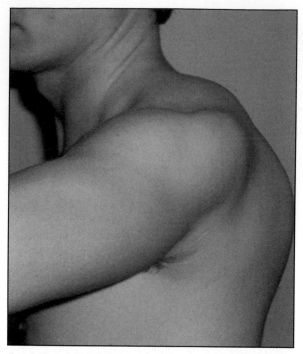

Figure 18 – Multi-directional instability. Patient showing how he can dislocate his shoulder posteriorly

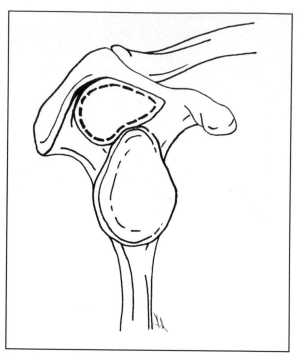

Figure 19 – Supraspinatus passes through the outlined area under the coraco-acromial arch

reconstruction undertakes an inferior capsular shift only. In both situations, the patient is immobilised in a neutral rotation brace for 6-8 weeks then placed on a graded rehabilitation programme extending over twelve months. Return to sports is not encouraged for at least twelve months.

TENDINITIS AND IMPINGEMENT

The supraspinatus is the most likely tendon to become inflamed as it passes under the coraco-acromial arch (Fig. 19). Tendinitis of the rotator cuff can occur because of overload/fatigue of the cuff tendons, trauma, and age-related degenerative changes. Occasionally, the acromion may have a shape which increases the crowding of the cuff tendons in the subacromial space that leads to impingement (Fig. 20). Tendinitis may also occur in patients with very lax shoulders as a consequence of the muscles overworking to stabilise the humeral head. It is important to beware of tendinitis in patients younger than 25 years as this may often be secondary to subtle instability.

Patients present with pain occurring in the anterior aspect of the **shoulder** with radiation into the deltoid. The pain is minimal at rest and rarely radiates down the arm or into the neck. The pain is aggravated with overhead and rotation activities. Night pain with waking is a feature of more severe cases. On examination, tenderness is located over the greater tuberosity and impingement signs are present (Fig. 21). Biceps provocation test may be positive as tendinitis of the biceps can occur coincidentally (Fig. 22). The acromioclavicular joint may also be tender if it is pathological. Range of motion and strength are usually normal, wasting may occur early (Fig. 23). There may be pain on loading the rotator cuff muscles and any weakness is due to inhibition from pain. As cervical conditions may refer pain into the shoulder, it is important to exclude any such causes for patients complaint. Patients with associated cervical irritation may hold the shoulder posture in a depressed or elevated position.

In most cases the diagnosis of tendinitis is made on **clinical grounds**. Ancillary tests, however, may assist in, or confirm the diagnosis. A plain X-ray is essential (also include a supraspinatus outlet view) (Figs. 24 &

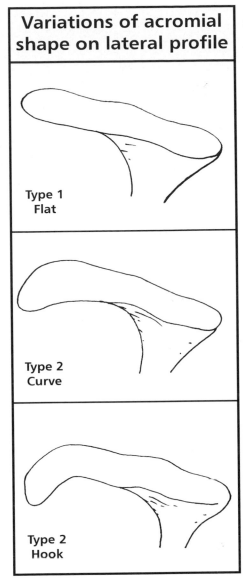

Variations of acromial shape on lateral profile

Type 1 Flat

Type 2 Curve

Type 2 Hook

Figure 20 – Variation of acromial shape on lateral profile. The more curved or hooked the acromion, the more likely that impingement may occur on the supraspinatus. Type 2 (hook) has a high correlation with rotator cuff damage

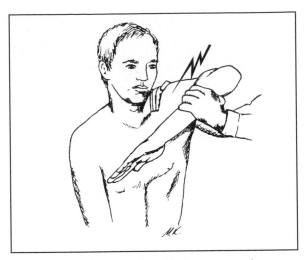

Figure 21 – Impingement sign. Tenderness over the greater tuberosity is noted on forward flexion and internal rotation

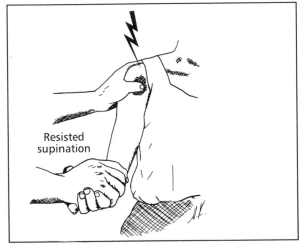

Resisted supination

Figure 22 – Yergason's test. Resisted supination of the flexed elbows causes pain in bicipital tendinitis

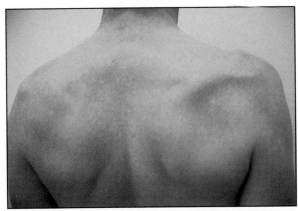

Figure 23 – Periscapsular muscle wasting noted may occur early in rotator cuff (suraspination) problems

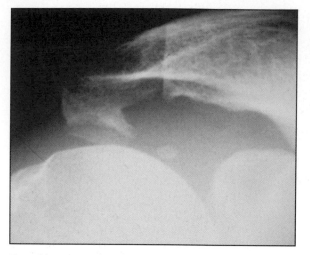

Figure 24 – X-ray (AP view) of shoulder with acromial spur

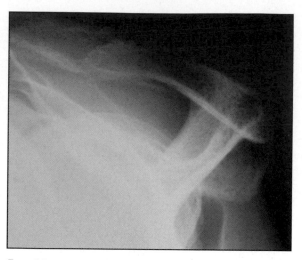

Figure 25 – The important supraspinatus outlet view which shows a curved acromion (on lateral projection)

25). The next investigation is the **impingement test**. Here, 5 - 10 ml of lignocaine is injected into the subacromial bursa and after waiting five minutes, there is a significant decrease in pain on forward elevation of the arm to perform the impingement sign.

Further test are indicated to demonstrate the presence of impingement and possible associated rotator cuff tears, either partial or full thickness. Ultrasound in **experienced** hands is reasonably accurate in predicting the presence of full-thickness tears and impingement. It is important to note that all shoulders which are stiff, e.g. adhesive capsulitis, will demonstrate impingement on ultrasound due to tightness of the posterior capsule limiting the inferior glide of the humeral head. Hence, investigations should be considered in the clinical context in which they are performed. Arthrography will show any cuff tears. MRI may show tendinitis changes in the supraspinatus as well as any rotator cuff tears.

Treatment includes activity modification, non-steroidal anti-inflammatory medications, and physiotherapy (consisting of stretching and strengthening of the rotator and scapular muscles). In most cases this should help the pain. If pain persists an injection of corticosteroid and local anaesthetic into the subacromial space is often diagnostic, and therapeutic. If conservative treatment does not help after 6 months, then acromioplasty (open or arthroscopic) is successful in 90% (Fig. 26).

ROTATOR CUFF TEARS

Normal tendons rarely tear. Younger patients require a violent injury (instability or direct trauma) to tear the cuff. In the older patient there is often underlying degenerative changes within the rotator cuff tendons so less significant trauma is required to disrupt the cuff. With repetitive overhead use of the arm, e.g. tennis or baseball, micro damage to the rotator cuff can progress to full-thickness tears.

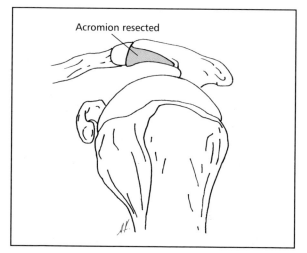

Figure 26 – Anterior acromioplasty. The shaded area is resected to convert the curved acromion to a flat under surface to minimise impingement of the tendons on the overhanging acromion

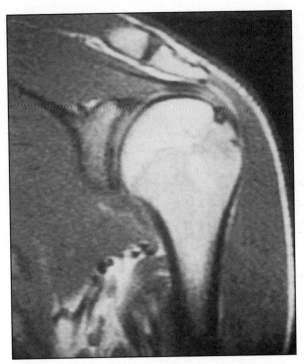

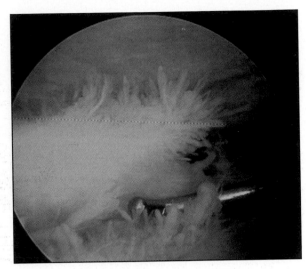

Figure 28 – Arthoscopic appearance of rotator cuff tear

Figure 27 – MRI of shoulder shows partial avulsion of deep surface of rotator cuff with small associated bone fragment

The symptoms are very similar to tendinitis. Pain is aggravated with overhead use of the arm, and at night. Weakness is almost always present, however in the majority of patients with full thickness tears there is a normal active range of motion. Only massive rotator cuff tears lose active range of motion. The long head of biceps may be torn.

Investigations include X-rays which may show an acromial spur. Narrowing of the acromiohumeral gap occurs where the tear is large. Other investigations should include either an arthrogram, ultrasound or MRI to confirm the diagnosis, extent of damage, atrophy of muscles and associated joint disease (Fig. 27).

In the younger patient (less than 50 years) surgery with acromioplasty and rotator cuff repair is recommended as there is a risk of increase in tear size and deterioration of shoulder function. In the older patient a short trial of activity modification, non-steroidal anti-inflammatory medications, physiotherapy and corticosteroid injection is reasonable. If pain persists then surgery with acromioplasty and rotator cuff repair is indicated (Figs. 28 & 29).

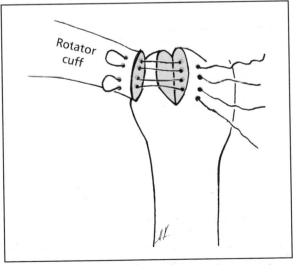

Figure 29 – Rotator cuff repair is usually done by direct suture into a bone trough

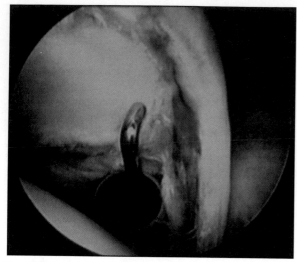

Figure 30 – Arthroscopic appearance of a SLAP lesion

INTERNAL DERANGEMENTS WITHIN THE GLENOHUMERAL JOINT

LABRAL TEARS, SLAP (SUPERIOR LABRAL ANTERIOR POSTERIOR) LESIONS, LOOSE BODIES

These are often caused by trauma, either direct or in association with instability. The labrum is most developed in the upper portion of the shoulder joint and tears in this area may extend into the biceps attach-

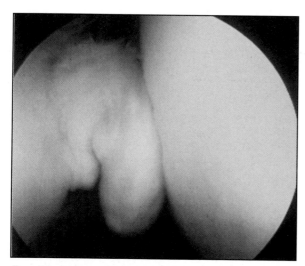

Figure 32 – Arthroscopic appearance of glenoid labrum tear

ment (anchor) (Fig. 32). Superior labral tears are referred to as SLAP (Superior Labral Anterior Posterior) lesions and there are four types (see Fig. 30 and Classification of SLAP Lesions, Fig. 31). Loose bodies may arise from trauma or synovial disease (as in synovial chondrometaplasia).

The patient experiences pain with sudden motion, clicking or catching with rotation of the shoulder. Pain is experienced with resisted elevation of the arm while it is forward flexed 90 degrees and slightly adducted across the body with the hand in internal rotation. When the hand is externally rotated in the same position then the pain decreases. There may be associated features of instability.

Diagnosis is **difficult** and often requires further investigation. The best test is an MRI scan with gadolinium arthrography. The treatment is usually arthroscopic with either resection or repair of the torn labrum and removal of loose bodies. It is also important to treat the underlying cause, e.g. instability.

ACROMIOCLAVICULAR JOINT INJURIES

The acromioclavicular joint (ACJ) is usually injured from a fall onto the point of the shoulder. The resulting injury may cause chondral or meniscal damage. More severe injuries may result in subluxation or dislocation of the joint. (*See - Classification of Acromioclavicular Joint Dislocation, Fig. 33*).

On examination, localised tenderness and swelling is often seen. In dislocations of the joint the outer clavicle appears superiorly displaced, though, in most cases, it is the shoulder that sags below the clavicle. Forced cross-body adduction may provoke discomfort.

X-rays of the joint should include standing weighted views of the ACJ with the weight tied to the wrists of the patient (Fig. 34).

For **undisplaced** or type 1 and 2 dislocations ice, rest and then gradual return to activity over a 2 - 6 week period is usually adequate. It is important to remember that seemingly minor ACJ injuries may give rise to grumbling discomfort for up to 6 months. **Major dislocations may require surgical stabilisation** in athletes if their dominant arm is involved, especially if they intend to participate in upper limb sports or are workers who use their arms overhead.

Classification of SLAP Lesions

Type 1
Fraying of the superior labrum.
Biceps anchor intact.

Treatment -
Debridement of frayed edge.

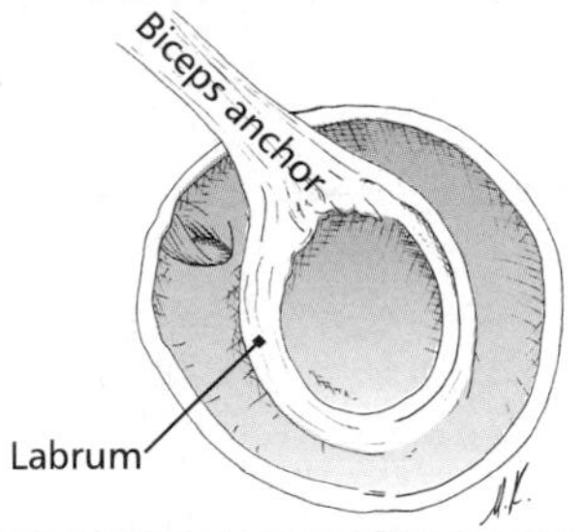

Type 2
Superior labrum detached with
detachment of the biceps anchor.

Treatment -
Debridement of superior glenoid rim
and reattachment of biceps and labrum.

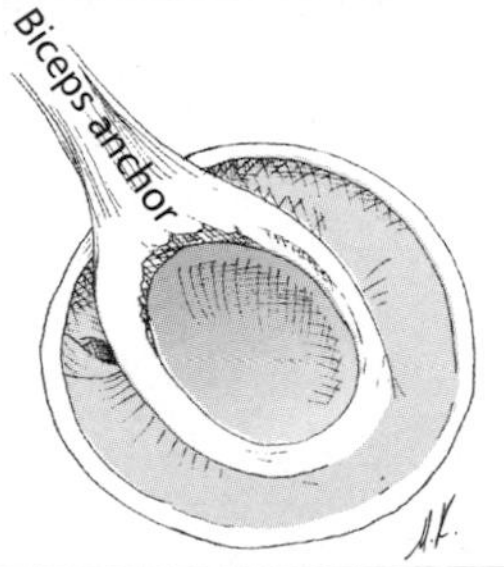

Type 3
Bucket handle type tear of the superior
labrum with the biceps anchor intact.

Treatment -
Resection of tear.

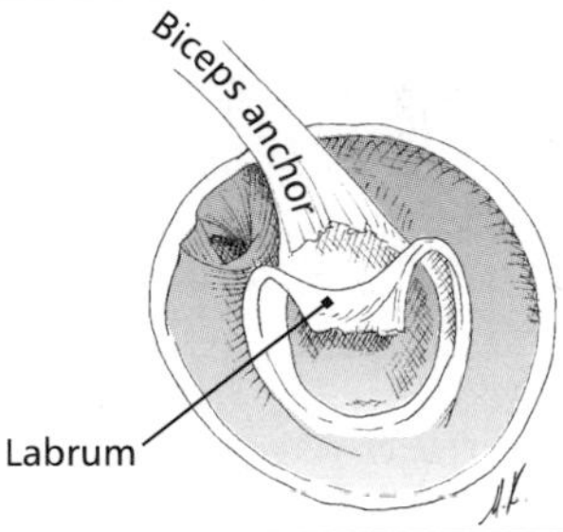

Type 4
Bucket handle tear of the superior labrum
with extension into the biceps tendon.
Part of the biceps anchor still intact.
Treatment -
Resection of tear and if greater than 50%
of tendon also involved, then tenodesis
is recommended

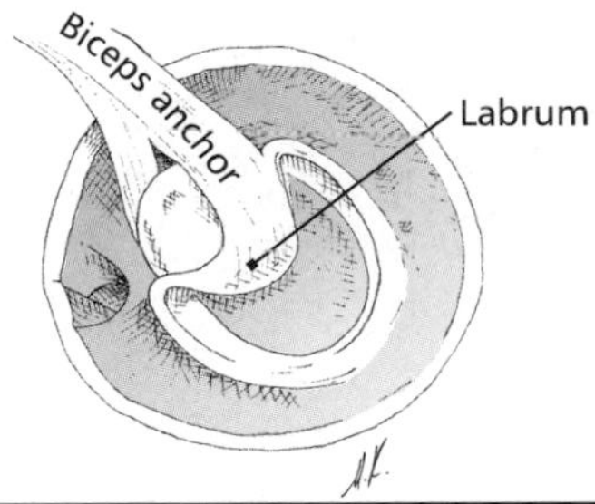

Figure 31 – Classification of SLAP lesions.

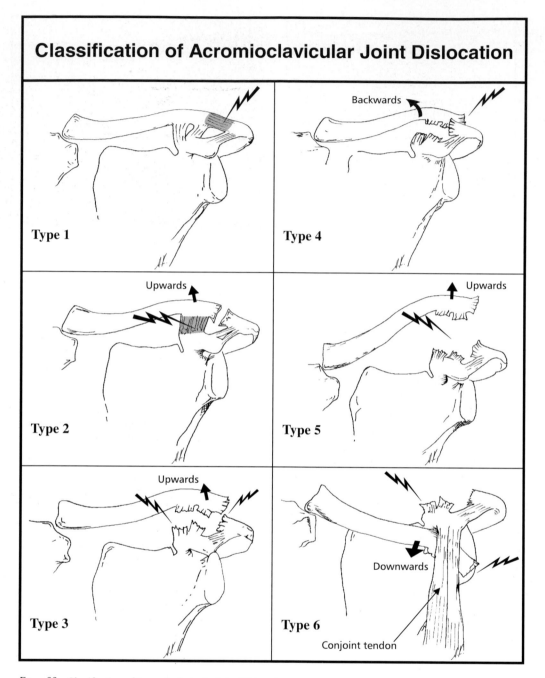

Figure 33 – Classification of Acromioclavicular Joint Dislocation.

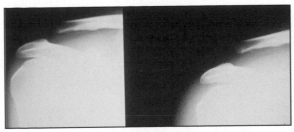

No weight   **With weight**

Figure 34 – X-rays of acromioclavicular joint with weights will reveal a clinically unapparent disruption

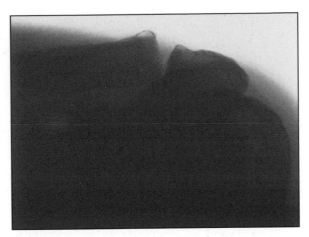

Figure 35 – Outer clavicle osteolysis

CLAVICLE FRACTURES

Fractures can occur with a fall onto the outstretched hand. Most of these fractures occur in the mid–shaft, though medial or lateral injuries also occur. Clinically there is pain with swelling and deformity over the site of the fracture. Neurological lesions are rare but may include brachial plexus injury. Vascular injuries are very rare.

The **majority** of fractures will go **on to union with little morbidity**, even with moderate shortening or angulation. Some patients however may develop symptoms with cross body actions if the clavicle is too shortened. Where the fractures are lateral and involve the coracoclavicular ligaments or ACJ, treatment may include stabilisation of the outer end of the clavicle. Most fractures are treated non-operatively with a sling for elbow support. Clavicle rings to pull shoulders back may decrease discomfort and help stabilise the fracture ends. Care is necessary to avoid skin pressure problems and axillary neurovascular compression. With marked displacement or shortening, early open reduction and internal fixation may be considered.

OUTER CLAVICULAR OSTEOLYSIS

This occurs from a **direct blow or fall**, but often develops in individuals who work out in the gymnasium on overhead machines or are involved in overhead sports. The probable pathology is a chondral or minor osteochondral fracture which initiates an inflammatory response and leads to resorption of the outer clavicle.

Patients complain of pain over the ACJ which may radiate to the deltoid or base of neck. On examination there is localised tenderness and swelling over the ACJ. In more advanced cases a palpable gap is evident at the site of the ACJ. X-rays show irregularity of the outer clavicle with osteolysis (Fig. 35). A bone scan, which is not always necessary, will be hot in the region of the outer clavicle.

Treatment includes rest, activity modification and non-steroidal anti-inflammatory medications. If the pain persists then surgical excision of the outer clavicle is indicated.

MEDIAL CLAVICULAR SCLEROSIS

(OSTEITIS CONDENSANS)

This is a rare disorder characterised by osteosclerosis of the medial end of the clavicle. The aetiology is unknown, though low grade osteonecrosis or osteomyelitis have been proposed, though never proven. Most commonly it occurs in middle aged females who present with a long history of insidious onset of pain and discomfort with elevating the arm.

X-rays show mild enlargement and sclerosis of the medial end of the clavicle without any bone destruction or periosteal reaction. Confirmation of the diagnosis is with CT scan though MRI can also be used.

Treatment is non-operative with analgesics and non-steroidal anti-inflammatory medications. Patients may be symptomatic for many years. Surgical excision has been described though the condition is rarely painful enough to warrant this.

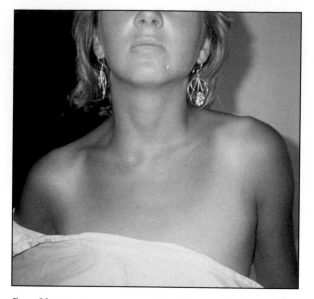

Figure 36 – Anterior dislocation of the right sternoclavicular joint

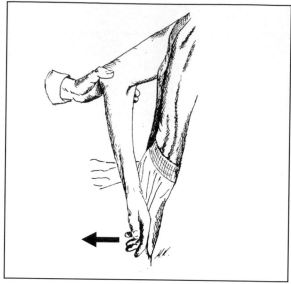

Figure 38 – Subscapularis lift-off test for subscapularis tendon distruption

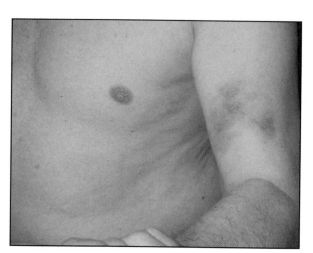

Figure 37 – Ruptured long head of biceps seldom requires surgery

be reduced closed, though many surgeons prefer to leave the dislocation and treat the patient symptomatically (Fig. 36). The diagnosis is best confirmed with a CT scan as X-rays of this region are difficult to interpret.

Posterior dislocation may cause pressure on structures in the neck with dysphagia, dyspnoea or great vessel compression. This can be a **surgical emergency**. Posterior dislocations should be reduced urgently if there is compromise of the thoracic outlet or mediastinal structures. A bolster is placed between the shoulder blades and posterior directed pressure is applied to the shoulders. If the clavicle doesn't reduce closed, then under sterile conditions a surgical towel clip may be hooked around the clavicle and pulled forward to reduce the clavicle.

STERNOCLAVICULAR DISLOCATION

Despite the limited ligamentous support of the inner end of the clavicle, dislocations are rare. It may be anterior or posterior. The dislocation usually occurs with a fall onto the side and compression of the shoulder from another player failing on top of the patient.

Anterior dislocation has a painful prominence of the medial end of the clavicle. In the acute situation it may

MUSCLE RUPTURES

Apart from the rotator cuff a number of muscles may rupture about the shoulder. These commonly include: **pectoralis major, long head of biceps** (Fig. 37); and **subscapularis**. The muscle tears when there is contraction of the muscle against an unexpected resistance. Weight lifters, trying to bench press large weights, are a common source of patients. If the arm is in 90 degrees of abduction and is force into extension subscapularis may tear.

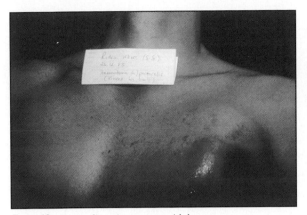

Figure 40 – Pectoralis major rupture with haematoma

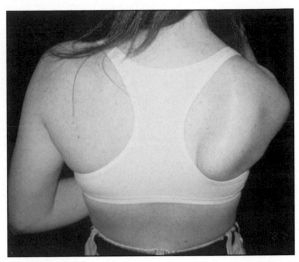

Figure 41 – Wing of the scapula following a shoulder dislocation (damage to the long thoracic nerve)

The patients complain of severe pain and tearing sensation at the time of rupture, and this is followed by swelling and bruising. The damaged pectoralis major bunches on contraction. Long head of biceps rupture may be associated to rotator cuff disease. Subscapularis rupture is difficult to pick, with weakness on the posterior lift-off test being the only sign (Fig. 38).

For the ruptured pectoralis muscle, surgical repair is recommended, as the patients will notice a deformity and weakness in the future (Fig. 39). For patients with a subscapularis tear there may be long term changes in rotator cuff balance and function, and so repair is recommended.

BICEPS TENDON INJURIES

The biceps may be injured with anterior instability or be associated with impingement and rotator cuff tears. Only 5% of biceps tendinitis is primary, whereas, 95% is secondary to other causes.

The patients complain of pain over the anterior aspect of the shoulder. Examination shows tenderness in the biceps groove. Sometimes a click from subluxation of the tendon may occur with rotation of the arm.

Treatment includes rest, non-steroidal anti-inflammatory medications and steroid injections in the biceps groove. If pain persists or there is dislocation of the biceps then surgical tenodesis is recommended. If the

long head of biceps ruptures after a period of tenodesis then the pain often subsides. The rupture is treated symptomatically and surgery is rarely recommended.

NERVE INJURIES

Nerve injuries about the shoulder can occur as a result of direct trauma, traction, compression or secondary to instability. The nerves may sustain a neuropraxia or division depending on the type of injury. Nerves which can be involved often include the axillary, suprascapular, musculocutaneous, long thoracic (Fig. 41) and radial nerve. A brachial plexus palsy (partial or complete) can occur with high energy trauma (Fig. 42).

The patient complains of pain related to the injury and this may be associated with weakness. Winging of the scapula occurs with long thoracic nerve injury. To localise the nerve damage, careful neurological examination is important.

In most cases the injury is a neuropraxia and will recover with time. EMG studies are recommended to help ascertain whether the lesion is complete and/or recovering. Exploration and repair of the nerves may be indicated if the lesion does not recover within 6 months. If suprascapular nerve compression is evident then an MRI scan may reveal a spino-glenoid notch ganglion cyst pressing the nerve. This requires surgical excision.

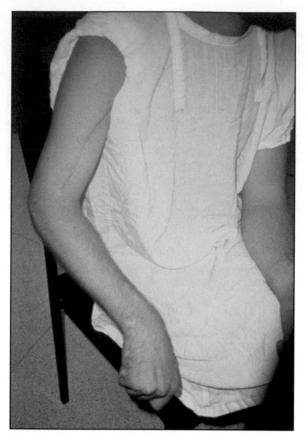

Figure 42 – Partial brachial plexus palsy following trauma (radial nerve affected)

PREVENTION OF INJURY TO THE SHOULDER

The most important step to prevent injury during sports participation is the implementation of **a general conditioning programme.** In those sports where upper limb activity is essential, the programme needs to encompass appropriate muscle strengthening and stretching about the shoulder and scapula. Appropriate strength and muscle length allows for optimal muscle function.

Prior to exercising or sports participation, **warm–up** is the first step. Stretching of the rotator cuff and posterior capsule and then gentle strengthening exercises with attention to the rotator cuff and scapular stabilisers is necessary.

Technique of throwing or other sports activity should be carefully developed under skilled supervision to optimise performance without causing undue strain on the shoulder capsule or muscles. At the first sign of fatigue or discomfort the athlete should cease the sport to prevent any injury progressing to a more serious level. After coming from the field the athlete should cool down the affected area and then reinstate a gentle stretching programme before rest.

It is important that all athletes recognise that **high level performance** at sport places **an extreme demand** on the bodies tissues and the off-season plays an important role in allowing micro damage to heal itself. Aside from the in-season conditioning appropriate complementary exercises are important in the off-season. These should not place the same strains on the tissues but should be directed at maintaining aerobic fitness in preparation for the next season.

With these thoughts in mind all athletes should be able to enjoy their sports for many seasons with a minimal risk of injury.

11

ELBOW

Des Bokor
David Duckworth

INTRODUCTION

The elbow has notoriously been a difficult joint to examine, diagnose and treat. This may be due to the fact that there is no particular predisposition for disease processes in this joint or that it is not a frequent site of trauma and injury. Despite these findings the elbow is slowly becoming better understood as more sportsmen participate in throwing or overhead sports resulting in an increasing number of elbow problems.

Overuse injuries in throwing or catching sports create the mainstay of chronic elbow problems and can either involve the ligaments, capsule, muscles or articular surfaces of the joint, subsequently impairing function (Fig. 1). It is important to understand the anatomy and biomechanics of the elbow joint to appreciate the predisposition of particular sports to specific injuries around the elbow (Fig. 2).

ANATOMY AND BIOMECHANICS

The elbow is a highly constrained hinge joint, whereby its stability is maintained by ligamentous, osseous and capsular structures. There is a slight degree of varus/valgus and rotational laxity (3-5 degrees) throughout the flexion - extension arc.

SPORTS SPECIFIC ELBOW PROBLEMS	
Golf	Medial epicondylitis
Tennis	Lateral epicondylitis
Baseball	MCL injuries Valgus extension overload Little leaguers elbow *OCD (Panner's disease) Ulnar neuritis/cubital tunnel Acute rupture MCL Medial epicondylitis
Gymnastics	OCD
Javelin	Acute rupture MCL Partial rupture MCL Epicondylitis

Figure 1 – Sports Specific Elbow Problems
★ OCD: osteochondritis dissecans.

There are 3 articulations at the elbow joint (Fig. 3):

1. Ulnohumeral - allows 0-150 degrees flexion.

2. Radiocapitellar.

3. Proximal Radio-ulnar joints (with radiocapitellar allows 75 degrees pronation and 85 degrees supination).

Most daily activity is performed through a 100 degree arc of flexion and extension usually **between 30 - 130 degrees.** Forearm rotation is also important occurring in an arc of **100 degrees,** essentially between 50 degrees supination and 50 degrees pronation. Any loss of this arc of movement can severely limit one's function (Fig. 4).

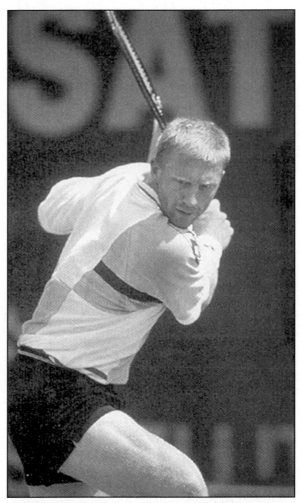

Figure 2 – A down-the-line backhand from Boris Becker. Overuse injuries are common in high-level sport. (Photograph courtesy of John Anthony, Sydney.)

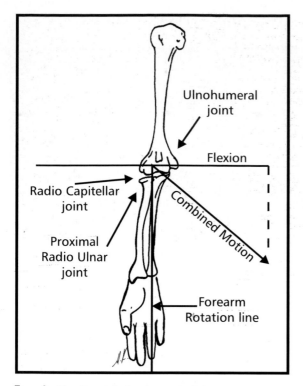

Figure 3 – The elbow joint has three articulations

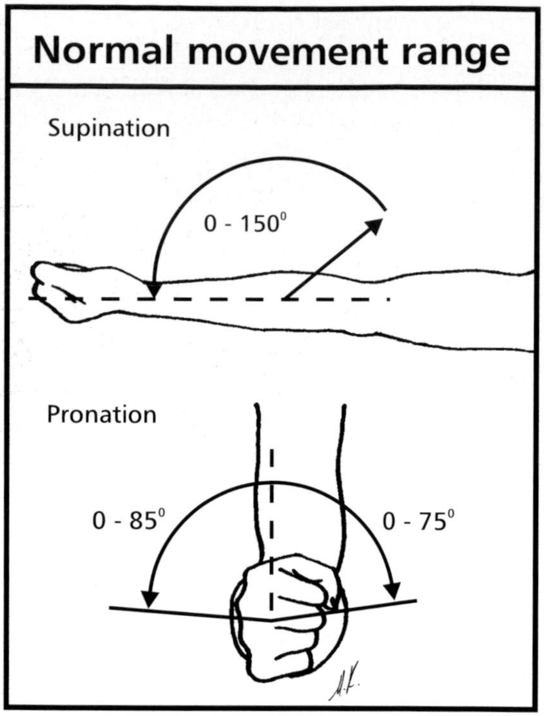

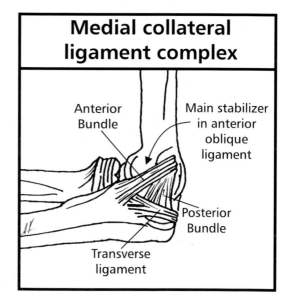

Figure 4 – Normal movement range of elbow but the range of motion required for most activities is 30 to 130° (flexion/extension) and 100° (supination/pronation)

ELBOW STABILITY

Ligamentous **stability** is provided at the elbow by both a medial and lateral ligamentous complex. The importance of these complexes is dependent on the position of the arm.

Medial Collateral Ligament: is formed by 3 bands (Fig. 5). The anterior oblique ligament being the most important of these bands originating from the medial epicondyle and inserting onto the medial aspect of the coronoid process. The anterior band is the primary constraint to VALGUS instability and the radial head is of secondary importance. Clinically, this function is observed in throwing as the repetitive valgus stress can result in microtrauma and attenuation of the anterior oblique ligament.

Lateral Collateral Ligament: is formed by 3 ligaments and offers varus stability which is rarely stressed in the athlete (Fig. 6). The lateral ulnar collateral is the most important of these ligaments playing an important role in rotational instability, it originates from the lateral epicondyle and inserts onto the tubercle of the

Figure 5 – The medial collateral ligament of the elbow. The anterior oblique ligament is the most important

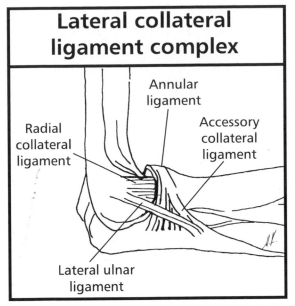

Figure 6 – The lateral collateral ligament of the elbow. The lateral ulnar ligament is the more important

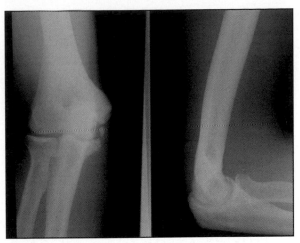

Figure 7 – Osseous bodies in MCL in baseball pitcher

supinator crest of the ulna. Its function is to prevent **Varus** and **Posterolateral** rotatory instability of the elbow.

The capsule is only an important constraint to instability in full extension.

NEUROLOGICAL ANATOMY

Neurological compression syndromes are common around the elbow due to the **close proximity of the nerves**. The ulnar nerve in particular is vulnerable and lies within the cubital tunnel which lies posterior to the medial epicondyle. The median nerve lies anterior deep within the cubital fossa, the radial nerve lies lateral and branches in the cubital fossa.

LIGAMENT INJURIES AND INSTABILITY

MEDIAL (ULNAR) COLLATERAL LIGAMENT INJURIES

This injury is predominantly related to the **throwing sports** whereby repetitive valgus stress results in small tears in the anterior band of the MCL and subsequent rupture. The mechanism of injury **is** generally sport related, occurring most commonly in javelin throwers

and baseball pitchers. Whilst throwing there is an enormous valgus stress on the elbow during the late-cocking phase, subsequently overloading the ligament leading to attenuation and then rupture. Occasionally there may be a single acute painful throw or a fall onto the outstretched hand.

Acutely, there is swelling and pain localized to the medial side and occasionally of paraesthesia in the ulnar nerve distribution. Valgus deformity and elbow contracture may develop. Valgus stress testing with the elbow at 30 degrees of flexion shows increased laxity and pain. Incongruity may develop between the olecranon process and its fossa with loose body formation at the medial aspect of the olecranon. X-rays may show osseous bodies in the MCL or fluffy calcification at the tip of the olecranon (Fig. 7).

Treatment initially includes rest, activity modification, NSAID and physiotherapy. If posteromedial pain continues then arthroscopy can be performed to surgically debride the osteophytes. If there is evidence of chronic UCL laxity or instability then surgical reconstruction (primary repair or use of palmaris longus).

ACUTE RUPTURE OF THE MCL

Isolated tears of the anterior oblique ligament can occur especially in javelin throwers. The mechanism of injury is almost pure valgus stress with the elbow flexed at 60-90 degrees. There is acute pain and the feeling that something popped on the medial side of the elbow. Ulnar nerve symptoms can also occur with ecchymosis around the elbow some 48 hours later. If

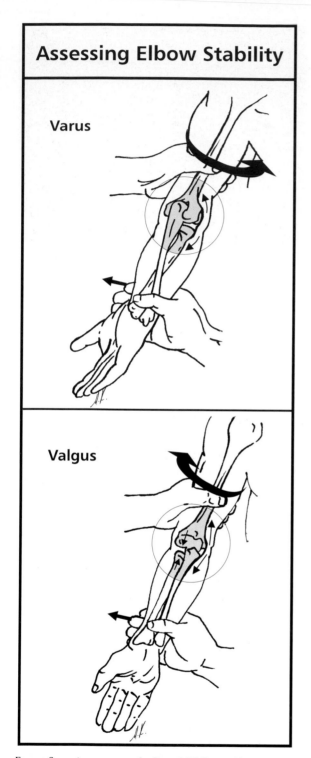

Assessing Elbow Stability

Varus

Valgus

Figure 8 – Assessment of elbow stability with varus and valgus loads

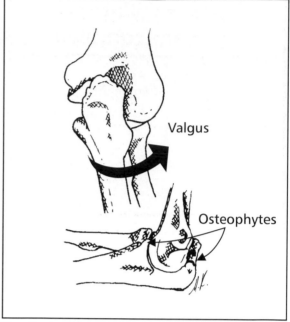

Figure 9 – Ostophyte formation in the posterior and posteromedial position secondary to valgus extension overload

the diagnosis is in doubt stress tests or stress X-rays can be performed (Fig. 8). Acute repair of the ligament is recommended in these circumstances.

VALGUS EXTENSION OVERLOAD

Usually a problem exclusively related to **pitchers** during the acceleration phase of pitching. In this early phase of acceleration, excessive valgus stress is applied to the elbow causing the impingement. This results in osteophyte formation both posterior and posteriomedial which can cause chondromalacia with loose body formation (Fig. 9).

The pitcher will often present with pain on pitching early in the game and complain they just cannot let go of the ball. Pain over the olecranon fossa in valgus and extension is common. Radiographs demonstrate a posterior osteophyte at the tip of the olecranon seen on routine lateral views.

Conservative therapy should be started early and includes increasing functional strength, heat and ultrasound. This rarely relieves symptoms when an osteophyte is present on X-ray (needs surgical excision).

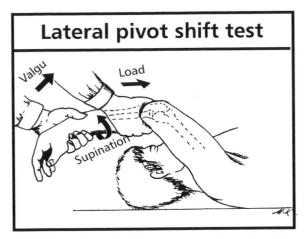

Figure 10 – Lateral pivot shift test for posterolateral rotary instability

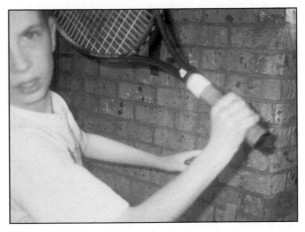

Figure 11 – Tennis elbow may result from improper grip size (here too big)

POSTEROLATERAL ROTATORY INSTABILITY

Should be distinguished from elbow dislocation. It is caused by a laxity or disruption of the ulnar part of the lateral collateral ligament which allows a transient rotatory subluxation of the ulno-humeral joint and a secondary dislocation of the radio-humeral joint.

Usually a history of preceding trauma such as a dislocation or something as subtle as a sprain from a fall on an outstretched hand causes the instability. Previous surgery may precede the instability and include procedures such as radial head excision or lateral release for a tennis elbow.

Presents with the history of a recurring click, snap, clunking or locking of the elbow. The feeling that ones elbow is giving way or about to dislocate may also be experienced. These instability episodes usually occur with a loaded extended elbow and supinated forearm. Examination is often unremarkable except for the diagnostic **"Lateral Pivot Shift"** (Posterolateral rotatory apprehension test). This test is performed with patient supine and preferably under general anaesthesia. The elbow is extended overhead and the forearm fully supinated. A valgus and supination force is then slowly applied to the elbow going from the extended to flexed position. This results in subluxation of the ulno-humeral joint and radio-humeral joint (Fig. 10).

Radiographically, the joint will look normal except if the film is taken with the joint subluxed, therefore the diagnosis is made from history and after an examination under anaesthesia. Generally, when symptomatic surgery is required (re-attach the avulsed lateral ulnar collateral ligament or reconstructing it with a tendon graft).

TENNIS ELBOW

(LATERAL EPICONDYLITIS)

A lateral tendinitis primarily involving the origin of **Extensor Carpi Radialis Brevis.** It is generally related to activities that increase tension and stress on the wrist extensors and supinator muscles. Such activities may include tennis however many cases do not (Fig. 11)

Clinically, it usually occurs between the ages of 35-55 years with pain being the usual complaint localized to the lateral epicondyle especially after a period of unaccustomed activity e.g. tennis 3-4 times a week. The pain is aggravated by movements such as turning a door handle or shaking hands. On examination, pain is localized to the lateral epicondyle with some radiation distally. This is aggravated by passive stretching of the wrist extensors or actively extending the wrist with the elbow straight (Fig. 12)

X-rays should be performed, although they are often normal. A bone scan may show increased uptake around the lateral epicondyle, whilst an ultrasound or MRI may show degeneration within the belly of ECRB. The **differential diagnosis** includes posterior interosseus nerve entrapment, which can be excluded due to a more distal localization of the pain and associated weakness.

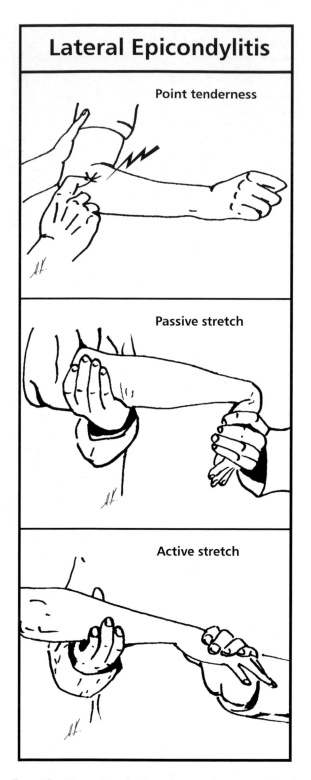

Figure 12 – Signs of tennis elbow. Point tenderness over lateral epicondyle; pain on passive and active stretching

The natural history is resolution over a 10–12 month period with a 30 % recurrence. Initial management is outlined (Fig. 13).

GOLFERS ELBOW

(MEDIAL EPICONDYLITIS)

Primarily an inflammation of the flexor tendinous origin from the medial epicondyle. Secondary to repetitive activity of wrist flexion and active pronation such as in baseball pitching or occasionally golf and tennis. The pathology at the interface between pronator teres and FCR.

Presents with localized tenderness over the medial epicondyle radiating down the forearm (Fig. 14). The pain is exacerbated by resisted palmer flexion and pronation. Ulnar nerve symptoms are demonstrated in 60% of cases.

The treatment is very similar to lateral epicondylitis, and once again it is important to exclude other causes such as ulnar neuropraxia, joint instability or cervical pathology. Treatment includes rest, activity modification NSAID and physiotherapy. Only rarely is surgical release necessary (release of the common flexor origin and occasionally a medial epicondylectomy).

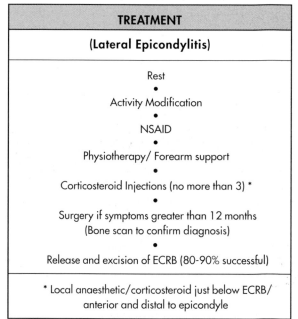

TREATMENT
(Lateral Epicondylitis)
Rest • Activity Modification • NSAID • Physiotherapy/ Forearm support • Corticosteroid Injections (no more than 3) * • Surgery if symptoms greater than 12 months (Bone scan to confirm diagnosis) • Release and excision of ECRB (80-90% successful)
* Local anaesthetic/corticosteroid just below ECRB/ anterior and distal to epicondyle

Figure 13 – Treatment of tennis elbow

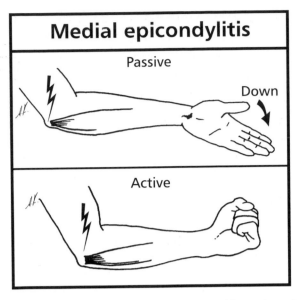

Figure 14 – Medial epicondylitis. Pain aggravated by passive and active stretching

OSTEOCHONDRITIS DISSECAN'S (OCD)

A spontaneous necrosis and fragmentation of the capitellar ossific nucleus. The aetiology is believed to be secondary to compression forces at the Radio-Capitellar joint producing focal arterial injury and subsequent bone death. Common relationship

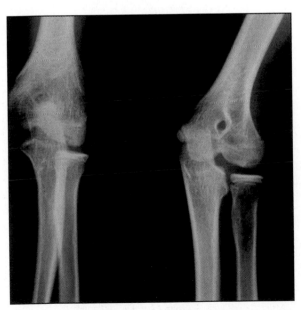

Figure 15 – Osteochondritis dissecans of the capitellum

between this injury, gymnastics and the throwing sports, particularly baseball pitchers, who most commonly present with lesions of the capitellum (Fig. 15).

There is lateral elbow pain after activity, generally occurring in the 10-15 year group, involving the dominant arm. Examination reveals an inability to extend the elbow fully and pain on forced extension. A similar condition is Panner's disease, the major difference being in the radiographic appearance and age of onset (Fig. 16). Early on in the condition the X-rays may be normal and if clinically suspected, a bone scan or CT Scan is appropriate to confirm the diagnosis. **Treatment** initially is rest for 6 weeks. However, if pain and contracture persist after this period of time then the likelihood of fragmentation should be considered. Arthroscopy is then performed and if the fragment is separate, removal is performed. Occasionally the fragment is reattached if large.

PANNER'S DISEASE

A form of 'Osteochondrosis' which affects the growth centres in children resulting in necrosis followed by regeneration. In this instance it involves the capitellum, resulting in fragmentation and then regeneration. Commonly confused with OCD due to similar symptomatology and signs although in contrast it usually occurs in boys between the ages of 7-12 years during active ossification of the capitellum. The process results in dull aching elbow pain aggravated by use, loss of full elbow extension and lateral swelling. Radiographically, fragmentation, irregularity and a smaller capitellum is seen in comparison to OCD and as growth progresses the capitellum begins to regain its normal appearance (Fig. 16).

As it is a self-limiting condition, no specific treatment is necessary apart from rest during the acute period. Treatment of these two conditions is outlined (Fig. 17).

LITTLE LEAGUER'S ELBOW

A medial epicondylar stress lesion or acute valgus stress syndrome seen in children. Classically results from repetitive valgus stress in a young throwing athlete which causes a flexor forearm muscle pull on the medial epicondyle epiphysis (Fig. 18).

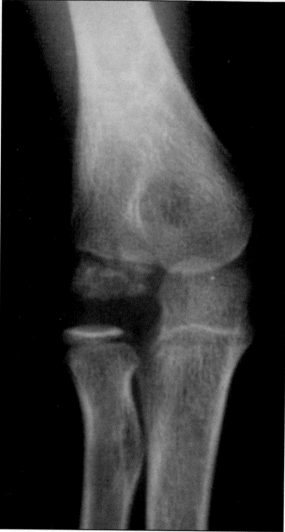

Figure 16 – Panner's disease – an osteochondritis of the capitellum resulting in necrosis, fragmentation and regeneration

Little League's elbow

1 Separation

Widened epiphysical secondary to repetative vulus stress

Valgus

2 Displacement

Fall resulting in displaced medial epicondyle fracture

3 Entrapment

Occasionally the fragment is caught in the joint

Figure 18 – Little Leaguer's elbow. Repetitive valgus stress results in separation, displacement and possible entrapment of medial epicondyle

	OCD	PANNER'S
Age	10 - 15 yr	< 10 yr
Onset	Gradual	Acute
X-ray	Island of subchondral bone	Fragmentation of entire capitellar ossific nucleus
Loose Bodies	Present	Absent
Residual Deformity of Capitellum	Present	Minimal

Figure 17 – The differences between OCD and Panner's

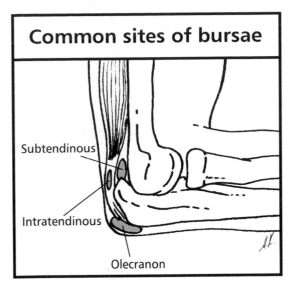

Figure 19 – Location of bursae about the elbow joint

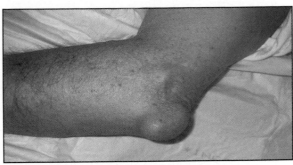

Figure 20 – Large olecranon bursa requiring excision.

There is medial sided elbow pain associated with decreased throwing effectiveness and throwing distance. On examination, signs of medial epicondylar tenderness and pain on loading the flexor muscles is apparent. An elbow flexion contracture may also be demonstrated.

X-rays may show separation and fragmentation of the epiphyseal lines. Usually a benign injury which responds to rest and activity modification. Return to throwing after 6 weeks can be expected and only occasionally if there is a large separation of the fragment medially is surgical fixation necessary.

MEDIAL EPICONDYLAR FRACTURES

A more substantial acute valgus stress such as from a fall or a violent muscle contracture when throwing can sometimes produce a fracture through the epiphseal plate.

There is a painful elbow and localized tenderness over the medial epicondyle. A 15 degree flexion contracture or more is usually present. X-rays can vary from a minimally displaced fragment to markedly displaced with the fragment occasionally caught in the joint.

Treatment: largely depends on the degree of displacement. Generally, if the fragment is undisplaced or displaced less than 1 cm, then only immobilization for 3-4 weeks is required. If grossly displaced, if the

fragment is caught in the joint or if ulnar nerve symptoms are present then open reduction is required (Fig. 18).

OLECRANON BURSITIS

• Acute

An inflammation of superficial olecranon bursa, usually results from direct trauma or repetitive stress around the elbow (Fig. 19). The most common nontraumatic cause is gout followed by rheumatoid arthritis.

There is an enlarged, nontender bursa which has minimal effect on elbow movement. Exclude a septic bursitis (the bursa is usually inflamed and tender; the patient may have systemic symptoms such as fever and malaise) (Fig. 20).

If concerned about sepsis then aspiration should be performed under aseptic conditions. For recurrent bursitis an X-ray may be of value looking for an **olecranon spur or calcification as seen in gout.** If the bursitis is associated with an inflammatory condition then control of the underlying condition is the obvious first step. Generally, on first presentation, commence the patient on a NSAID, and try to identify the precipitating cause. Rest, activity modification and NSAID will generally relieve the bursitis over a few months.

• Chronic

Persistent olecranon bursitis, if severe enough, may require operative intervention. This is performed via a posterior incision and the bursal sac is removed.

• Septic

Infection of the bursa does not imply elbow joint infection as it does not communicate with the joint. Of those that develop septic olecranon bursitis, one-third give a history of a previous non infected bursitis.

Symptoms vary from an acute onset of cellulitis to a low grade process of 2 or more weeks duration. Classically, the bursa is erythematous and tender and one may have signs of generalized sepsis. Diagnosis is confirmed by aspiration looking for organisms and an increased white cell count consistent with infection. The presence of crystals in the aspirate generally indicates gout or pseudogout. Treatment initially requires aspiration and antibiotics however, if this fails, surgical drainage is required (Fig. 17).

TENDON INJURIES AROUND THE ELBOW

Other than epicondylitis, injuries to the tendons around the elbow are uncommon. The tendons that can rupture, although rarely are the distal biceps from the radial tuberosity or the distal triceps from the insertion into the olecranon.

DISTAL BICEPS RUPTURE

Accounts for 3 – 10 % of all biceps ruptures and commonly occurs in the dominant arm of a well developed male in his 40's-50's. It is usually the result of a single traumatic event, whereby one has a sudden extension force whilst flexing (contracting) the biceps.

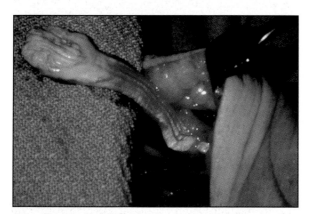

Figure 21 – Distal biceps rupture needs to be reattached

There is sudden sharp pain with discomfort in the antecubital fossa and notable weakness with elbow flexion and supination (with the elbow flexed). The muscle contracts proximally and a defect is palpable (Fig. 21).

In most cases surgical treatment is recommended as conservative management leads to moderate weakness especially noticeable in manual workers. Complications relevant to surgery should be discussed with the patient: these include cross union between the radius and ulna or a posterior interosseous nerve palsy.

RUPTURE OF THE TRICEPS TENDON

Can occur spontaneously or after trauma. The most common event is a decelerating force on the arm during extension, such as during a fall. It can also result from sudden forced extension whilst the elbow is being flexed.

There is a sudden onset of pain and local swelling with a corresponding defect in the triceps tendon. There may be a small bony fragment related to avulsion of the tendon from the olecranon. Some loss of extension power is also present.

An X-ray maybe beneficial due to the potential of an avulsion injury In most cases surgical repair is indicated.

FRACTURES AND DISLOCATIONS

SUPRACONDYLAR FRACTURES

The majority occur in children with 97% being posteriorly displaced or angulated. This generally results from an extension injury due to a fall on an outstretched hand, causing the distal fragment of the humerus to be pushed backwards (Fig. 22).

Presents with a painful, swollen elbow and a S-deformity. Check the pulse and circulation which can be affected due to swelling and fracture configuration. Check the nerves as 10 to 15% have a neuropraxia (the median, anterior interosseous or the radial nerves).

Treat undisplaced fractures in a collar and cuff for 3 weeks (carefully monitor the position with serial X-rays). Most displaced fractures require at least a closed reduction and occasionally percutaneous K-Wires if unstable (Fig. 23).

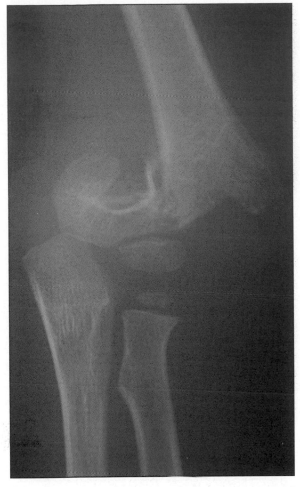

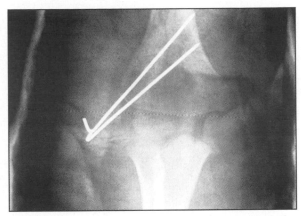

Figure 23 – Supracondylar fracture reduced and held with two K-wires

Figure 22 – Supracondylar fracture; humerus markedly displaced. There may be neurovascular compromise

Complications with such a fracture are mainly cosmetic resulting in cubitus varus (gun-stock deformity) or neurological mainly involving the median or anterior interosseous. Vascular insufficiency resulting in Volkmann's ischaemia and later myositis ossificans can occur. **Adult** supracondylar and intercondylar fractures are not nearly as common (generally require open reduction and internal fixation).

LATERAL CONDYLAR FRACTURES

The lateral condyle epiphysis begins to ossify by one and then fuses to the shaft by 12 to 14 years of age. It is during these years (in particular from 4 to 10) that fracture separations occur. **It is important** to recognize such a fracture as it can lead to growth plate damage and involves the joint, making accurate

reduction necessary (Fig. 9). If undisplaced then splinting the arm in a backslab at 90 degrees is required. Displaced fractures generally require accurate reduction and fixation with K- wires (see Fig. 13, Chapter 18).

FRACTURES OF THE RADIAL HEAD

Are much more common in adults than children . They usually result from a fall on the outstretched hand pushing the elbow into valgus and compressing the radial head. **If undisplaced** it can be treated in a backslab; **displaced** fractures generally require open reduction if possible or occasionally excision if grossly comminuted (Fig. 24).

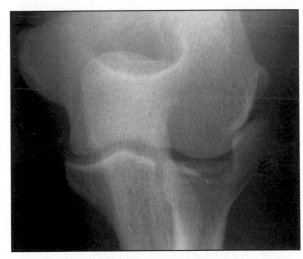

Figure 24 – Displaced fracture of the radial head

FRACTURES OF THE NECK OF RADIUS

Result from a similar mechanism of injury as radial head fractures. In adults, one is more likely to fracture the radial head whereas in children, due to the cartilaginous epiphysis, one is more likely to fracture through the radial neck. Up to 20 degrees of radial tilt is accepted; beyond 20 degrees requires closed reduction and occasionally open reduction if difficult. **Monteggia fractures** result from a fall on an outstretched hand resulting in a fracture of the ulna with dislocation of the radial head. This fracture requires a closed reduction and immobilization **closely monitoring the position of the radial head** (Fig. 25).

ELBOW DISLOCATIONS

Occur commonly and are more frequent in adults than children. Dislocations without fracture are called simple and are classified according to the direction of the displacement of the olecranon (79% are posterior or posterolaterally) (Figs. 18 & 19, Chapter 18).

Dislocations usually result from a fall on the outstretched hand with the elbow in extension. The anterior capsule usually tears as may brachialis. The surrounding ligaments may stretch or rupture depending on the direction of the dislocation and an associated fracture may occur.

Clinically, one presents with obvious deformity, pain and swelling. The bony landmarks formed by the epicondyles and olecranon look abnormal and there maybe associated vessel and neurological damage. Neuropraxia is seen in 20% of cases and generally involves the ulnar or median nerves, these are usually transient. X-rays should be performed to document the direction of dislocation and possible fractures.

Closed reduction is performed. Apply longitudinal traction and with the free hand move the olecranon back onto the trochlea (ideally under general anaesthetic so as to assess the elbow stability post reduction). If stable postoperatively, can return to protected motion as soon as possible (may lose the last few degrees of extension and supination).

Associated injuries and complications (should be noted) include fractures (or avulsion of the medial epicondyle), head of radius, olecranon process, heterotopic ossification, recurrent dislocations and vascular or neural injury.

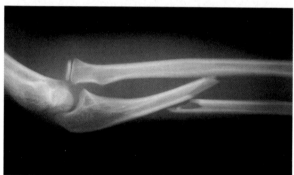

Figure 25 – Nerve compression about the elbow

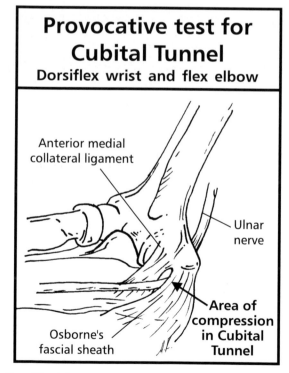

Figure 27 – Cubital Tunnel. The provocative test is to dorsiflex the wrist and flex the elbow

---

NERVE COMPRESSION ABOUT THE ELBOW

- Ulnar nerve - (Cubital tunnel syndrome)
- Radial nerve and Posterior interosseous nerve
- Median nerve - (pronator syndrome)
- Anterior interosseous syndrome

Figure 26 – Nerve compression about the elbow

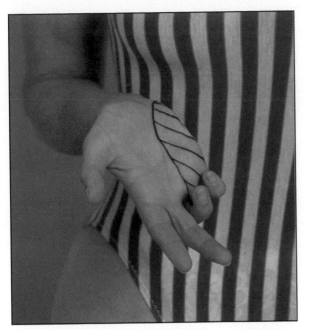

Figure 28 – Claw hand of low ulnar nerve palsy (less clawing when at level of elbow)

NERVE COMPRESSION SYNDROMES

Numerous nerves can be compressed around the elbow (Fig. 26). Nerve compression may be secondary to a fracture or have gradual onset (no injury) from degenerative change around the joint, a space occupying lesion (ganglion or bursa) or musculo tendinous anomalies.

Clinically localised sensory and motor changes specific for a particular nerve are generally present.

CUBITAL TUNNEL SYNDROME

An irritation or compression of the ulnar nerve within the cubital tunnel at the elbow. In the athlete, ulnar neuritis usually results from physiological as well as from pathological responses to chronic activity. Chronic valgus strain can cause traction neuritis, scar formation, spurs, calcification in the MCL or osteophytes which can all contribute to ulnar nerve pathology.

Presents with pain along the medial side of the forearm which may migrate proximally or distally.

Paraesthesia in the little and ring fingers are encountered early and usually precede any detectable motor weakness of the hand. One may have a positive percussion test over the ulnar nerve at the elbow, abnormal mobility of the nerve over the medial epicondyle and a positive provocative test. Clumsiness of the hand especially after pitching a few innings may be the main complaint (Figs. 27 & 28).

Before treating, be sure of the diagnosis which can be confirmed on clinical examination, X-ray and nerve conduction studies. Differential diagnosis would include cervical spine pathology, thoracic outlet or pathology involving the ulnar nerve at the wrist. Treatment is initially an elbow splint and correction of the underlying pathology. If this fails then surgical decompression with transposition of the ulnar nerve (or medial epicondylectomy).

RADIAL NERVE

The radial nerve is vulnerable to compression along its path from the lateral head of triceps to mid forearm (where it branches into the posterior interosseous nerve) and from trauma. There is lateral elbow pain (similar to lateral epicondylitis pain). Neurological symptoms and signs include weakness of wrist and finger extension and paraesthesia dorsally over the base of the thumb (differentiate it from epicondylitis) (see Fig. 42, Chapter 10). After diagnosis, surgical decompression is usually required.

MEDIAN NERVE (PRONATOR SYNDROME)

The median nerve is susceptible to compression from the supracondyloid process (proximally) to the flexor superficialis arch (distally).

Pronator syndrome – symptoms are often vague consisting of discomfort in the forearm. Numbness of the hand in the median nerve distribution is often secondary. Repetitive strenuous motions such as industrial activities, weight training or driving, often provoke the symptoms. Signs include proximal forearm pain on resisted pronation, elbow flexion and wrist flexion. **Anterior interosseous syndrome**— pain in proximal forearm, weakness of pinch and in the FPL, and index finger FDP (see Fig. 38, Chapter 12). Treatment requires surgical release.

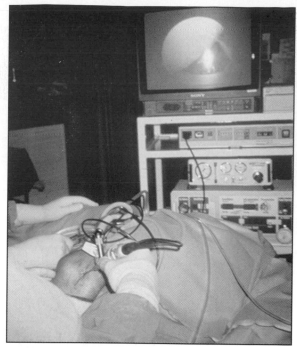

Figure 29 – Arthroscopic removal of loose body from elbow

INTRA-ARTICULAR DERANGEMENTS

LOOSE BODIES

Common in the elbow from old trauma, degenerative arthritis, osteochondritis dissecans and synovial chondromatosis.

Clinically, extension is reduced and there is pain and locking or grating. X-rays are useful.

If troublesome then surgical removal is required, performed arthroscopically. However if there are multiple loose bodies, an arthrotomy should be performed (Fig. 29). Specific conditions may require specific treatments (synovectomy for synovial chondromatosis).

OSTEOARTHRITIS OF THE ELBOW

A primary form of involvement of the elbow joint from trauma, OCD or synovial disease (chondrometaplasia). There is pain with loss of range of motion with or without locking, localised tenderness, joint thickening and crepitus and sometimes a flexion contracture with associated ulnar nerve irritation (Fig. 30).

Rest, physiotherapy and NSAID with modification of activity are the main treatment. Later, arthroscopic

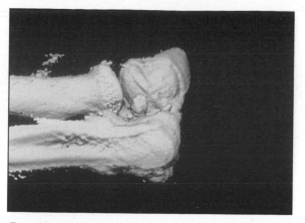

Figure 30 – CT of early OA elbow with loose bodies

debridement, radial head excision or arthroplasty may be necessary.

SEPTIC ARTHRITIS

Children are more commonly affected and septic arthritis is common in rheumatoid arthritis. There is an acutely tender elbow joint held in flexion. Any movement is painful and generalised symptoms of sepsis are present. The differential diagnosis (in the child) includes rheumatoid arthritis, trauma, acute rheumatic fever and transient synovitis and (in the adult) gout or pseudogout.

Patients have a leucocytosis, an increased ESR and X-rays which may show the fat pad sign early and later subtle bone erosion. Blood cultures are positive in 40-60% (normally **staph. aureus**). Treatment is surgical drainage with antibiotics.

SUMMARY

A useful clue to the diagnosis of elbow pain is the location of the pain and tenderness (Fig. 31).

CAUSES OF ELBOW PAIN BY LOCATION	
Medial Elbow Pain	**Lateral Elbow Pain**
Partial/Complete MCL tear	Posterolateral instability
Ulnar neuritis	Radial/PIN irritation
Medial Epicondylitis	Lateral Epicondylitis
Valgus Extension Overload	Synovial Impingement
Little Leaguers Elbow	OCD/Panner's Disease

Figure 31 – Causes of elbow pain by location

12

HAND AND WRIST

David Dilley
Beverley Trevithick

INTRODUCTION

The hand and wrist are often injured in sport. Careful assessment and refined investigations have improved diagnosis and management. The essential functions of the hand are touch and firm grip. The thumb opposes the fingers and provides precise grip. The wrist is the stable platform for the hand and fine tunes grasp. Hunter, tool maker, soldier and athlete alike depend upon their hands.

ANATOMY AND BIOMECHANICS

Anatomy, biomechanics and function are inextricably linked. This balance and interplay are nowhere more evident or finely tuned than in the hand. Tendons, intrinsic muscles, nerves and vessels are packed together in an intricate, delicate, yet robust unit capable of delivering a knockout punch or coordinating with brain and body to project a ball with pinpoint accuracy from the cricket boundary or baseball outfield to the gloves of the catcher or 'keeper. A freestyle rockclimber can support their entire body weight with one or two fingers; a golfer's 'touch' with a putter accurately sends the ball to the cup.

A knowledge of surface anatomy is essential to an accurate assessment of injury (Fig. 1). Awareness of the more common anatomic variations is also important, e.g. flexor digitorum superficialis to the small finger is absent in a significant number of people. An extensor digitorum manus brevis may be confused with a ganglion.

The hand and fingers are capable of adapting to an extraordinary range of shapes and sizes, yet a relatively small amount of oedema in the finger is enough to significantly restrict movement (Fig. 2).

ASSESSMENT OF INJURY

The assessment of any injury begins with the history. What is the **chief complaint?** Usually this falls into one or more of three broad areas. **"It doesn't feel right; it doesn't work right; it doesn't look right."** Key questions include asking about the position of the hands and fingers at the time of the injury, as well as what was being attempted. An understanding of the mechanism of injury combined with the chief complaint will often be enough to make the diagnosis which then need only be confirmed by

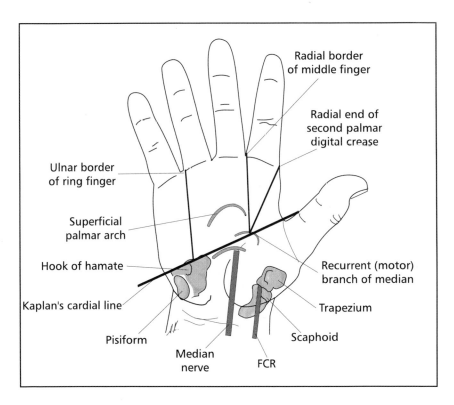

Figure 1 – Surface landmarks for underlying anatomy with reference to Kaplan's line

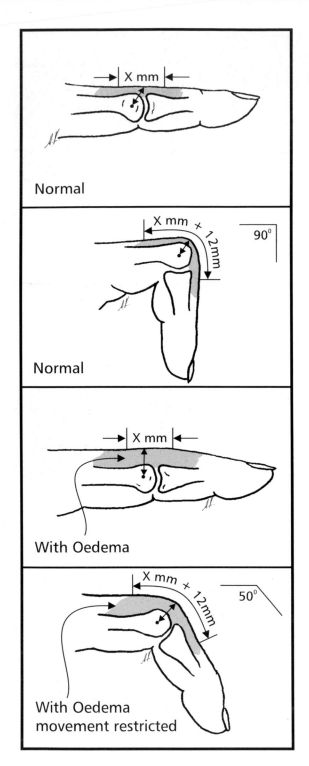

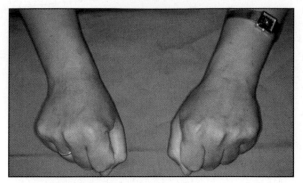

Figure 3 – Overview of hand: preliminary inspection of hands and wrist. Flexion fingers (make fist)

Figure 2 – How oedema restricts joint motion (same 12 mm dorsal skin lengthening only allows 50° PIP flexion)

examination and X-ray. The team doctor is often in the privileged position of witnessing the injury as it occurs.

Clinical assessment of the hand and wrist includes an appraisal of each anatomic structure and its function. Skin and nails cover and protect. Each joint should be stable (ligaments) and mobile (musculotendinous unit for each joint movement). Nerves subserve sensation and motor supply. Vessels bring to, and take blood from, the part. Bones provide stability.

Unless otherwise obvious, the examination begins by asking the patient to localise precisely (point, with one finger, to one spot!) the site of the problem. The site of **maximal tenderness** is sought, but near the end of the exam so as not to begin by hurting the patient. The exam should proceed in orderly sequence, examining all structures to exclude other injuries. **Look, move, feel,** then apply any special manoeuvres that may be appropriate to the clinical situation. **Always compare sides.**

Look. Inspect the dorsal and palmar surfaces of the wrists, hands and fingers. Look from the side, above, and end on (Figs. 3-8). Assess the position of wrists, hands and fingers. Is there an abnormal posture suggestive of a fracture, ligament or tendon injury (Fig. 9)? What are the site and extent of swelling, lacerations, bruises, and sweat patterns?

Move. Ask the patient to make a complete fist and fully extend, abduct and adduct, all fingers and both thumbs. Check wrist dorsiflexion, palmarflexion, radial and ulnar deviation, as well as pronation and supination.

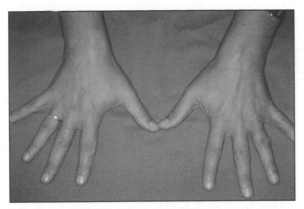

Figure 4 – Extension fingers

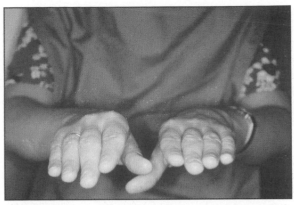

Figure 5 – Pronation (also check supination)

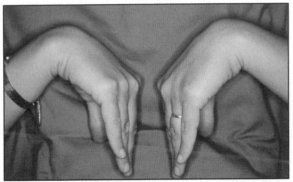

Figure 6 – Wrist palmar flexion

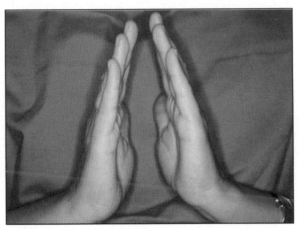

Figure 7 – Wrist dorsiflexion

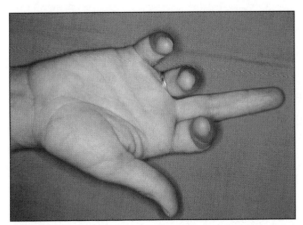

Figure 8 – Abnormal posture of long finger due to missed division of both flexor tendons

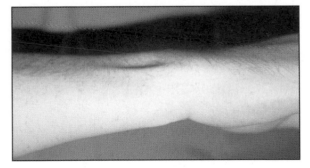

Figure 9 – Unusual injury: isolated volar dislocation of distal raio-ulnar joint. (Apparent from careful inspection)

Feel: Palpate the areas in question, gently seeking sites of tenderness, instability, masses, etc. Routinely assess sensation and circulation. Finally, perform any relevant provocative manoeuvres. Assessment of grip and pinch strengths should generally be made and recorded to aid in later monitoring of recovery.

When X-rays are ordered specific views and sites must be requested. Request a minimum of two views at right angles. If the injured part is a finger, specify views of that finger, **not just the hand**. Special views are particularly useful in assessing wrist injury. PA clenched fist (to assess scapholunate gap), carpal tunnel (hook of hamate fracture) and pisotriquetral views often add valuable information. At the very least PA views in neutral, ulnar and radial deviation and direct lateral are required.

CT scanning can provide additional anatomic information in trauma to the wrist, particularly in the setting of difficult or unusual fractures, or fracture dislocations around the bases of the metacarpals and carpus.

Bone scans are helpful in telling "where," but not what. They are particularly useful in the assessment of chronic wrist pain.

Ultrasound is "operator dependent", but when performed and interpreted by skilled, experienced people, can localise non radio-opaque foreign bodies, as well as give much valuable information regarding soft tissue masses, tendons and ligaments.

Magnetic resonance imaging is still finding its niche in the hand and wrist. It can be of value in assessing the triangular fibrocartilage complex.

GUIDELINES FOR THE MANAGEMENT OF AN ISOLATED HAND INJURY

Initial priorities are important and outlined here (Fig. 10). Bleeding is controlled by direct pressure on the wound. Artery clips and tourniquets have no place in the control of bleeding as the potential for iatrogenic damage is great. An artery clip can turn a relatively simple arterial anastomosis into an interposition vein graft and nerve repair. Incorrect use of tourniquets can be limb threatening.

INITIAL PRIORITIES
• Stop bleeding (direct pressure)
• Relieve pain (digital/wrist block)
• Assess injury (and splint)

PATH TO RECOVERY
• Pain relief
• Protection
• Physiotherapy

Figure 10 – Initial priorities in management of isolated hand injury; and path to recovery

At the time of injury a **digital, or wrist block** is the most effective way of relieving pain. Lignocaine 2% without adrenaline is used in doses not exceeding 5mg/kg. Obviously any nerve injury must have been assessed and documented prior to the administration of nerve block.

Splinting the injured part is a simple, and sadly often forgotten, means of providing effective and rapid pain relief. This is more effective if a deformity has been reduced, but is effective even if the part is splinted as it lies. Unless there is a specific reason for doing otherwise the hand should only be splinted in the **"safe"** position.

The safe position holds the wrist in about 30° extension, metacarpophalangeal joints 70-90° flexed, and the interphalangeal joints fully extended. The thumb, if included in the splint, is held parallel to the index finger (Fig. 11). In this position the collateral ligaments are at their longest. If the joints are splinted otherwise, for any length of time, the ligaments tend to shorten and joint stiffness which is difficult (near impossible) to treat ensues.

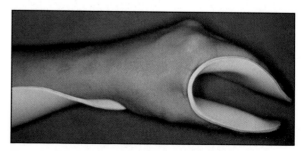

Figure 11 – The hand splinted in the "safe" position

The injured athlete is the **key member** of the team whose aim is to speed a safe recovery from injury. Interaction between athlete, surgeon, sport physician, hand therapist, and team coach is essential to achieve this aim. The surgeon and physician can, usually, restore anatomy, relieve pain, and advise when various treatments and activities are appropriate. **The coach can correct faulty technique** and advise the medical team on the demands of the sport. It is emphasised that **the patient is primarily responsible for their own recovery. Only the patient can do and carry out the advice given.**

Pain relief, protection, and physiotherapy are the three "Ps" on the path to recovery (Fig 10).

Pain relief. The use of ice, crepe, and elevation are standard methods to reduce pain and swelling. Analgesics are used as required. The use of NSAID has been somewhat illogical in that the doses usually prescribed are analgesic but not anti-inflammatory in their effects (the prolonged use can lead to gastro-intestinal and occasionally renal side effects). Ice, heat, laser and TENS (transcutaneous electrical nerve stimulation) may also reduce pain.

Steroids such as betamethasone ("Celestone") or methylprednisolone ("Depomedrol") have little role in the acute traumatic injury. They are useful in chronic inflammatory conditions but rarely should more than two or three injections be given in the one area. Complications with prolonged or repeated use include skin atrophy, fat necrosis, infection, and tendon rupture.

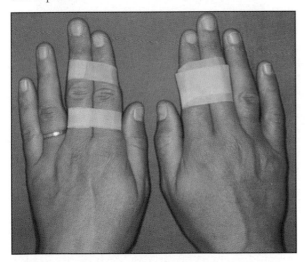

Figure 12 – Buddy tapping. The fingers of the left hand correctly taped to allow unimpeded joint movement, those on the right have been incorrectly taped

When the athlete is considering a return to activity they may request a **"pain killing injection"** in order to play or train. The injection of local anaesthetic in these circumstances is rarely, if ever, indicated. If the part is too painful to stand up to the rigours of competition it is not ready for them.

Protection. Continuation of splinting from the acute stage of injury is often required to stabilise and protect the injured part. The splint should allow protected movement ("buddy taping" to a healthy digit is easy and most useful). Apply tape so as not to interfere with joint movement (Fig. 12). Use caution when buddying an injured small finger to the ring finger as deforming rotatory forces may be applied to the injured digit. Buddy taping is a form of dynamic splinting. As a **general rule dynamic** splinting is preferred but is often used in combination with static splints (at night).

On occasion, surgery is necessary to obtain stability and protection.

Physiotherapy. This emphasises early active movement and should begin as soon as possible. As pain settles, stability established, and movement returns, stretching and strengthening are added to the treatment regimen. Any impediment to movement should be removed (pain, instability, and oedema).

Oedema is removed by movement, elevation, ice, and pressure from elastic bandages (Coban or similar) or tailor made gloves. Massage, laser, and intermittent positive pressure (Masman pump) are also useful.

FRACTURES

The biology and biomechanics of fracture and soft tissue healing are no different in the athlete than in anyone else. Athletes do not heal more quickly because they seek the advice and treatment of a "sports doctor", or any other physician or therapist for that matter. Fracture union in the upper limb can be expected in approximately six weeks in the adult, about half this time in the child. Fracture consolidation takes about twice the time for union. What is often different is the **attitude to injury**. The demands of competition, especially at the elite level, often result in an athlete trying to return to training and competition too early, thus running the risk of further injury. Financial considerations may also bear on the decision to return early at the risk of later long term problems. The athlete must make the ultimate decision. It is the role of the medical team to advise what the risks are and how they may be eliminated or minimised.

The **clinical hallmarks** of fracture are important (pain, swelling, deformity and loss of function). Diagnosis is confirmed by X-ray. In the hand, early movement is the key to a swift return to full function and for this to happen the fracture must be of a stable pattern, or it must be rendered stable by splinting or surgical fixation. The outcome deteriorates if active range of motion is delayed beyond 3 weeks.

The fracture is reduced under appropriate anaesthesia by closed or open means and rendered stable. The adequacy of reduction is confirmed by X-ray and this should be checked with further X-rays one week post injury. Later X-rays may be necessary depending on the situation.

Those fractures that cannot, by splinting, be rendered stable enough to immediately mobilise should be considered for **surgical fixation.** There are numerous techniques described for the fixation of phalangeal and metacarpal fractures and the treating surgeon should have a good knowledge of the options available. A discussion of these techniques is without the scope of this text. The interested reader should refer to the numerous articles and standard operative texts in hand and orthopaedic surgery.

Displaced fractures involving joint surfaces will nearly always require reduction and surgical fixation. Be wary of so called "chip" or "avulsion" fractures as these are often the bony equivalent of a tendon or ligament rupture (Fig. 13). These will usually require surgical repair.

DISTAL PHALANX FRACTURES

Most distal phalangeal fractures result from a direct blow, often with the finger being "crushed" between bat and ball. The hallmark of this injury is a subungual haematoma. Occasionally the nail plate is lifted out of the nail fold, an indication that the fracture is, or was, displaced and significant injury to the nail bed has occurred. As first aid, a painful **subungual haematoma** under pressure may be relieved by drilling the nail plate with a sterile 18 or 19G needle, X-rays should then be taken to rule out underlying fracture (Fig. 14). These injuries are open fractures and should be treated as such. Surgical cleaning of the fracture site, with accurate repair of the nail bed, assisted

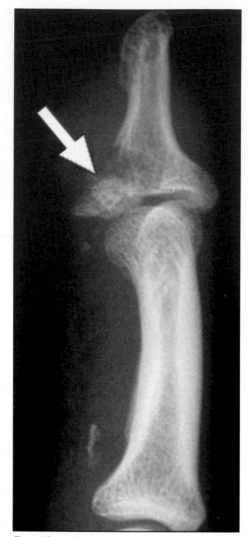

Figure 13 – "Chip" fracture of the volar surface of the distal phalanx representing avulsion of the profundus tendon. Note the bone sliver just distal to PIPI indicating the level to which the tendon has retracted

by the use of magnification, and fracture fixation where appropriate, give the best results. Some surgeons feel a haematoma involving more than 25% of the nail plate is an indication for its removal to allow nail bed repair even in the absence of an underlying fracture.

BONY MALLET

Jamming a finger on the ground, ball, or opponent can result in avulsion fractures of the extensor tendon (bony mallet) (Fig. 15), or less commonly avulsion of the flexor tendon. This latter injury is more serious

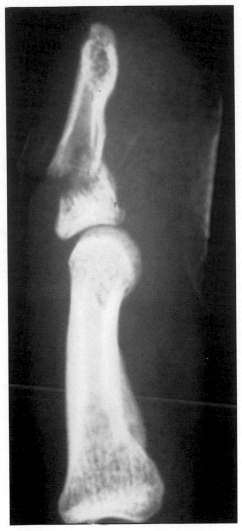

Figure 14 – Fracture to the distal phalanx suggested clinically by displacement of the nail plate from beneath the nail fold. Irrigation, nail bed repair and pinning or the fracture was performed.

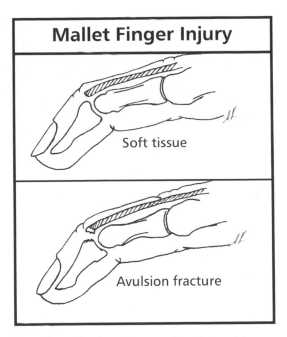

Figure 15 – Mallet finger injury may be soft tissue injury or bony avulsion.

and unfortunately less recognised. It will nearly always require surgical treatment. Occasionally the tendon will pull away from the bone chip and be found in the palm.

The bony mallet, provided no more than 30% of the joint surface is involved and there is no joint subluxation, can be treated in a hyperextension splint which must be maintained for at least 6 weeks, probably 8. Appropriate instruction in skin care and changing splints must be understood by the patient (Figs. 16 & 17).

MIDDLE AND PROXIMAL PHALANGES, METACARPALS

Transverse fractures of the middle phalanx distal to the insertion of flexor superficialis result in extension of the distal fragment, those proximal to its insertion are flexed. Transverse fractures of the proximal phalanx usually result in the interossei flexing the proximal fragment. Transverse fractures of metacarpals tend to have the distal fragment flexed by the long flexors. Reduction and neutralisation of the deforming forces may be possible using various combinations of buddy and extension block splinting (Figs 18-22)

Short oblique, and to a lesser extent, spiral fractures of the phalanges and metacarpals may shorten and rotate. They are thus more likely to require surgical fixation. Rotation is assessed with the fingers in flexion. The fingers should not cross and the tips should individually point to the tubercle of the scaphoid (Fig. 23).

The common, so called, **"boxer's fracture"** (a fracture of the neck of the small finger metacarpal and a result of untrained or unskilled punching) is usually best treated in a resting splint with the hand in the safe position until pain and swelling subside (7-10 days) followed by active mobilisation. These fractures generally do not require fixation despite what appears to be marked X-ray deformity.

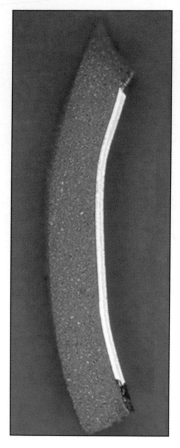

Figure 16 – Mallet finger splint

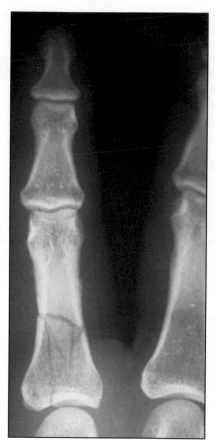

Figure 18 – Fracture of the proximal phalanx (AP view). A stable pattern treated by buddy tape and immediate mobilisation

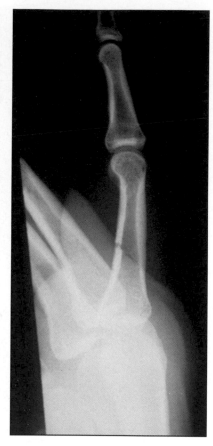

Figure 19 – Same fracture lateral view

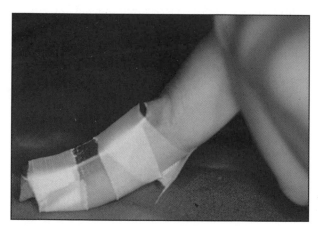

Figure 17 – Sequence of application. Tape is prepared, placed in readiness and skin care attended. Note the joint is maintained in flexion by not allowing the finger to leave the table top at any stage

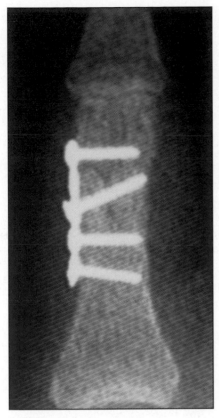

Figure 22 – Fracture internally fixed.

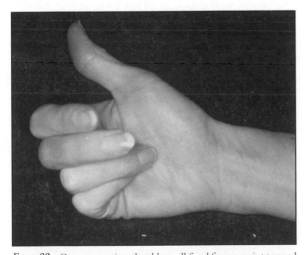

Figure 23 – Correct rotation should see all fixed fingers point toward tubercle of scaphoid.

DISLOCATIONS AND COLLATERAL LIGAMENT INJURY

Dorsal dislocation of the PIPJ is the most common of these lesions. Closed reduction is usually possible either immediately, on the field, or later, under digital block. Following reduction, joint stability should be gently assessed. The volar plate is avulsed from the middle phalanx, sometimes with a bony fragment. Splinting the joint straight for 7-10 days followed by protected motion by "buddy taping" or dorsal block splint for a further 3 weeks is recommended. Protect the finger by buddy taping during strenuous activity for a further 6-8 weeks.

Occasionally a dislocation will not reduce easily by closed means. This is often because of **soft tissue interposition** or entrapment of the dislocated phalangeal or metacarpal head. If dislocations will not reduce easily with gentle closed manipulation, rougher efforts are avoided and open reduction performed.

Partial collateral ligament ruptures are treated by immediate motion protected by buddy taping for 6-8 weeks depending on residual tenderness. The treatment of complete ruptures is a little more controversial, with advocates of both splinting and operative repair.

Metacarpophalangeal joint dislocations are rare and may require open reduction. Besides the thumb, collateral ligament injuries of this joint are likewise rare.

SKIER'S THUMB
(GOAL KEEPER'S THUMB)

This common injury is caused by sudden forced radial deviation of the thumb phalanx on the metacarpal. Seen in skiers (the ski stock handles do not protect from it) and football. There is ulnar sided pain, swelling and instability (Fig. 24a). X-rays may show a bony avulsion. Athletes are often reluctant to seek treatment for such a "minor" injury. Rupture of the ulnar collateral ligament of the thumb may require open exploration and repair as it is almost impossible to tell clinically whether or not the avulsed ligament has come to lie superficial to the adductor aponeurosis (Stener lesion) (Fig. 24). Exploration of older injuries has also revealed the ligament folded back on itself beneath the adductor aponeurosis. Treatment is outlined in Figure 25.

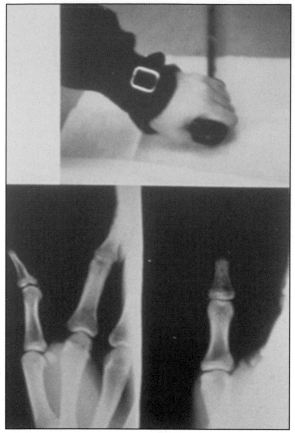

Figure 24 – Skier's thumb is a common sports injury from forced hyperabduction/extension (X-rays may show a bony avulsion)

SKIER'S THUMB	
Type 1	- sprain - splint
Type 2	- partial tear - splint
Type 3	- complete tear * - surgery (* > 30° abduction)

Figure 25 – Skier's Thumb Classification and treatment

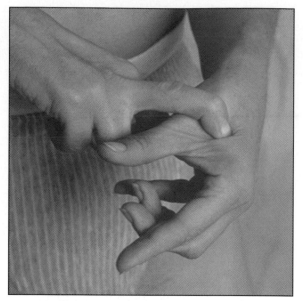

Figure 26 – Mallet finger (extension lag at DIP)

MALLET/BASEBALL FINGER

Closed rupture of the distal extensor tendon results in the "mallet", or "baseball" finger (Fig. 26). Provided there is no joint subluxation, or a fracture involving one third or greater of the articular surface, these are best treated by splinting the distal interphalangeal joint in slight hyperextension for 6-8 weeks (even if presentation is delayed beyond 7-10 days). Splints are changed at least daily to allow care of the skin, which can become reddened and tender over the dorsum of the joint. It is important that these splint changes be carried out so that flexion of the DIPJ is prevented at all times (Fig. 15). In particularly supple fingers a secondary swan neck deformity may rapidly develop at the PIPJ necessitating inclusion of this joint in the splint for 3-4 weeks (in slight flexion). Commercial splints are available for treatment of this injury, but if they are poorly fitted they will not properly position the joint.

RUPTURE OF MIDDLE SLIP

Rupture of the middle slip of the extensor mechanism over the PIPJ is a commonly missed injury resulting ultimately in a boutonniere deformity which is extremely difficult to correct. This injury should be suspected in a "jammed" PIPJ, particularly when the joint is swollen, and most tender over its dorsum. There are specific tests; these include inability to actively extend the last 10- 15 degrees at the PIPJ and the Elson test (flex the PIPJ to a right angle, "over the edge of a table" and ask the patient to attempt extension of the PIPJ). A central slip rupture will result in no pressure being felt by the examiner over the middle phalanx and the distal phalanx will tend to extend. The lack of full extension, in the presence of full passive extension, of the PIPJ by tenodesis when the wrist and metacarpophalangeal joints are fully passively flexed is also indicative of rupture. Later signs include fixed flexion of the PIPJ associated with decreased passive DIPJ flexion with PIPJ fully extended.

Splinting is the most effective form of treatment. The first step is to correct PIPJ flexion and then DIP flexion. The splinting programme may take a minimum of 8 weeks or longer to achieve the desired results (Fig. 27).

Ruptures of the extensor mechanism at the level of the MPJ occur occasionally. Most often these take the form of a ruptured sagittal band, usually on the radial side of the long finger. The patient presents with localised pain and swelling and an inability to actively extend the MPJ. It is possible for the patient to maintain full extension of the joint if it is passively extended. A type of triggering (extensor tendon subluxing between the metacarpal heads) of the finger at MPJ rather than PIPJ level may be a later presentation. If seen acutely, these injuries respond well to splinting the MPJ in extension for 3 weeks. Other joints are left free. If not seen acutely, the tear is best repaired surgically.

A rarer form of extensor injury at MPJ level is a longitudinal split in the tendon and rupture of the dorsal MPJ capsule. This is usually the result of a direct blow, as in boxing or other forms of martial arts. Surgical repair is usually indicated.

FLEXOR TENDON AVULSION ("JERSEY" FINGER)

Flexor tendon avulsion is less common than extensor injury and less well recognised. The usual mechanism of injury is an attempt to grab the jersey or equipment of an opposing player ("jersey" finger). The DIPJ loses its ability to actively flex, bruising is often present and there may be a tender lump in the palm. The ring finger is most commonly affected (Fig. 27). Players of "Oztag", a variation of touch football in which a "tackle" is effected by ripping a velcro fastened tag from the shorts of an opponent, seem to be at particular risk of this injury.

If seen acutely, an attempt to repair the tendon is made. Repair becomes increasingly difficult after only a few days because of swelling in the injured tendon and collapse of the flexor sheath. Those who present late may not require intervention if there is no pain and little functional deficit. Hyperextension of the DIPJ with or without "weakness" in the finger may best be treated by DIPJ fusion. Two stage tendon reconstruction has more complications and is more demanding of surgeon and patient. It requires prolonged rehabilitation and long absences from training and competition which the athlete may not tolerate.

WRIST FRACTURES

SCAPHOID FRACTURE

The most common carpal fracture occurs in the scaphoid. Volumes have been written about the appropriate management of this fracture. The diagnosis should be suspected following a fall onto the hand and tenderness is located over the scaphoid or in the anatomic "snuff box" (Fig. 29). Swelling and "thickening" in the AP length of the wrist may be present. Resisted pinch is painful. The X-ray request should include a "scaphoid view" (PA in ulnar deviation).

It is not uncommon to have the above clinical scenario and negative X-rays. Standard orthopaedic teaching is to place such patients in a "scaphoid cast" and X-ray at two weeks. If there is still pain in the presence of negative X-rays, consider the possibility of a truly

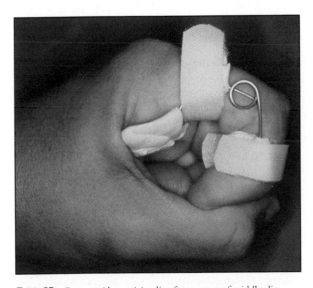

Figure 27 – Capener (dynamic) splint for rupture of middle slip.

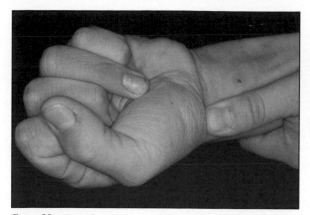

Figure 28 – Ring fingerflexor profundus avulsion. The patient has been asked to make a fist

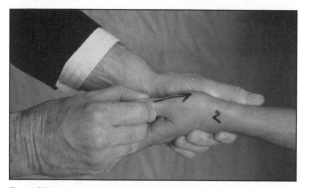

Figure 29 – Scaphoid fracture is suspected where there is anatomical snuff box tenderness (or positive scaphoid impaction test in cast)

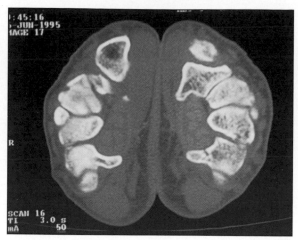

Figure 30 – Fracture hook of hamate with point tenderness (seen on CT carpal tunnel view, lower view)

(including the thumb up to, but not including the IP joint) with the thumb pulp opposed to the pulp of the middle finger for 6 weeks. If there is no evidence of union progressing the fracture is fixed with **a Herbert screw**. Displaced waist and proximal third fractures are fixed per primum with a Herbert screw. If early mobilisation is desired, as is often the case with athletes, the fracture is also fixed *per primum*. Return to training or competition may be possible as early as 3 weeks after surgery in non contact sports. Contact and collision are not permitted until union has occurred and definitely not before 6-8 weeks post fracture.

OTHER CARPAL FRACTURES

Fractures of the triquetrum are reportedly the second or third most common carpal fracture. Usually these are avulsions from the dorsum of the bone. Immobilisation in a splint for 3-4 weeks is usually sufficient to allow pain to settle enough for resumption of activity. Occasionally, they may be the source of ongoing pain and fragment excision and ligament repair may be required.

FRACTURE OF THE HOOK OF HAMATE

Fractures of the hook of the hamate constitute approximately 2% of carpal fractures and are more common in "club" or "racquet" sports such as hockey, golf, baseball and less common in cricket and tennis (Fig. 30). The mechanism of injury is impact between the base of the club, bat or racquet and hypothenar eminence. The handle of a cricket bat is sprung to

"occult" fracture, or a scaphoid-lunate ligament injury and obtain stress X-rays and a bone scan.

Controversy also exists regarding how a scaphoid fracture should be immobilised (long arm versus short arm cast), and also how many of the thumb joints require immobilisation. The indications for surgery are also controversial. Some authors advocate fixation of the majority of fractures. Arthroscopic techniques have been developed for surgical reduction and fixation.

The median time to union of a scaphoid fracture is 12 weeks. The more proximal in the bone the fracture is, the more likely is avascular necrosis and/or non-union. It should be borne in mind that there is little literature to show the expectation of decreased rates of avascular necrosis with fracture, fixation is borne out in practice.

It is best to immobilise tubercle or undisplaced (**no displacement**) wrist fractures in a short arm cast absorb impact and thus a "batsman" is less likely than a "batter" to suffer this fracture.

Tenderness is located over the hook of the hamate. A carpal tunnel view may show the fracture, but they are often best seen on CT scan. Treatment is to either fix the fracture or excise the fragment. Not holding the base of the bat adjacent to the hypothenar eminence may lessen the risk of this injury.

CARPAL INSTABILITIES AND LIGAMENTOUS INJURIES

SCAPHO-LUNATE LIGAMENT

The scapho-lunate ligament is commonly injured and presents like a scaphoid fracture. A fall on the out-stretched hand is usual, but the author has seen patients present with a story of a painful "pop" follow-ing an attempt to play a backhand volley. Pain is locat-ed over the dorsal aspect of the ligament. Tenderness located over the ligament just distal to Lister's tubercle may be the only clinical sign. Kirk Watson has report-ed a provocative manoeuvre to assess the stability of the scaphoid. X-rays show a scapho-lunate gap; the

Terry Thomas sign. Clenched fist PA views, especially when compared with the uninjured side, may be helpful. Arthrography will usually demonstrate the tear. MRI is as yet too unreliable for diagnosis. Arthroscopy can make the diagnosis and occasionally be the avenue of treatment.

Treatment is difficult and recovery often prolonged. (Controversial: whether limited intercarpal fusion or capsulodesis.)

Chronic tears may lead to a dorsal intercalated seg-ment instability (DISI) with eventual degenerative change throughout the carpus (Figs. 31 & 32).

Tears of the lunotriquetral ligament present with ulnar wrist pain. Stress across this joint by balloting the bones with respect to each other causes pain and reproduces the patient's symptoms. X-rays may show a step off in the curve formed by scaphoid, lunate and triquetrum as assessed at mid carpal level (Fig. 33). Later changes may result in a volar intercalated insta-bility. Assessment of the midcarpal joint and triangular fibrocartilage complex is imperative since these injuries may be associated with, or mimic, each other. Arthroscopic debridement, reduction and pinning of

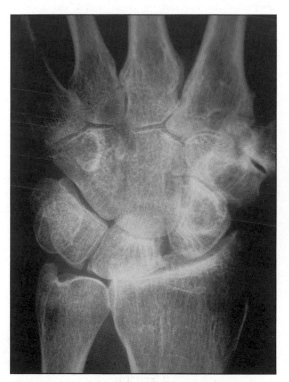

Figure 31 – Scapho-lunate gap and flexed scaphoid seen on AP X-ray

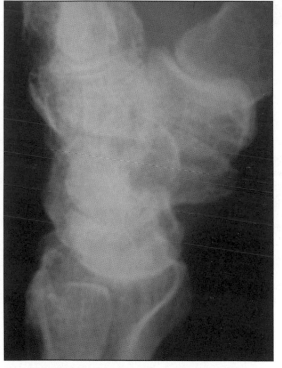

Figure 32 – Lateral X-ray shows dorsiflexed lunate in chronic scapho-lunate ligament tear

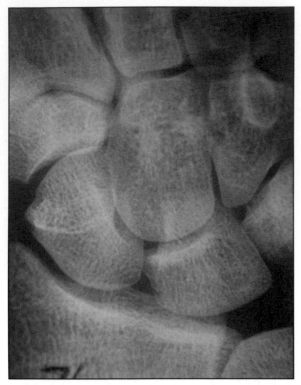

Figure 33 – Subtle step in line up of lunate and triquetrum in mid-carpal instability

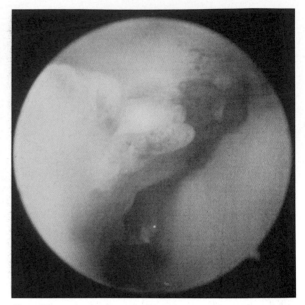

Figure 34 – Arthroscopic view of TFCC tear

the joint has been tried with small numbers of patients and has had some success.

Midcarpal instabilities may present with a painful clunk and this can be reproduced by Lichtman's manoeuvre where the patient is asked to make a tight fist and move the wrist from radial to ulnar deviation.

TRIANGULAR FIBROCARTILAGE COMPLEX (TFCC) INJURY

Triangular fibrocartilage complex (TFCC) injuries also cause ulnar sided wrist pain (Fig. 34). Tenderness can often be elicited just distal to the tip of the ulna and "grinding" of the TFCC by compressing the dorsiflexed and ulnar deviated carpus against the complex will usually reproduce symptoms. The incidence of degenerative tears of the TFCC increases with increasing age. "Congenital tears" have also been described.

If pain is worsened by pronation and supination the **distal radio-ulnar joint (DRUJ)** may also have been injured. Compress the joint as the patient pronates and supinates the forearm. Stability of the DRUJ is

assessed by stressing the dorsal and volar radio-ulnar ligaments in neutral, as well as the fully pronated and fully supinated forearm. In full supination the volar ligaments are taut and there should be no volar translation of the ulna with respect to the radius compared with the uninjured side. The reverse occurs with forearm pronation.

Arthroscopy is the best means of investigating these problems and in many cases provides a treatment option with debridement or suture of tears.

SOFT-TISSUE WRIST PAIN

A common cause of chronic wrist pain in the athlete, that is diagnosable only by arthroscopy, is injury to the chondral surfaces. Some authors have reported good relief of symptoms with debridement of isolated lesions, those with associated pathology did less well. Occult ganglion should also be a suspect in cases where diagnosis is difficult. These may be detected by ultrasound or MRI.

DE QUERVAIN'S TENOSYNOVITIS

Other, more common, causes of radial sided wrist pain include de Quervain's tenosynovitis (Fig. 35), not uncommon in tennis, squash, racketball players, and weight lifters. Causes tenderness over the first extensor compartment of the wrist. **Finkelstein's sign** is posi-

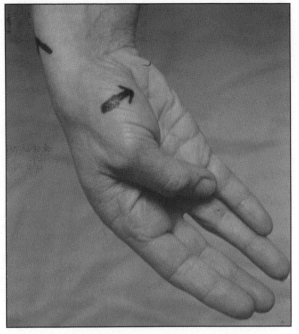

Figure 35 – Finkelstein's test is positive in de Quervain's tenosynovitis (ulnar deviation of hand with flexed thumb causes pain)

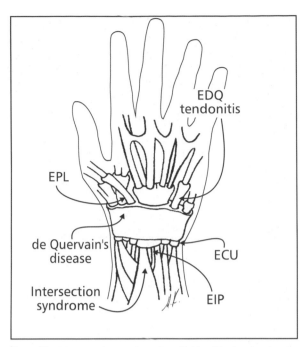

Figure 36 – Not uncommon sites of tendinitis of the hand and wrist

tive. Initial treatment consists of rest, splinting and one or two injections of steroid and local anaesthetic into the compartment. If this management fails, operative release gives good results.

WARTENBERG'S SYNDROME

Neuritis of the radial sensory nerve (Wartenberg's Syndrome) may mimic de Quervain's synovitis or be associated with it. Forearm pronation causes an increase in symptoms with paraesthesia in the distribution of the radial sensory nerve. This too usually responds to steroids and splinting, or (rarely required) a neurolysis.

Occasionally the **tendon of extensor pollicis longus** is subject to inflammation. This is one circumstance where steroid injection is contraindicated since rupture of the tendon in this instance is not uncommon. Surgical release of the tendon sheath is the preferred treatment.

INTERSECTION SYNDROME

Intersection syndrome, in which there is inflammation in the area between the crossover between the first and second dorsal compartments, may occur in row-

ers, weightlifters and skiers (Fig. 36). Splinting the wrist in extension is usually effective and surgical "release" rarely required.

SCAPHOID IMPACTION SYNDROME

The scaphoid impaction syndrome has been described in weightlifters and gymnasts. This presents with dorsal wrist pain reproduced by forced dorsiflexion. It is thought to be caused by impingement of the scaphoid against the radius. X-rays may show an osteophyte on the dorsoradial aspect of the scaphoid. Operation to remove any osteophytes is usually successful; an initial trial of splinting for 6 weeks is an alternative.

Injury to the growth plate of the distal radius may occur particularly in young, elite, female gymnasts. Premature closure of the physis may occur in severe cases. The only treatment is cessation of activities which aggravate the pain. Interruption of activity may be needed for up to 6 months.

Other causes of ulnar sided wrist pain in the athlete include ulnar abutment syndrome, subluxing extensor carpi ulnaris tendon, extensor carpi ulnaris tendinitis, and acute calcific "tendinitis", among others.

ULNAR ABUTMENT PAIN

Ulnar abutment pain is reproduced by forced ulnar deviation and X-ray demonstrates an ulnar plus variant. Later changes may be seen in the lunate where chondral lesions are often noted at arthroscopy. Surgical treatment includes arthroscopic excision of the ulnar head and debridement of chondral flaps, or ulnar shortening.

Subluxation of ECU can be detected on pronation and supination of the forearm. Surgical reconstruction is required to correct the pathology. Tendinitis is treated with splinting, anti-inflammatory drugs, and occasionally, local infiltration of steroids. Acute calcific tendinitis may be confused with infection and acute rheumatic conditions. It usually settles with a few days of splinting and anti-inflammatory drugs.

NERVE COMPRESSIONS

THE MEDIAN NERVE

The median nerve may occasionally be compressed in the arm by the ligament of Struthers, or in the forearm at the level of the lacertus fibrosus, pronator, or at the origin of the flexor digitorum superficialis. Activity related discomfort in the forearm and median nerve paraesthesia are the chief complaints. Forced repetitive pronation, as in weight training, has been implicated as a cause in athletes. The **"true" Tinel's sign** (sustained pressure directly over the nerve) reproduces paraesthesia, and what is now regarded as Tinel's sign may also be positive at the site of compression and so defines the exact level of compression. Symptoms may

also be reproduced by resisted elbow and wrist flexion (**at lacertus**), resisted pronation (**at pronator**), or resisted long and ring finger PIPJ flexion (**at superficialis arch**). Nerve conduction studies are "often normal (90%)".

Treatment is rest and avoidance of aggravating factors. Surgical release is occasionally needed.

CARPEL TUNNEL

Carpal tunnel (Fig. 37) has no special treatment in the athlete. Mild symptoms may be controlled by splinting the wrist in neutral. Surgical release gives excellent relief, but the athlete should be warned of the persistence of "pillar pain" at the incision site with forcible grip for about 3 months. Remember that **Kienböck's** disease can sometimes present as carpal tunnel syndrome.

ULNAR NERVE

The ulnar nerve (Fig. 38) may be compressed at the level of **Guyon's space** in cyclists as a result of wrist hyperextension and direct pressure from handlebars. Numbness in the ulnar one, or two, and half fingers is the usual preitial priorities in management of isolated hand injury. Motor signs are often present. Avoidance of prolonged riding for a time, use of padded gloves and handlebar modification, will usually resolve the problem though it can persist for several months. In other situations, the most common cause of ulnar nerve compression at this level is a ganglion which if not clinically obvious may be picked up on ultrasound.

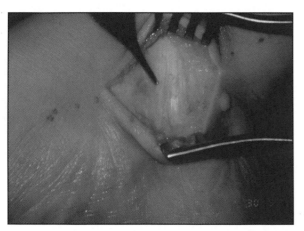

Figure 37 – Surgical release of transverse carpal ligament in carpal tunnel syndrome

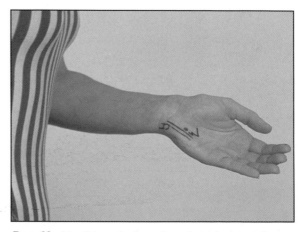

Figure 38 – Handlebar palsy in cyclists where ulnar nerve is compressed in Guyon's canal

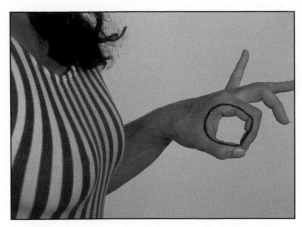

Figure 39 – The ring sign (flexion of IPL and index FDP) is negative (not possible) in anterior interosseous nerve compression

ANTERIOR INTEROSSEOUS NERVE COMPRESSION

Anterior interosseous nerve compression may result in vague forearm pain and occasionally weakness of flexor pollicis longus, index profundus and pronator quadratus (Fig. 38). Anatomic variations in vessels, muscle origins and nerves may be contributing factors. Space occupying lesions such as ganglia and lipoma should not be forgotten. Management is similar to pronator syndrome.

RADIAL NERVE

Radial nerve compression may mimic or be associated with lateral epicondylitis. Provocative manoeuvres for lateral epicondylitis produce pain over the extensors a few centimetres distal to the lateral epicondyle. Rest and splinting the forearm in neutral generally resolve symptoms. Numbness in the radial sensory nerve is rarely seen in runners who maintain marked elbow flexion throughout their gait cycle. Technique modification is usually all that is required. **Wartenberg's syndrome** is manifest by numbness and pain over the dorsum of thumb and finger. Tight bands (weightlifters) or prolonged, forced phonation and supination may play a role in this syndrome. Again, rest and splinting are the mainstay of treatment, with neurolysis rarely needed.

A rare cause of dorsal wrist pain, and a diagnosis of exclusion is **"distal posterior interosseous nerve syndrome"**. Diagnosis may be suspected if injection of local anaesthetic into the fourth dorsal compartment completely resolves symptoms. Should the usual measures fail, transaction of the nerve is effective. Repetitive trauma to the **ulnar digital nerve** of the thumb may occur in ten pin bowlers, and is also sometimes seen in racquet sports. Equipment and technique modification are essential early or permanent damage can occur. Neurolysis may be needed in more severe cases.

CHRONIC COMPARTMENT SYNDROME

Reproducible exertional pain over the first dorsal interosseous muscle and flexor forearm compartments can rarely be due to a chronic compartment syndrome. Diagnosis is confirmed by careful examination and compartment pressure studies. Treatment is activity modification or fasciotomy.

Acknowledgements

Cathryn Dilley for writing assistance and Dr Richard Honner for his advice and guidance on script preparation

13

HIP, THIGH AND PELVIS

John Ireland

INTRODUCTION

Injuries of the hip, thigh and pelvis are common from sport. They may be subtle in presentation making diagnosis difficult. Careful examination and investigation will help (possibly arthroscopy). Contusions, strains, tears and avulsion fractures may form a continuum of injuries to this region. The more obvious fractures and dislocations may be limb or life threatening.

BIOMECHANICS OF THE HIP

The hip is a ball and socket joint with simultaneous motion in all 3 planes (up to 120° of flexion, 20° of abduction and 20° of external rotation). The joint reactive forces are 3 to 6 times body weight due to contraction of the large muscle groups about it.

The acetabulum has a fibro cartilaginous rim (labrum) to deepen it and so add further stability. The postero-superior surface of the acetabulum is thickest to accommodate weight-bearing. The neck forms an angle of about 125° with the shaft and is 20° anteverted. The hip capsule drops down across the front of the neck but only part-way at the back. It is re-inforced by three ligaments (the ilio-femoral ligament of Bigelow is the strongest). The major blood supply to the head is

from the medial circumflex branch (of the profunda femoris) which is at risk from fractures of the neck of femur and dislocations.

CONTUSION OF QUADRICEPS (CORK THIGH, CHARLEY HORSE)

Contusion is the general result of a direct blow during contact sports and vary from mild to severe. They are often worse when the muscle is relaxed. The injury commonly occurs in the musculo tendinous junction of the rectus femoris (Fig. 1).

The clinical features include pain, stiffness, a limp, and progressive swelling and bruising. The pain is exacerbated by resisted knee extension and hip flexion. Due to bleeding in the soft tissues the pain and limitation of movement often becomes worse over the subsequent 48 hours.

These injuries can be classified according to that of Jackson and Fagin (1973) (Fig. 2).

Treatment– Jackson and Fagin initially described three phases in the treatment. The first phase was limitation of motion to minimise haemorrhage. This included rest, ice, compression and elevation. The leg

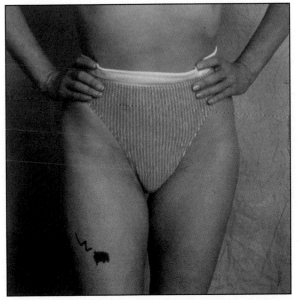

Figure 1 – Contusion of the quadriceps (cork thigh, Charley Horse) commonly occurs at the musculo tendinous junction of the rectus femoris

CLASSIFICATION OF CONTUSIONS	
Mild	Characterised by localised tenderness in the quadriceps, knee motion of 90 degrees or more, non alteration of gait. The athlete is able to do a deep knee bend.
Moderate	Characterised by swollen tender muscle mass, less than 90 degrees of knee motion and antalgic gait. The athlete is able to do knee bends, climb stairs, or arise from a chair without pain.
Severe	Thigh is markedly tender and swollen and the contours of the muscle cannot be defined by palpation. Knee motion is less than 45 degrees and there is a severe limp. The athlete prefers to walk with crutches and frequently has an effusion in the ipsilateral knee.

Figure 2 – Classification of contusion of the thigh (Jackson BW, Fagin JA. Quadriceps Contusions in Young Athletes. JBJS. 55A; 95–105, 1973)

was maintained in extension and quadriceps isometric exercises were allowed. This lasted for a period of 24 hours, in mild contusions, 48 hours in severe contusions. A more recent study advised maintaining hip and knee in as flexed a position as could be tolerated.

Phase 2 was the restoration of motion and this depended upon the condition of quadriceps stabilising and the patient being pain-free at rest. Continuous passive motion; gravity assisted motion. Supine and prone inactive knee flexion was encouraged along with isometric quadriceps exercises. Once a pain-free passive range of motion of 0 to 90 degrees had been achieved, along with good quadriceps control, the programme progressed to static cycling with increasing resistance. The conclusion of this phase was marked by restoration of motion of more than 90 degrees, and normal crutch-free gait.

Phase 3 was functional rehabilitation with progressive increasing resistance exercises to help with strength and endurance.

The essence of this program is that it should always be pain-free.

MYOSITIS OSSIFICANS TRAUMATICA

This is a severe contusion or tear in the quadriceps mainly with haematoma formation followed by acute inflammation. Fibroblasts may then form osteoid (Fig. 3). In 1991, a 3-year study found 17 quadriceps contusions in Westpoint cadets and found an instance of myositis ossificans of 9%. The majority of these occurred in moderate or severe contusions. It was interesting to note that no cadet with a knee range of motion greater than 120 degrees at initial evaluation developed myositis ossificans. Specific risk factors were identified:

1.   Knee motion of less than 120 degrees
2.   Injury associated with football
3.   A previous quadriceps injury
4.   Delay in treatment greater than three days
5.   Ipsilateral knee effusion

Clinical features – pain was localised to the anterior aspect of the thigh associated with fluctuant mass which evolved into a hard mass at the 2-4 week mark. This can resolve after 6 months if the injury is low grade and in the muscle belly involvement of the musculo tendinous region.

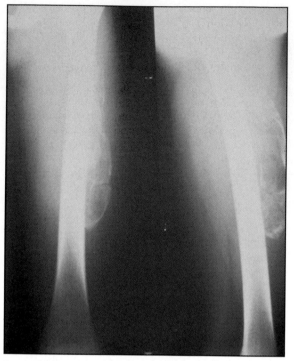

Figure 3 – Myositis ossificans of the quadriceps with mature osteoid formation

Treatment as for contusion of the quadriceps. Aspiration or open drainage of the haematoma may be necessary. The use of femoral nerve blocks, NSAID and radiotherapy have been advocated with some success.

QUADRICEPS STRAINS AND RUPTURES

These injuries are the result of a severe contraction when either accelerating or kicking. The rectus femoris is the most commonly affected with the injuries usually more distal than the thigh.

Clinical features include localised tenderness or a defect (Fig. 4). The pain is exacerbated by resistance of hip flexion in extension and full knee flexion in a prone position. MRI will often confirm the site with a high signal on a T2 weighted image corresponding to the area of inflammation and oedema.

Pain in the anterior aspect of the thigh needs to be differentiated from an L3 nerve root lesion.

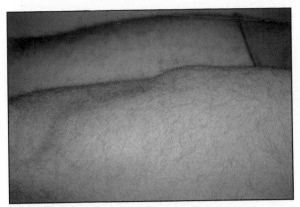

Figure 4 – Defect in quadriceps from quadriceps rupture

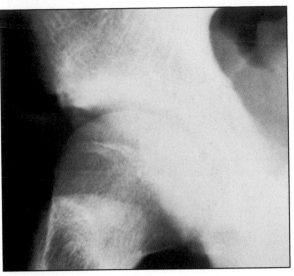

Figure 6 – Bony avulsion of the rectus femoris from the anterior inferior iliac spine

Treatment follows that already outlined for quadriceps contusions.

AVULSIONS OF THE ILIAC SPINES – SUPERIOR AND INFERIOR

Mechanism of injury is a sudden severe contracture of the rectus femoris muscle, occasionally the sartorius muscle. (Most common in soccer players) (Fig. 5). Players tend to be in their mid teens.

Clinical features – include significant pain, tenderness and bruising, and the X-ray is usually diagnostic (Fig. 6). Treatment includes rest, ice, compression and elevation. If there is persisting functional impairment then surgery may be necessary to fix the apophysis or avulsed fragment. On occasions, and often at a later date, the bone fragment may need to be excised.

HAMSTRING STRAINS

In the late swing phase of the gait cycle, hamstrings decelerate the limb. With sudden acceleration from the stabilising flexion to active extension, strain is put on the hamstring muscles. This injury is most likely to occur with sudden hamstring contraction in athletes when they are cold or have not done adequate stretching. Common situations are at the starting blocks, sprinters at take off, (or high jumpers and long jumpers) and sudden acceleration or resisted extension by football players (Fig. 7).

The short head of the biceps femoris is most commonly affected. Occasionally, dystrophic calcification is seen.

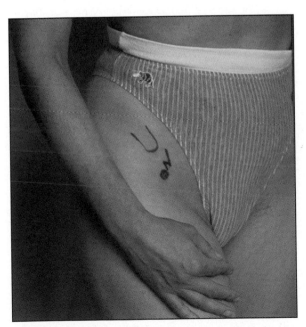

Figure 5 – Marked demarcated area of tenderness over the anterior inferior iliac spine

The patient may describe a twinge or a snap and localise an area, quite often the region of the short head of the biceps, as the most tender. Swelling and a palpable defect are common.

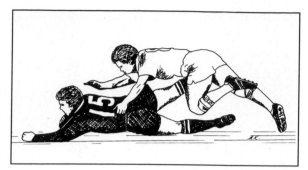

Figure 7 – Hamstring strain (usually involves short head biceps) from sudden contraction as in resisted extension in football tackle (Number 15)

Treatment includes rest, ice, compression, elevation and physiotherapy (local cryotherapy and ultrasound). A stretching programme is commenced once pain has subsided.

The recovery time can be from days to weeks depending upon the severity of the injury.

The **key to treatment is to remedy poor training techniques and improve flexibility**. The athlete must carry out an adequate warm-up and stretching programme prior to a return to sporting activities. The significant imbalance between quadriceps and hamstrings and adequate return of hamstring strength needs to be overcome before returning to sport. The use of a firm elasticised support is a desirable adjunct.

ISCHIAL APOPHYSITIS (WEAVER'S BOTTOM, ISCHIAL BURSITIS) AND AVULSIONS

This is the result of excessive running, especially in adolescents. Repetitive strain is put upon the apophysis and is compounded by tight hamstrings. Severe contracture of the hamstrings musculture may avulse the tuberosity (*See Fig. 22, Chapter 18*).

There is a dull ache and tenderness in the area of the apophysis and often associated tightness of hamstrings. Ecchymosis and a palpable defect may also be present.

An X-ray may show fragmentation or avulsion of the apophysis.

Treatment includes rest, ice, compression, elevation and physiotherapy and a flexibility programme as per a hamstring strain. Significant displacement or functional disability may necessitate surgical fixation of the apophysis.

GROIN STRAINS (ADDUCTOR STRAIN)

The groin is an **ill-defined area** but for the most part injuries in this area involve the adductor muscles. Exclude fractures, avulsions, hip joint injuries, inflammation of the pelvic joints, bursitis about the hip, snapping hip, nerve entrapment and various forms of referred groin pain from hernias, prostatitis, urinary infections, gynaecological disorders, rheumatological diseases, bone infections and tumours.

Groin strains occur in sports where cutting, side stepping or pivoting are required, especially in soccer and rugby players. There is a violent external rotation with the leg in a widely abducted position (Fig. 8). Generally occurs at the musculo-tendinous junction. Injuries are often acute-on-chronic disruptions due to increased collagen at the musculo-tendinous junction, and thereby reducing extensibility.

The injured athlete often describes a sudden knife-like pain in the groin area, and bruising and swelling may be noted but tenderness is well localised. The pain is exacerbated by adduction against resistance (Fig. 9). In chronic cases the symptoms may be somewhat vaguer and diffusely located. Renstrom (1980) described pain with exercise as most common but also at rest often associated with stiffness in the morning, and some weakness.

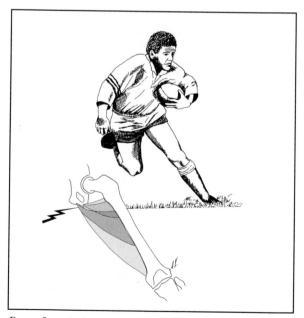

Figure 8 – Groin strains commonly occur in sports where cutting, side stepping or pivoting are necessary

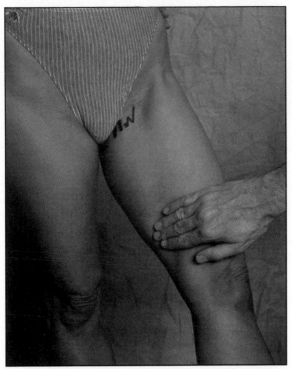

Figure 9 – The pain of groin strain is exacerbated by adduction against resistance

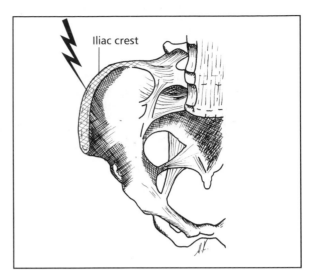

Figure 10 – Hip pointer injury occurs from a direct blow to the iliac crest

MRI confirms the adductor longus as the only muscle affected .

Treatment includes rest, ice, compression and elevation. After the initial 24 to 48 hours haemorrhage should have ceased and physiotherapy modalities (cryotherapy and ultrasound) can begin. Anti-inflammatory medication may be useful for short periods in chronic cases. A stretching programme should be commenced and isometric contractions of the muscles without resistance followed by the gradual introduction of resistance within the limits of pain.

Some attention should be paid to a lack of flexibility and improved training techniques. Use of an elasticised tape for support may be beneficial. Steroids are occasionally of benefit in a chronic situation.

Surgery should not be contemplated without a prolonged period of conservative management of a minimum to six to twelve months. A release of the adductor longus tendon is carried out with the hip in a flexed and abducted position. If a degenerate nodule is identified this should be debrided; failing this a tenotomy is often sufficient.

A Grade III complete rupture is very uncommon (it occurs at the femoral attachment). In selected cases surgical repair is desirable.

HIP POINTER AND FRACTURE OF THE ILIAC CREST

This is the result of a direct blow to the iliac crest resulting in bruising, a fracture or muscle fibre separation (Fig. 10)

Seen in contact sports either from a tackle or due to a fall on to the area of the iliac crest.

Clinical features include maximum tenderness that is frequently over the mid point of the iliac crest, corresponding to the divergence of abdominal and lumbar musculature where there is muscle fibre separation. Otherwise, the area of tenderness may be anywhere along the iliac crest. Swelling and ecchymosis are progressive over the subsequent 24 hours. X-rays are important to rule out a fracture and later X-rays may show periostitis or exostosis formation.

Treatment includes rest, ice packs, compression and elevation in the first 24 hours. Occasionally aspiration and injection of local anaesthetic can give good symptomatic relief. After the phase of bleeding has ceased, ultrasound and other physical therapy modalities may be introduced. Protective padding should be used if returning to contact sports.

ILIAC CREST APOPHYSITIS AND AVULSION

Mechanism – This may result from repetitive stress in adolescents especially running with a cross-over style of arm swing. Severe contraction or a direct blow may avulse the iliac crest.

Clinical features – tenderness may be anteriorly or posteriorly in the iliac crest depending upon whether tensor fascia lata, gluteus medius or oblique abdominal muscles are responsible for the increased strain. Resistance to abduction and contralateral flexion of the trunk frequently exacerbates the pain.

X-rays are essential to exclude avulsion of the iliac apophysis.

Treatment includes rest, ice, compression and elevation and physical therapy. It may be necessary to change the athletes running action and gradually re-introduce activities. Occasionally surgery is necessary to relocate the avulsed iliac crest.

TROCHANTERIC BURSITIS AND SNAPPING HIP

Trochanteric bursitis is inflammation of the bursa over the greater trochanter region as a result of increased shear stress created by the ilio-tibial band over the trochanter (Fig. 11). This is often associated with a broad pelvis and large quadriceps angle (Q-angle). Leg length discrepancies, pelvic tilt or cross-over type running style may also be implicated. A snapping hip is due to thickening of the posterior part of ilio-tibial band which produces a painless snapping sensation.

Clinical features include pain over the lateral aspect of the thigh when lying on the affected side (in the posterior and lateral aspect of the trochanter). Abducting against resistance in an internally rotated position can exacerbate the pain. A snapping sensation may be noted with the patient standing with the knee extended and pushing the hip into an abducted and flexed position.

Another form of snapping hip is derived from repetitive rubbing of the capsule in running or ballet which involves the iliopsoas tendon (Fig. 12).

Clinical features include pain around the medial aspect of the groin which occurs with rotation of the hip. Resistance to flexion of the hip from 90 degrees of flexion leads to increased pain and tenderness in the groin. (Fig. 13). Clicking may be reproducible in some instances. It is important to note that pain can sometimes be referred from the lumbo-sacral spine or sacro iliac joint to this area and must be differentiated from these condition.

Treatment includes rest, ice, compression and elevation followed by ultrasound and stretching of the ilio-tibial band and iliopsoas to overcome contractures. It is important to correct any leg length discrepancy or abnormal running style and orthotics will occasionally be warranted. Steroid injections and anti inflammatories may be useful in an acute bursitis. Surgery has a limited place and should not be contemplated without a prolonged period of conservative management. Surgical technique involves Z plasty of the ilio-tibial band.

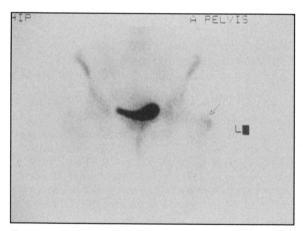

Figure 11 – Hot bone scan in trochanteric bursitis

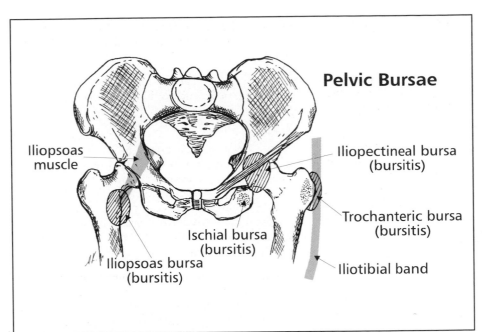

Pelvic Bursae

Iliopsoas muscle

Iliopectineal bursa (bursitis)

Trochanteric bursa (bursitis)

Ischial bursa (bursitis)

Iliopsoas bursa (bursitis)

Iliotibial band

Figure 12 – Snapping of the hip may occur from repetitive rubbing of the hip capsule by the iliopsoas tendon in running or ballet. Trochanteric bursitis and other possible sites of bursitis shown about the pelvis and hip

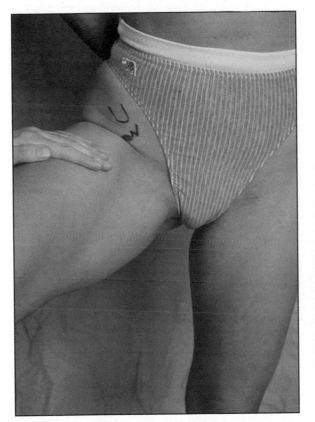

Figure 13 – In snapping hip, increased pain and groin tenderness occurs with resisted flexion of the hip beyond 90°

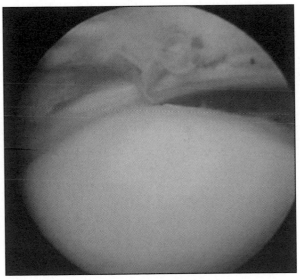

Figure 14 – Synovitis of the hip seen at arthroscopy

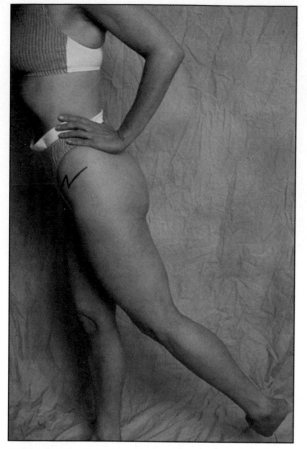

Figure 15 – In hip joint strain, groin pain is exacerbated by extension and internal rotation of the hip

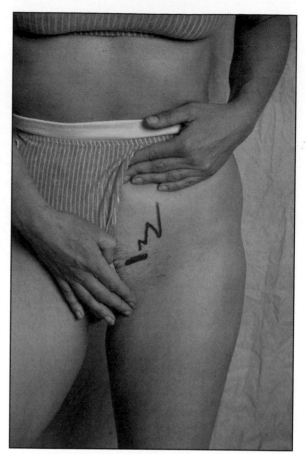

Figure 16 – Conjoint tendon strain of the hip is characterised by tenderness over the superior pubic ramus

HIP STRAIN (PERICAPSULITIS, SYNOVITIS, IRRITABLE HIP)

The result of a direct blow, twisting injury, or from overuse of the hip. Inflammation of the lining or a strain of capsular ligaments occurs (Fig. 14).

This results in pain in the groin, radiating into the thigh. The position of comfort is flexion, abduction and external rotation. Pain is exacerbated by extension and internal rotation (Fig. 15). Antalgic gait may be noted.

Exclude infection (especially in children). X-rays may show some joint widening and a bone scan is often positive.

Treatment includes rest, ice, compression and elevation (RICE) and non-weightbearing. Often complete bed rest (with springs and slings) in children, until complete resolution of symptoms. If capsular tightening occurs then a flexibility programme is required.

CONJOINT TENDON STRAIN OF THE HIP

This injury results from stress on the abdominal musculature, as in a mark in football or heading in soccer.

The athlete experiences pain and tenderness over the superior pubic ramus (Fig. 16). Hip movements are full. X-rays are normal. The bone scan is occasionally diagnostic.

Treatment is RICE, physical therapy and a flexibility programme. Only occasionally is surgical repair necessary.

OSTEITIS PUBIS

This is a non-suppurative self-limiting necrosis in the bone of the pubis and synchondrosis.

It occurs from repetitive shear stress across the symphysis in running and kicking sports which leads to a subacute periostitis.

Clinical features include a gradual onset of groin discomfort which deteriorates with further activity. Severe pain may be experienced when jumping. Tenderness is maximal over the symphysis and the body and rami of the pubis. Pain is aggravated by pelvic compression, full flexion, wide abduction of the hips and even sit ups. Exclude hernias, groin strains and prostatitis in males. X-rays changes are delayed for at least a month but manifest with periosteal reaction and demineralisation of the subchondral bone leading to a "moth eaten" appearance around the symphysis. In the most severe cases, erosion can lead to instability which can be detected in single leg weight bearing views of the pelvis.

Bone scans are often positive in the early stages (Gallium scans may be useful to exclude an infection).

Treatment includes rest, NSAID and occasionally steroid injections in chronic cases. After cessation of symptoms, gradual re-introduction of a flexibility programme and a progressive increase in weight bearing should be instituted. It may take up to 12 months for complete recovery.

NERVE ENTRAPMENT

The commonest nerves involved are the ilioinguinal nerve, obturator nerve, genito-femoral nerve and lateral cutaneous nerve of the thigh (Figs. 17 and 18). Although the mechanism is unknown in most cases, hypertrophy of muscles (hypertrophied abdominal muscles may construct the ilio-inguinal nerve; enlarged hip adductors in skaters may constrict the obturator nerve) or scarring as a result of previous injuries are the most likely causes. A thorough knowledge of the distribution of the nerves will help in making a diagnosis and these areas are likely to exhibit

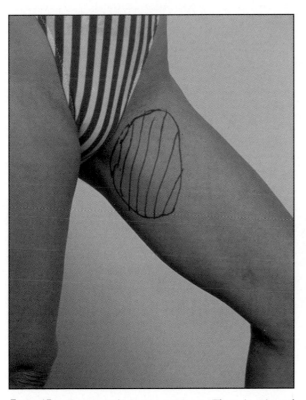

Figure 17 – Ilio-inguinal nerve entrapment. There is pain and paraesthesia in the groin and hypo-aesthesia in the inguinal ligament area. The nerve may be tender at its exit

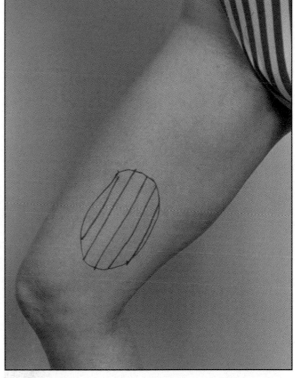

Figure 18 – Obturator nerve entrapment. Pain about inner aspect thigh with reduced sensation

pain and paraesthesia. Tenderness may be experienced over the sub cutaneous emergence of the nerve. EMG may occasionally be helpful in confirming nerve entrapment.

Rest and the occasional introduction of local steroid injections are the first line of treatment, but if symptoms persist then surgical release may be necessary.

LABRAL TEARS

These are seen in dysplastic hips where there is abnormal shear and strain on the acetabular labrum. It may also occur with excessive twisting in sports.

There is sharp pain or a catching sensation on a background of a dull ache. It is aggravated by flexion and internal rotation of the hip. X-rays may show evidence of acetabular dysplasia. Tears are confirmed by arthrography or arthroscopy (usually in the posterior aspect of the hip joint) (Fig. 19).

Treatment is rest and surgical excision or repair.

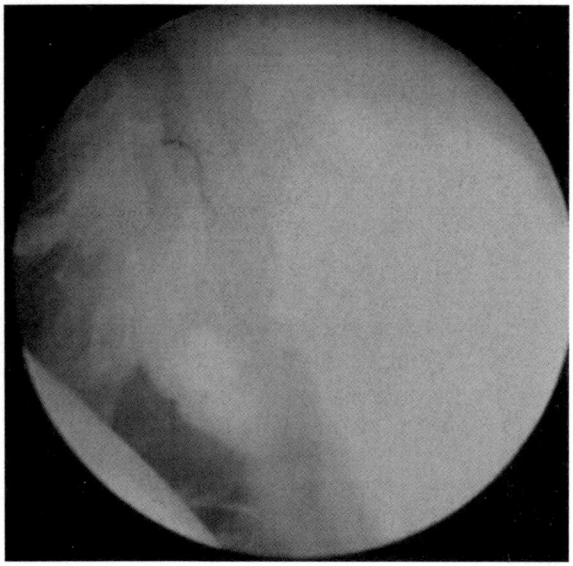

STRESS FRACTURES

This entity was first described by Briethaupt in 1855 in German soldiers. Stechow first noted these on X-rays in 1897. Stress fractures of the neck of femur were first described by Blecher in 1905. Much of the early literature relating stress fractures was from the military. There is an increasing prevalence of stress fractures in athletes and this, interestingly, is more often found in highly motivated athletes who are in peak condition and following a period of maximal performance. Commonly identified risk factors in athletes are endocrine disorders, particularly in amenorrhoeic female athletes (see Chapter 18).

They are a process of partial or complete fracture of bone due to an inability to withstand non violent stress that is applied in a rhythmic repeated sub maximal mode.

There is controversy as to whether or not the condition is due to fatigue of muscles leading to increased load or, as Stanitski believes, an increased muscular force plus increased rate of remodelling leading to resorption and rarefaction and ultimately to stress fractures. This will manifest itself as a periosteal or endosteal response giving an appearance of a stress fracture which may ultimately progress to a linear fracture and in time displace.

The clinical and X-ray criteria for diagnosis of a stress fracture are outlined (Fig. 20).

Figure 19 – Labral detachment at arthoscopy

CLINICAL AND X-RAY CRITERIA FOR DIAGNOSIS OF STRESS FRACTURES

- Premorbid normal bone

- No direct trauma/inciting activity

- Pain and tenderness (on percussion and antalgic limp) prior to X-ray changes)

- Subsequent X-rays show resolution and modelling

- Positive bone scan

Figure 20 – Clinical and X-ray criteria for diagnosis of stress fractures

STRESS FRACTURES FEMUR
Femoral Neck (Hajeck, 1982)
• Compressive inferior cortex – young patients/ early internal callus/fracture/sclerosis (Fig. 22)   • Non-weight bear/modify training transverse superior cortex – older patients/initial crack in superior cortex/fracture/displaced fracture   **Operate**
Femoral shaft (Blickenstaff, Morris)
• Medial proximal femur   • Displaced spiral oblique   • Transverse distal   **Operate**

Figure 21 – Classification of stress fractures femur and treatment. (Hajck MR, Noble HB, Stress fractures of the femoral neck in joggers. *Am J Sports Med* 1982;**10**:112. – Bickenstaff LD, Morris JM Fatigue fracture of the femoral neck. *JBJS* 1966; **48A**:1031)

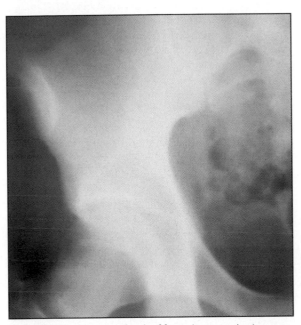

Figure 22 – Stress fracture of neck of femur (young patient)

Assess the opposite side both clinically and by X-ray to exclude a stress fracture (as not always symptomatic). Differential diagnosis includes tumour (particularly osteosarcoma and Ewing's tumour), osteomyelitis or periostitis from TB or syphilis. Jumping sports have a strong association with injuries to the femur and pelvis

but stress fractures have been noticed amongst hikers and fencers especially in the pelvic bones.

These injuries can be classified into those affecting the femoral neck and the femoral shaft (Fig. 21).

Treatment involves decreased weight bearing and modifying training. This may be sufficient in early femoral shaft stress fractures and the compressive variety of femoral neck fractures. In the older patient it is wise to pin these at an early stage as there is a risk of progression. A degree of suspicion by medical and training staff is necessary to ensure that both elite athletes and amateurs do not suffer significant stress fractures. From finite element analysis it is recommended that a maximum 100 miles over a three month period be the limit for a first time jogger.

FRACTURED HIP; ACUTE SLIP OF THE UPPER FEMORAL EPIPHYSIS (SUFE)

These injuries occur from a severe impact while the foot is planted and the hip twisted. They may occur in cross country and downhill skiers from a low velocity fall ("Skier's hip", Fig. 23). (Hip fracture may occur or SUFE in child) (see Figs. 23-25, Chapter 18).

There is severe pain and an inability to weightbear, with shortening and external rotation in the hip. Exclude a past history of ache or an antalgic gait with an acute or chronic slipped upper femoral epiphysis.

Treatment is immediate immobilisation and then immediate operative stabilisation and drainage of the capsular haematoma.

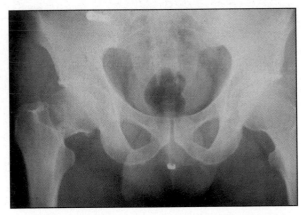

Figure 23 – Fractured neck of femur in 46 year old skier from fall

DISLOCATION OF THE HIP

Dislocations are the result of a direct impact to the flexed knee and hip (anterior or posterior).

The athlete has severe pain and deformity with the leg in a flexed and internally rotated position (posterior dislocation) or externally rotated (anterior dislocation) (Fig. 24 and 25). There may be associated sciatic nerve injury.

Immobilise the athlete and plan immediate reduction (open if necessary) of the hip to reduce the likely development of AVN.

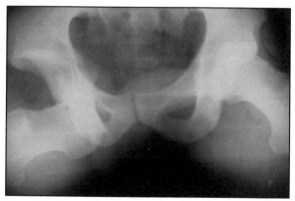

Figure 24 – Skier with right anterior hip dislocation (23 year old male). An emergency which requires immediate reduction (closed or possibly open). The leg is externally rotated

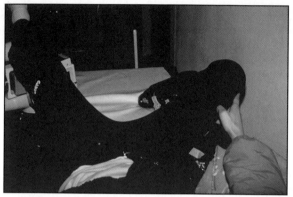

Figure 25 – The X-ray of the anterior hip dislocation

FRACTURED FEMUR AND PELVIS

These are high velocity injuries (Figs. 26 and 27).

Significant pain and deformity occurs. Exclude neurological or vascular compromise. There are associated head, neck, chest and abdominal life threatening injuries which must be found and treated.

Resuscitate the athlete with special attention to head injury, immobilise the neck, exclude need for chest tube/peritoneal lavage/exploratory laporatory. Optimise volume replacement (up to 40 units of blood can disappear into a fractured pelvis) and give adequate analgesia. Surgery is almost always required to reduce and hold fractures of the femur and quite often for the pelvis (external fixation to tamponade bleeding in displaced and unstable pelvic fracture (Figs. 28 and 29).

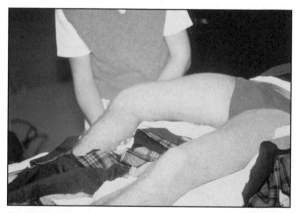

Figure 26 – Fractured femoral shaft in skier. Note the obvious shortening and deformity

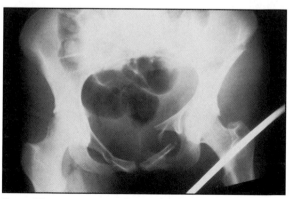

Figure 27 – Fractured anterior pelvis from skier colliding with thigh-high ski pole (staunching blood at tip of penis from ruptured urethra – *See Fig. 8, Chapter 16.)*

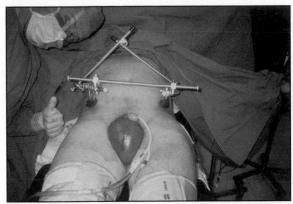

Figure 28 – External fixator applied to open book fracture of pelvis to tamponade pelvic bleeding and so haemodynamically stabilise

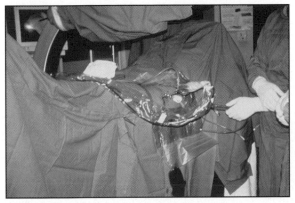

Figure 30 – Arthoscopy of the hip allows evaluation of unexplained hip pain and removal of loose bodies and lavage of the hip in OA

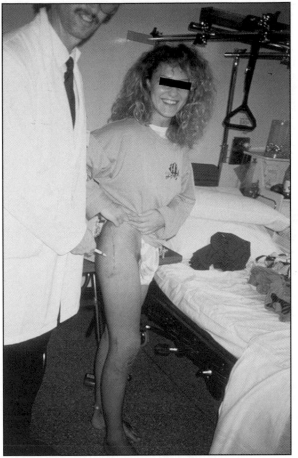

Figure 29 – Early surgical stabilisation of femoral sharf patients in young athletes allows rapid rehabilitation

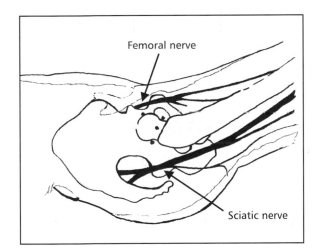

Figure 31 – It is important to place the hip arthroscopic incisions carefully to protect the sciatic and femoral nerves

Hip arthroscopy – Bowman first reported hip arthroscopy being performed in 1937. It has only recently become more widely used but even to this day, the uses, apart from diagnostic, are fairly limited (Fig. 30).

It is frequently used where there is unexplained hip pain, in situations of synovitis or osteoarthrosis. It may be used for lavage in early osteoarthrosis and for treatment of labral tears, removal of loose bodies (from fractures, osteochondromatosis and villonodular synovitis). Several techniques have been described (Fig 31).

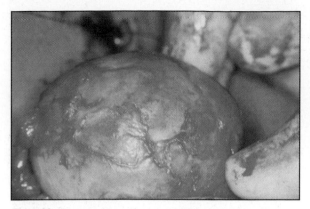

Figure 32 – Segmental avascular necrosis of the hip, as seen at surgery

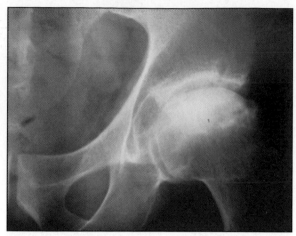

Figure 33 – X-ray appearance of segmental avascular necrosis with collapse in 4th year male

AVASCULAR NECROSIS OF THE FEMORAL HEAD

This is a partial or complete disruption of the blood supply to the femoral head resulting in necrosis of a segment which may undergo collapse before revascularisation has occurred (Figs. 32 & 33).

This condition most commonly follows a fracture of the head or femoral neck or dislocation, especially if associated with some delay in reduction. Posterior dislocations in particular disrupt the superior retinacular vessels. Perthes' disease, results from an increased intracapsular pressure following a synovitis which compromises the vascular supply to the femoral head. This condition is classified according to that of Ficat (Fig. 34) with diagnostic and surgical intervention noted.

FICAT'S CLASSIFICATION OF AVN						
Stage	Pain	Exam	XR	Bone Scan	MRI	Treatment
0	None	Normal	Normal	Normal	Normal	Normal
1	Minimal	↓ I.Rot.	Normal	No help	Some changes	? core decompression
2	Moderate	↓ ROM	Porosis/sclerosis	Positive	Positive	Graft
3	Advanced	↓ ROM	Flat, crescent sign	Positive	Positive	Joint replacement
4	Severe	Pain	Acetabular changes	Positive	Positive	Joint replacement

Figure 34

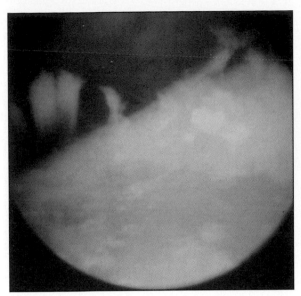

Figure 35 – Osteoarthritis of the hip, as seen at arthroscopy

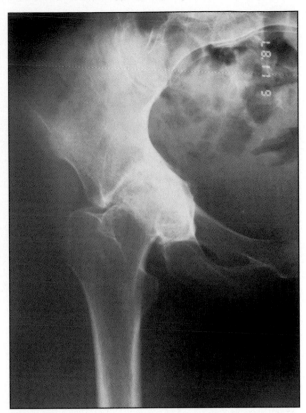

Figure 36 – X-ray appearance of osteoarthritis of the hip which requires a total hip replacement

OSTEOARTHROSIS

This condition has a high correlation with high impact sports especially track and field and racquet sports (Figs. 35 & 36). Work performed by Radin shows that compression of the joint with oscillating repetitive high impact loads leads to microfractures. Obviously, conditions associated with avascular necrosis can advance the onset of osteoarthrosis. Athletes with intensive sports participation have a 4 to 5 fold increased incidence of OA (up to 8.5 if also involved in an occupation at risk of OA). Patients who have had hip replacements should not play impact sports.

14

KNEE

Jim Sullivan

INTRODUCTION

The knee is the most commonly injured joint in sport. Its size, lack of stability and forward prominence make it prone to contact and injury (Fig. 1).

BIOMECHANICS

The knee is a complex hinge joint which allows free flexion, and some rotation in flexion. With progressive flexion there is roll-back of the femur on the tibial surface, controlled by tension in the posterior cruciate ligament.

The articular surfaces of the tibo-femoral joint have relatively poor congruity and little inherent stability, as is evident on examination of dried bones. The articular congruity is improved by the menisci, but stability is dependent on ligaments, capsule and muscle control.

The knee is vulnerable to high torsional and deceleration forces often encountered in running sports, as well as to contact forces. The key to diagnosis of injury rests with history and clinical examination. A description of the mechanism of injury often gives a clear indication to the likely diagnosis (Fig. 2). A sportsman who describes that he felt his knee dislocate or slip, with pain and a pop when he stepped off it, is providing a fairly classical history of an isolated rupture of the anterior cruciate ligament.

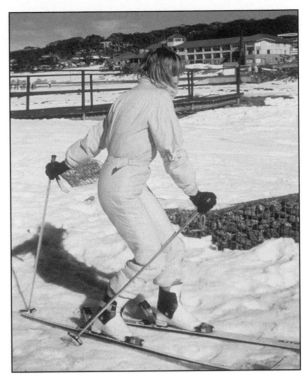

Figure 2 – Most ligament injuries of the knee occur when the athlete (skier) falls forward with an abduction and external rotation force applied to the knee

LIGAMENTOUS INJURY

The medial and lateral collateral ligaments, and the anterior and posterior cruciate ligaments constitute the four major ligamentous structures about the knee. Integrity of these ligaments is important for normal stability and kinematics of the knee. Altered kinematics may lead to degeneration of the knee.

MEDIAL COLLATERAL LIGAMENT

The medial collateral ligament extends from the medial femoral epicondyle, widens and inserts onto the tibia 8 to 10 cm below the joint line. It is orientated in a posterior to anterior direction and is taut in extension. It is susceptible to contact and non-contact injuries involving a valgus force and external rotation force to the knee.

Examination reveals swelling over the medial aspect of the knee, and later bruising may be seen. The knee is **typically held flexed** and there is a **painful soft end**

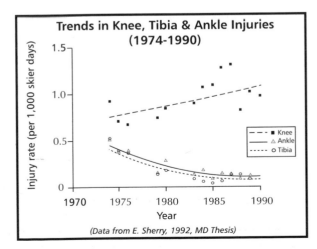

Figure 1 – The incidence of knee injuries has increased in many sports despite equipment modification (here skiing)

point limiting extension (pseudo-locking). There is tenderness along the course of the medial ligament, most commonly at the site of femoral insertion. **Laxity** is assessed with the knee in 30 degrees of flexion and is graded I to III (Figs. 3 & 4). Grade III injury has greater than a centimetre of opening of the medial joint line. If there is instability in extension a more complex ligamentous disruption should be suspected.

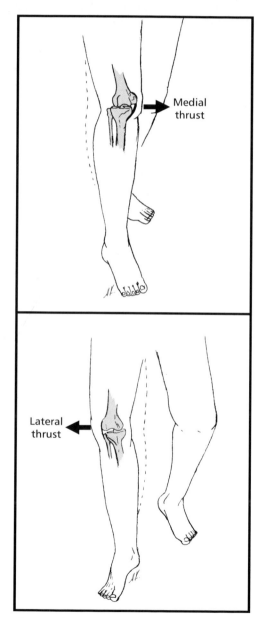

Figure 3 – Loss of integrity of the medial collateral ligament produces a medial thrust in the stance phase; a lateral thrust for lateral collateral injury

X-rays are usually normal, although an avulsion fragment is rarely seen. Later, calcification may be seen at the site of femoral insertion (Pellegrini-Stieda lesion).

All isolated medial collateral ligament injuries can be treated conservatively. Early treatment involves RICE with graded quadriceps strengthening. In normal gait there is a closing force on the medial joint line, and so early weightbearing can be allowed and bracing is not always required for Grade I to II injury. Bracing is indicated in Grade III injuries and where the patient feels instability on weightbearing. Recovery from a Grade I to II injury is usually between 3 and 4 weeks, and for a more significant injury 6 to 8 weeks.

LATERAL COLLATERAL LIGAMENT INJURY

The lateral collateral ligament extends from the lateral femoral epicondyle to the head of the fibula. Isolated ruptures are rare and the ligament is more commonly injured in association with disruption of the postero-lateral corner. Usually require surgical reconstruction.

ANTERIOR CRUCIATE LIGAMENT

Rupture of the anterior cruciate ligament is the commonest major ligamentous knee injury in athletes. The anterior cruciate runs from the postero-superior aspect of the lateral wall of the intercondylar notch in

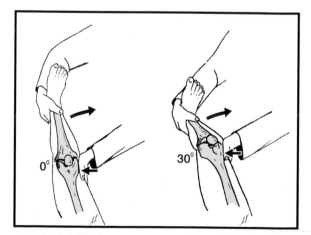

Figure 4 – Integrity of the collateral ligaments is best tested in 30° of flexion and then graded (Grade III > 1 cm opening of joint line)

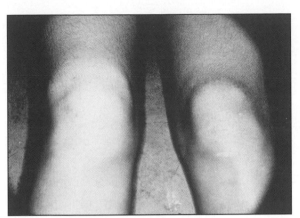

Figure 5 – An immediate large knee effusion (haemarthrosis) is pathognomonic of a torn anterior cruciate ligament injury (80%)

the femur to the tibial spines. The ligament averages 12 mm in thickness and has 2 major bundles, the antero-medial and the postero-lateral. The anterior cruciate ligament is a primary stabiliser to anterior tibial translation and also controls the rotational screw-home mechanism in terminal knee extension.

Eighty percent of anterior cruciate ligament ruptures are as a result of non-contact injury. The ligament is ruptured by an internal rotational and anterior translation force to the tibia caused by pivoting or cutting or landing awkwardly from a jump. It is also ruptured by hyper-extension of the knee and will fail with progressive valgus in combination with a medial collateral ligament tear.

In isolated non-contact injuries the patient will describe stepping off the knee at speed and feeling pain associated with a pop and giving way. **Swelling is almost immediate**, consistent with a **haemarthrosis** (Figs. 5 & 6). In the absence of fracture, 80% of acute knee haemarthroses are due to rupture of the anterior cruciate ligament.

Examination reveals an **effusion** and the knee is **often held flexed.** There may be tenderness over the antero-lateral joint line where there is commonly an associated capsular injury. The dynamic Lachman test is positive (Fig. 7), and depending on the amount of pain and spasm static Lachman and pivot shift tests may also be elicited.

Plain X-ray may reveal an avulsion fracture involving the tibial spine, particularly in younger patient groups. There may also be avulsion fracture from the antero-lateral tibia, so called Segond fracture. An MRI scan will usually demonstrate the ruptured ligament.

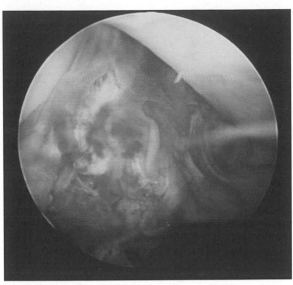

Figure 6 – A fresh rupture of the anterior cruciate ligament seen at arthroscopy

Treatment of anterior cruciate ligament ruptures is **determined by associated injuries** (meniscal, ligamentous), degree of instability and patient expectation. All patients can be managed initially conservatively with treatment directed at settling the effusion, regaining range of motion and a muscle strengthening programme. Patients who have persistent joint line symptoms or locking may have meniscal pathology which requires arthroscopy. Patients who have an associated Grade III rupture of the medial collateral ligament are probably better served by early cruciate reconstruction. Otherwise, anterior cruciate reconstruction is reserved for patients intending to return to high demand sports or those with symptomatic ongoing instability.

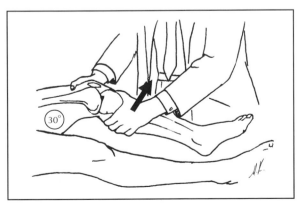

Figure 7 – Lachman's test is highly specific for ACL tear. The knee is flexed 30° and the upper tibia is found to move forward (sublux) on the lower femur

CHRONIC ANTERIOR CRUCIATE INSUFFICIENCY

Following isolated rupture of the anterior cruciate ligament, most knees settle down over 6 to 12 weeks. Although the ligament does not heal, up to **one third** of patients may be asymptomatic. Another group may only have symptoms with high demand sports such as football, netball or skiing. A smaller group of patients have marked instability such that they are at risk even crossing the road. Symptoms of anterior cruciate insufficiency include giving way, associated with pain, and recurrent swelling with repeated episodes of giving way. There may be injury to the menisci and osteochondral trauma with an increased likelihood of the development of degenerative arthritis.

Examination reveals usually good muscle tone and often no effusion. The range of motion is preserved. The Lachman, pivot shift, and anterior draw tests are positive. McMurray's test will indicate whether there is associated meniscal pathology.

For a patient who suffers occasional instability with high demand sports, modification of activity and an intensive lateral hamstring strengthening programme may be all that is required. Other patients with symptomatic instability can be offered anterior cruciate reconstruction (Fig. 8). The results following surgery

suggest that up to 85% of patients will be able to return to their pre-injury level of sport. Laxity of the graft has been shown to gradually increase over the years following reconstruction, but the patients often remain asymptomatic. There is not strong evidence at this stage that reconstruction influences the development of osteoarthritis.

POSTERIOR CRUCIATE LIGAMENT RUPTURE

The posterior cruciate ligament courses from the anterior portion of the medial wall of the intercondylar notch of the femur to insert into the central posterior tibia, approximately 1 cm below the joint line. The ligament is composed of antero-lateral and postero-medial bands. The posterior cruciate ligament is the primary restraint to posterior tibial translation.

The posterior cruciate ligament can be ruptured by a direct blow onto the anterior upper tibia, such as a heavy fall on a flexed knee or a dashboard injury. It will also fail in hyperextension and in more complex postero-lateral or postero-medial disruption.

The acute symptoms may be mild and isolated ruptures may be missed (Fig. 9). Examination should elicit a posterior sag with tibial drop back (Fig. 10).

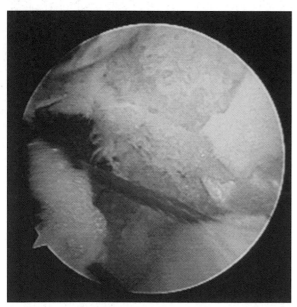

Figure 8 – Arthroscopic ACL reconstruction using hamstrings (here new ligament being passed through knee and about to be anchored in femoral tunnel)

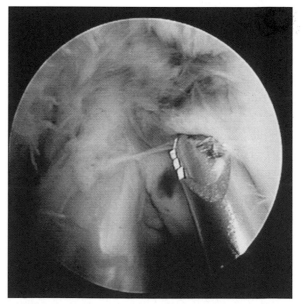

Figure 9 – Isolated PCL tear seen at arthroscopy (behind the instrument)

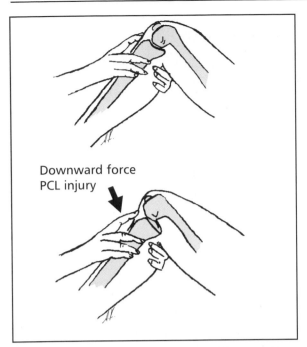

Figure 10 – PCL rupture. There is posterior sag of the upper tibia on the lower femur at 90° knee flexion

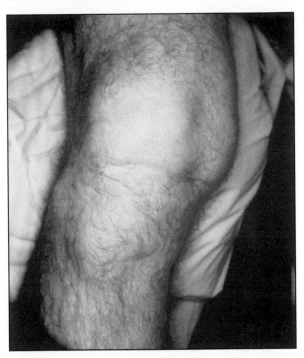

Figure 11 – Complete (lateral tibio-femoral) knee dislocation is a surgical emergency with injury to popliteal artery and lateral common peroneal nerve. Immediate reduction is necessary with careful assessment of circulation

Plain X-rays may show an avulsion fracture involving the tibial insertion (this type of rupture should be treated operatively). An MRI scan will demonstrate the ligament tear.

Treatment of mid-substance ruptures has been non-operative involving intensive quadriceps strengthening. However, a posterior cruciate deficient knee may develop osteoarthritis (due to the altered kinematics). Patients develop patello-femoral pain with degeneration of the patello-femoral and medial compartments. Early reconstruction is probably better for young patients.

KNEE DISLOCATION

Complete knee dislocation is an orthopaedic emergency with injury to the popliteal artery and common peroneal nerve (when lateral). Both the anterior and posterior cruciate ligaments are torn as well as the collaterals (Figs. 11 & 12).

Immediate reduction is necessary and then splinting. Close monitoring of circulation is essential and angiography performed if there is any doubt concerning circulation. (Delayed occlusion of the popliteal artery may occur due to an intimal flap tear.) Surgical reconstruction of the knee is usually required.

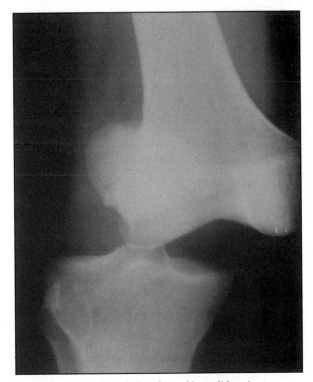

Figure 12 – X-ray of lateral tibio-femoral knee dislocation

MENISCAL TEARS

The menisci are fibrocartilaginous semi-lunar structures on the tibial surface. Their function is to improve the congruity of the tibio-femoral articulation and to transmit load. They also function as shock absorbers and improve knee joint stability. Following meniscectomy the contact area in the compartment is reduced and contact pressures may be increased by more than 350%. Shock absorbing capacity is reduced, and as a result of these factors meniscectomy has been shown to lead to development of osteoarthritis. The menisci are relatively avascular with blood supply limited to the peripheral one quarter to one third (*See Fig. 33, Chapter 18*). (Tears in the vascular region have the potential for healing.) Medial meniscal tears are 5 times more common than lateral meniscal tears.

A meniscus is torn by being **trapped** between the two bone surfaces when a rotary force is applied to a loaded knee (twisting when rising from a full squat) (Fig. 13).

There is **pain, delayed effusion, and with a bucket handle tear** the knee will be **locked**. With less dramatic tears there is usually a history of recurrent clicking and catching and joint line pain.

The signs include effusion, wasting of the quadriceps, pain on forced extension, pain on forced flexion, and a positive McMurray's test.

An MRI scan will exclude other pathology.

Arthroscopy allows good visualisation and partial meniscectomy (Fig. 14). Peripheral bucket handle, and incomplete bucket handle tears (in young patients) should be repaired (Fig. 15). Where there is an associated anterior cruciate ligament rupture this may need to be reconstructed to decrease the risk of recurrence of the meniscal tear. (Unhappy "Triad" is medial collateral/anterior cruciate ligament/medial meniscal injury combination.)

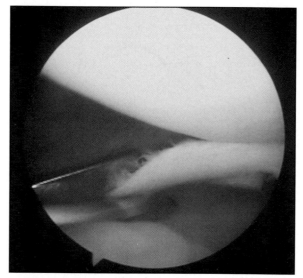

Figure 14 – Arthroscopic partial medial meniscectomy of the displaced bucket-handle tear of the medial meniscus

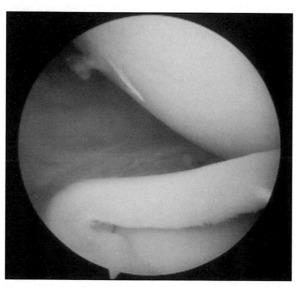

Figure 13 – A displaced bucket-handle tear of the medial meniscus (from football) which locked the knee (seen at arthroscopy)

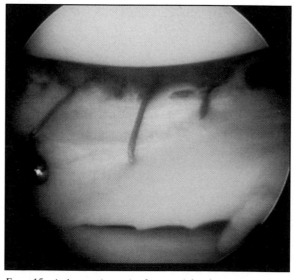

Figure 15 – Arthroscopic repair of torn peripheral meniscus

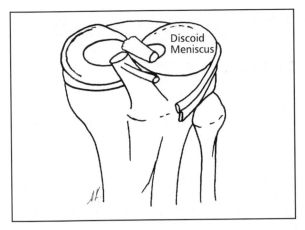

Figure 16 – A discoid meniscus (usually of the lateral compartment) may be complete or incomplete (as here) with mechanical symptoms

DISCOID MENISCUS

A meniscus, usually the lateral, which is not the usual C-chaped but nearly covers the whole plateau (2 types: complete/incomplete). There may be mechanical symptoms of joint-line pain and "clunking". Partial menisectomy may be required (Fig. 16).

MENISCAL CYST

Usually arise from a horizontal cleavage tear of the lateral meniscus (Fig. 17).

PATELLO-FEMORAL JOINT PROBLEMS

The patella is a **sesamoid bone** in the quadriceps tendon (present at seven and a half weeks gestation). It functions to **improve the efficiency** of the quadriceps mechanism by lengthening the moment arm, decreasing friction, improving stability, and centralising the quadriceps muscle pull and to protect the anterior aspect of the joint. The stability of the patella is provided by the bony anatomy of the trochlear groove and patella, static tension in the soft tissues of the medial and lateral retinaculum, and the dynamic control of the quadriceps mechanism. The vastus medialis obliquus muscle is particularly important in maintaining patello-femoral balance and normal tracking. **Acute injuries** to the patello-femoral joint **include** direct trauma, subluxation or patellar dislocation, patellar fracture, quadriceps tendon or patellar ligament rupture. Many patients, however, present with anterior knee pain without a history of specific traumatic incident.

ANTERIOR KNEE PAIN SYNDROME

Anterior knee pain is the commonest sports knee complaint. The pain may be well localised (patellar tendinitis), but more usually vaguely anterior. and aggravated by loading a flexed knee (as in climbing stairs or inclines). There is sharp retropatellar pain after sitting for prolonged periods, crepitus, catching, weakness and giving way and an effusion. The causes of anterior knee pain syndrome are **myriad,** and often physical examination is unremarkable other than for retropatellar crepitus (Fig. 18).

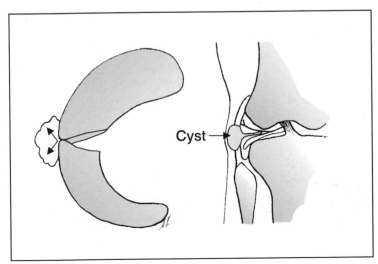

Figure 17 – A meniscal cyst originates from a torn (usually lateral) meniscus and presents with a joint line bulge (prominent in slight flexion)

ANTERIOR KNEE PAIN SYNDROME

- **Trauma** (Osteochondral injury)
- **Mal-alignment**
  Anatomical pre-disposition
  Muscle imbalance
  Patellar subluxation
  Patellar dysplasia
- **Compressive**
  Excessive lateral pressure syndrome
  Hamstrung patella
- **Over-use**
  Patellar tendinitis
  Medial plica syndrome
  Retinacular irritation
  Osgood-Schlatter's disease
  Bipartite patella
- **Degenerative/Inflammatory**
- **Idiopathic**
  Primary chondromalacia

Figure 18 – The causes of anterior knee pain

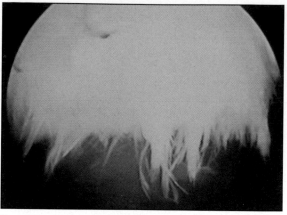

Figure 19 – Chondromalacia patellae. The crabmeat appearance of the patella seen at arthroscopy

CHONDROMALACIA PATELLAE

(Fig. 19)

This is softening of the patellar cartilage either from a direct blow or mal-alignment (with patellar subluxation) (Fig. 19). Typically seen in young overweight girls with knock-knees. The cartilage damage can be classified (Fig. 20).

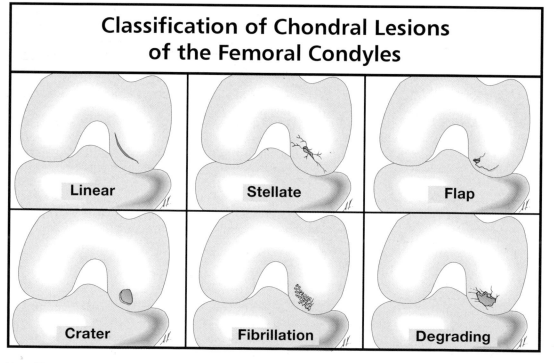

Figure 20 – Classification of chondral lesions (chondromalacia) of the patella showing the stages/progression

ACUTE DISLOCATION OF THE PATELLA

The mechanism of injury usually involves an **external rotation and valgus force with** the knee in near extension or a direct blow to the patella. The patient may present with the patella dislocated, in which case the diagnosis is obvious and reduction is usually readily achieved by gentle extension of the knee. However, spontaneous reduction often occurs soon after injury. The clinical signs include haemarthrosis, tender medial patellar retinaculum, a positive patellar apprehension test and patellar instability. An X-ray is essential to exclude a significant osteochondral fracture. If this is present arthroscopy and excision of the fragment is indicated.

A tense haemarthrosis may be drained for pain relief. The knee should be immobilised in extension and a removable splint is usually adequate. The patient is instructed in isometric quadriceps exercises and may weightbear as comfort allows. As the effusion resolves graduated flexion may be commenced and the knee immobiliser can usually be discarded by 3 weeks. The patient should not return to sport until they have regained normal quadriceps muscle tone and bulk and a negative apprehension test.

RECURRENT DISLOCATION

Recurrent dislocation is usually clear on history and if there is not a response to an extensive quadriceps strengthening programme, surgery is indicated (a lateral release and repair or advancement of the medial retinacular tissue and vastus medialis; if intra-operatively, this does not achieve stability, a distal bony realignment may be indicated).

RECURRENT SUBLUXATION

Symptoms include anterior knee pain and giving way. Examination may reveal anatomical features predisposing to patellar subluxation, including increased **Q angle** (line of pull of the quadriceps) due to valgus or rotational factors, out-turned patellae or patellar alta. The patella may track in a J-curve (Fig. 21). The patella may be subluxable or dislocatable, and lateral retinacular tightness may be evident. X-rays (with skyline views) and CT scan may show patellar dysplasia or subluxation. If there is no improvement with a protracted conservative programme, surgery is necessary (with soft tissue or bony realignment).

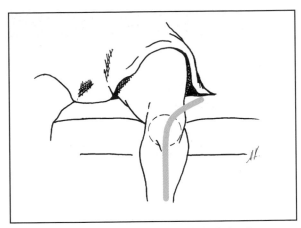

Figure 21 – The unstable (subluxable) patella tracks in a J-curve

PATELLAR TENDINITIS (JUMPER'S KNEE)

This is an **over-use injury**, commonly seen in basketball. There is anterior knee pain (with exertion). Examination reveals point tenderness over the central insertion of the patellar ligament into the patella, and there may be some swelling over the overlying soft tissues with palpable crepitus. The hamstrings and gastrocnemiae should be assessed for tightness. An MRI scan will confirm altered signal at the site of the degenerate tendon. A bone scan may show increased uptake at the site of tendon insertion.

Treatment includes rest with modification of aggravating activities (such as jumping). A graduated exercise programme should be provided to strengthen the quadriceps, combined with intensive stretches for the hamstrings and gastrocnemiae. The over-lying bursa may be injected with corticosteroid and local anaesthetic in protracted cases. If symptoms extend beyond one year despite conservative management, surgical debridement of the degenerate tendon with a segment of patellar bone may be considered.

PATELLAR FRACTURE

Caused by **direct impact** on the patella as in a fall on a flexed knee or a dashboard injury. May also occur following violent resisted contraction of the extensor mechanism. If there is disruption of the extensor mechanism (indicated by a **lag** on examination or a significant gap on X-ray) surgical repair is essential

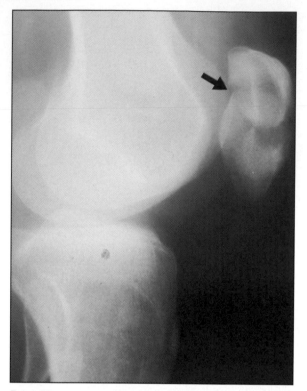

Figure 22 – Patellar fracture with displacement (gap). Surgery required.

(Fig. 22). Undisplaced or minimally displaced fractures with preservation of the extensor mechanism may be treated non-operatively, by splinting in extension for 6 weeks.

QUADRICEPS TENDON RUPTURE

Caused by sudden resistance to a strong quadriceps contraction. Seen in the older patient group (as with other tendon degeneration conditions). There is pain with loss of quadriceps function, a lag, and a palpable gap. When the diagnosis is unclear, and particularly when presentation is delayed, MRI can define the integrity of the tendons. To restore good quadriceps function, operative repair is required.

PATELLAR LIGAMENT RUPTURE

Occurs in younger patients by the same mechanism as quadriceps tendon rupture. Caused by penetrating injuries (dashboard). There is pain and loss of quadriceps function with a significant lag. The defect is usually palpable. Surgical repair is indicated.

PRE-PATELLAR BURSITIS

The **bursa** over the anterior aspect of the patella is prone to injury and inflammation from repetitive contact (seen in football players and gymnasts). Once a significant episode has occurred there is a tendency to become recurrent. Examination reveals enlargement of the thickened bursa with crepitus. Acute cases have signs of inflammation and there may be secondary infection with cellulitis.

Inflammatory bursitis is treated with RICE and NSAID. Padding and protecting the area on return to sport is important to minimise the risk of recurrence. Where there is secondary sepsis, antibiotics are needed and surgical draining of an abscess. Recurrent or chronic bursitis will eventually require excision of the thickened bursa.

BIPARTITE PATELLA (ACCESSORY OSSIFICATION CENTRE)

Present in <15% of patellae and usually asymptomatic and usually at **the superio-lateral corner**. Symptoms may occur after direct contact injury or over-use. Symptoms include anterior knee pain and tenderness. There is tenderness over the site of the pseudarthrosis. X-rays show the bipartite patella (a bone scan may be helpful in cases following significant trauma). Most cases settle with a conservative programme as in the Management of Anterior Knee Pain Syndrome. Rarely is excision of the fragment required.

PLICA SYNDROME

Synovial plicas are common and often seen at arthroscopy (Figs. 23 & 24). They may become a source of symptoms following a direct injury causing thickening and scarring of the plica, or from over-use. There is anterior knee pain syndrome with occasional clicking and snapping and tenderness over the medial femoral condyle.

Those that do not settle with rest and a conservative programme may be treated by arthroscopic resection.

Common Plica about the Knee

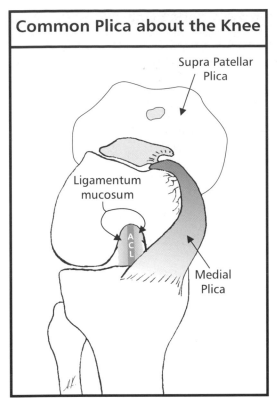

Figure 23 – The three common plicas of the knee (medial, supra patellar and ligamentum mucosum)

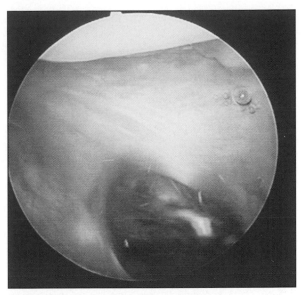

Figure 24 – Supra-patellar plica seen at arthroscopy

ILIO-TIBIAL BAND FRICTION SYNDROME

Seen in joggers and distance runners. There is inflammation over the lateral epicondyle caused by rubbing of the ilio-tibial band (Fig. 25). Examination reveals point tenderness over the lateral epicondyle, pain is reproduced as the ilio-tibial band passes back and forth over the lateral epicondyle. There may be tightness of the tensor fascia lata and hamstring muscles.

Treatment involves rest and a set of exercises to stress the ilio-tibial band and hamstring muscles. A break of 3 months from distance running is usually required.

SEMIMEMBRANOUS TENDINITIS

This is seen in male athletes and may be difficult to diagnose (postero-medial knee joint pain with hamstring spasm). A cyst may occur which is difficult to excise (Fig. 26).

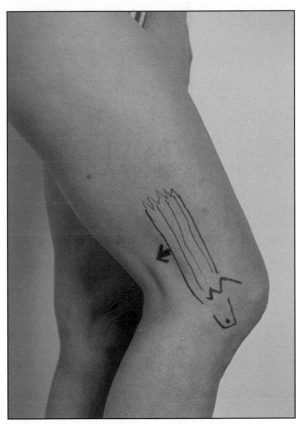

Figure 25 – Ilio-tibial band friction syndrome where there is inflammation over the lateral epicondyle of the knee from rubbing of the ilio-tibial band

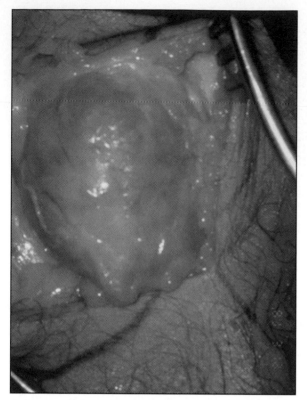

Figure 26 – Large semi-membranous cyst at time of surgical excision

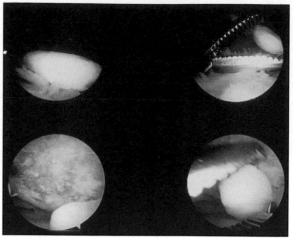

Figure 27 – Loose body being removed arthroscopically

LOOSE BODIES

Loose bodies cause mechanical symptoms of locking and recurrent effusions. Occasionally they can be palpated. They can be due to a meniscal fragment or osteochondral fragment (traumatic, degenerative, osteochondritis dissecans) or synovial chondromatosis (Fig. 27). X-rays will demonstrate radio-opaque loose bodies. Treatment by arthroscopic removal is usually successful.

15

FOOT AND ANKLE

Eugene Sherry

INTRODUCTION

The **evolution** of the human foot has allowed us to stand and move upright, so freeing our hands to explore and control our environment. The foot has changed from **an arboreal grasping organ** to an **agent for motion** - the big toe has fallen into line with the little toes (which shortened); a stiffer subtalar joint; a medial arch and bigger heel occurred. Our current foot **shape dates from 40 to 100,000** years ago. We now stand perched on a ledge (the sustentaculum tali of the calcaneus) and topple frequently on the sporting field to sprain the lateral ligament complex (Fig. 1). Design problems remain.

The foot and ankle is commonly injured in sport; such injuries account for 25% of all sporting injuries (Fig. 2).

BIOMECHANICS

The **tibio-talar articulation** allows 25° dorsiflexion, 35° plantar flexion and 5° of rotation. The instant centre of motion lies on a line along the tips of the malleoli and postero-laterally on the talar dome. Up to 5 times our body weight is transmitted across this joint.

Stability is gained by the talar mortise and ligament support. The subtalar joint functions like a hinge and

SPORTS SPECIFIC FOOT AND ANKLE INJURIES	
Sports	**Specific Foot and Ankle Injury**
Skiing	Peroneal tendon subluxation Nerve entrapment Plantar fasciitis
Running	Lateral ligament sprains Stress fractures Shin splints
Ballet	Os trigonum FHL impingement Sesamoiditis Stress fracture Hallux valgus
Football	Turf toe Ankle and mid-foot fractures
Tennis	Gastrocnemius strains TA injury Stress Fractures
Soccer	Ankle sprains Stress fractures
Basketball	Lateral ligament sprains Plantar fasciitis Jones fracture
Gymnastics	Sever's disease

Figure 2 – Sports Specific Foot and Ankle Injuries

allows eversion and inversion. The mid-foot permits abduction and adduction, the forefoot flexion and extension. Pronation of the foot (5°) is coupled dorsi flexion, eversion and abduction, supination (up to 20°) is coupled plantar flexion, inversion and adduction. The foot transmits 3 times the body-weight with running and has 3 arches (medial, lateral, transverse). The second metatarsal is the keystone of the mid-foot in gait (the first metatarsal in the stance phase).

Gait (walking - one foot is always on the ground; running - both feet off the ground at one point) has two phases (stance and swing) (Fig. 3).

Video analysis allows documentation and correction of abnormal running postures (Fig. 4).

Injuries in the region occur for the following reasons: the athletes physical and personality traits; training techniques, playing environment and equipment. Weekly running distance has been found to be the critical factor for injury among runners (>64 km per week).

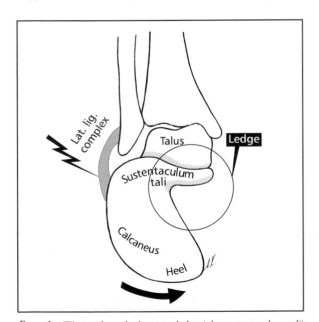

Figure 1 – We stand perched upon a ledge (the sustentaculum tali) held by the lateral ligament so it is not suprising that we topple frquently and damage the lateral ligaments

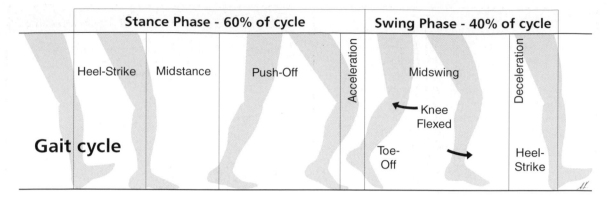

Figure 3 – The gait cycle is divided into stance (60% cycle; heel/mid-stance, push-off) and swing (40%, toe-off/toe clear/heel strike) phases .

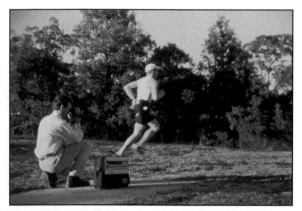

Figure 4 – Video analysis on the "field" allows careful scrutiny of faulty running postures

Certain athletes are prone to injury and certain body types confer a biomechanical advantage (Fig. 5).

STRESS FRACTURES

Bone pain with a normal X-ray in an athlete suggests a stress fracture. There are two types: **fatigue type** (abnormally increased load on a normal bone) or the **insufficiency type** (normal loads on deficient bone (such as osteoporosis). They typically occur 3 to 5 weeks into an intensive training programme. Exclude steroid use (decreases trabecular bone). Muscles are able to adapt faster than bone and after 2 weeks of new intensive training the fracture occurs. A small cortical crack occurs and spreads by subcortical infarction. Periosteal and endosteal new bone (callus) is seen at 2 to 3 weeks. X-rays may show the dreaded **"black**

ATHLETES PRONE TO INJURY	
Postural defects • Muscle weakness/imbalance • Lack of flexibility • Mal alignment problems (pronated feet, LLD with pelvic tilt)	
ATHLETES WITH BIOMECHANICAL ADVANTAGE	
Pigeon toed	Good for sprinters, tennis and squash.
Sway back	Increased lumbar, lordosis with anterior pelvic tilt – good sprinters, jumpers and gymnasts.
Duck feet	Everted feet – good for breaststroke.
Inverted feet	Good for backstroke and butterfly.
Double jointed	Ligamentous laxity — gynmnasts.
• Exception... Peter Snell (NZ) had body build of sprinter rather than middle-distance athlete – (gold medal 800, 1500m Rome, Tokyo, 1960, 1964).	

Figure 5 – Certain athletes are prone to injury and some to victory

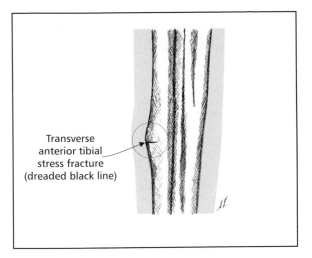

Figure 6 – The "dreaded black line" may herald an impending fracture (from a stress fracture)

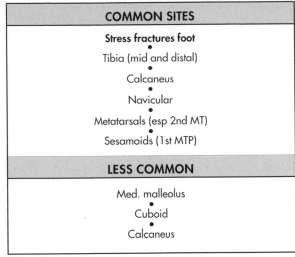

Figure 7 – Common sites of stress fractures of the lower limb

COMMON SITES
Stress fractures foot
•
Tibia (mid and distal)
•
Calcaneus
•
Navicular
•
Metatarsals (esp 2nd MT)
•
Sesamoids (1st MTP)
LESS COMMON
Med. malleolus
•
Cuboid
•
Calcaneus

line" of impending complete fracture (Fig. 6). Bone scans are positive early and diagnostic. **Common sites** are described (Fig. 7).

There is localised bone pain and tenderness relieved by rest. The athlete limps. Examine the sports shoes for excessive wear.

Treatment should be comprehensive (Fig. 8).

SPECIAL CONSIDERATIONS

Stress fracture of the neck of the femur need crutches for 3 to 4 weeks. If pain persists at 1 to 2 months (groin pain with rotation of the thigh) seriously consider surgical fixation of the fracture.

Navicular fractures are slow to be diagnosed and to heal. Immobilise for 6 to 8 weeks and surgically fix (and bone graft) if symptomatic at 1 to 2 months.

ANKLE SPRAINS

LATERAL LIGAMENT

Little wonder ankle sprains are common in sport. We stand **perched upon** the sustentaculum tali with the calcaneus bowed back under the ankle joint and all balanced (in tension) by the lateral ligament complex (Fig. 1). Inversion (with supination and plantar/dorsi flexion) causes injury of the lateral ligament complex; usually (2/3 of cases) the anterior talo-fibular ligament (**ATFL** - the weakest), sometimes the extra-articular calcaneo-fibular ligament (CFL) seldom the PTFL -

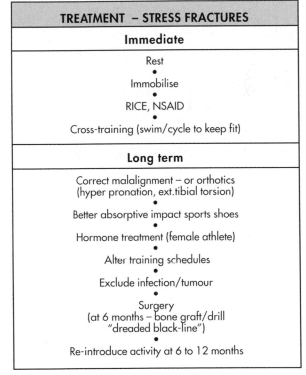

Figure 8 – Management of stress fractures

TREATMENT – STRESS FRACTURES
Immediate
Rest
•
Immobilise
•
RICE, NSAID
•
Cross-training (swim/cycle to keep fit)
Long term
Correct malalignment – or orthotics (hyper pronation, ext.tibial torsion)
•
Better absorptive impact sports shoes
•
Hormone treatment (female athlete)
•
Alter training schedules
•
Exclude infection/tumour
•
Surgery (at 6 months – bone graft/drill "dreaded black-line")
•
Re-introduce activity at 6 to 12 months

the strongest. Those at risk are large athletes, those with pes cavus (high medial arches) and a history of similar injury. High-top shoes and good splints may protect the ankle.

I   ATFL Sprain (⅔ cases)

II   ATFL, CFL spains (¼ cases)

III AFTL, CFL, PTFL tears

⬇

Or simply use

Incomplete: end-point to anterior draw

Complete: no end-point to anterior draw

Figure 9 – Grading of lateral injuries of ankle

There is immediate pain and swelling with resultant anterior and inversion instability. The severity of the injury can be graded (Fig. 9). Careful examination in the post-acute phase can delineate the ligament components injured (Figs. 10–12).

In the acute phase treat with RICE, NSAID, ankle splint (S-Ankle), early rehabiliation/peroneal eversion exercises, water jogging, proprioceptive wobble board exercises (Fig. 13). Elite athletes may elect for early surgical repair of complete ruptures (controversial).

X-rays are necessary to exclude fractures with good talar dome views to exclude osteochondral fractures (ignore bony avulsion of the ligaments). Do not miss a high fibular fracture with syndesmotic injuries (Maisonneuve fracture) (Fig. 14). Stress X-rays are unreliable but possibly helpful in the chronic phase where the patient does not give a clear history of instability ("going over" on the ankle).

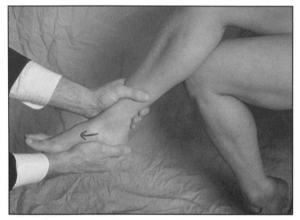

Figure 10 – Anterior draw test - important test for lateral ligament instability where tear of ATFL allows talus to be drawn forward on lower tibia

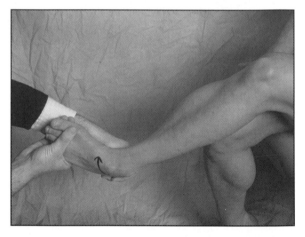

Figure 12 – The inversion test, for CFL damage (also for subtalar instability; difficult to differentiate)

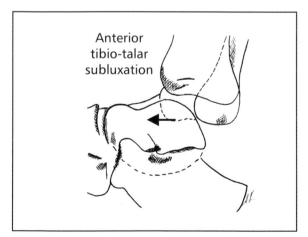

Anterior tibio-talar subluxation

Figure 11 – Talus is drawn forward in anterior test for ATFL tear

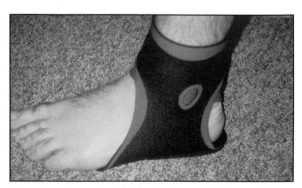

Figure 13 – S-ankle splint for lateral ligament injury supports in both swing (outer strap) and stance phases (heel wedge)

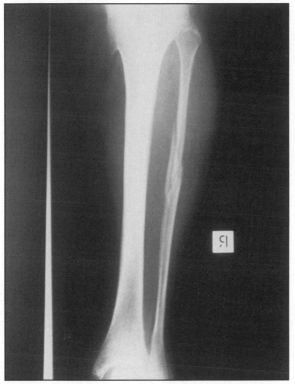

Figure 14 – Maisonneuve fracture where there is a high fibular fracture (may be out of X-ray view) and lower syndesmotic injury (needs surgery)

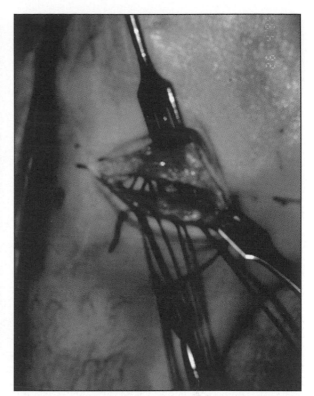

Figure 15 – Lateral ligament reconstruction using the Bröstrom procedure (capsulorrhaphy) works well

LATERAL LIGAMENTOUS LAXITY

Chronic unsuccessful treatment of the acute lateral ligament injury may result in chronic lateral ligament laxity from "stretched-out" ligaments. There is chronic lateral pain (over anterior border of the lateral malleolus sinus tarsi) exacerbated by repeated inversion injuries on irregular terrain. Too often athletes are left to persist with months of unsuccessful physiotherapy instead of a quick effective lateral ligament reconstruction. I favour the **Bröstrom** capsulorraphy with reinforcement from the inferior extensor retinaculum (Fig. 15).

MEDIAL LIGAMENT INJURIES

These are rare (usually with (lat.lig) sprain or fractures) and need to be differentiated from lesions of the nearby tibialis posterior or FHL tendons and syndesmotic injury. Careful examination (for localised tenderness) with ultrasound examination is useful (see tib. post. section). It is a strong ligament.

X-rays with bone scan and CT maybe necessary to exclude osteochondral fractures where there is severe,

localised pain about the talar dome. Weight-bearing X-rays may be useful (Fig. 16). Chondral damage (sometimes seen after lateral ligament injuries with medial impingement) may require arthroscopic attention (Fig. 17).

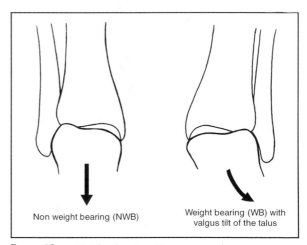

Non weight bearing (NWB)

Weight bearing (WB) with valgus tilt of the talus

Figure 16 – Weight bearing X-rays may demonstrate tear (i.e. incompetent) medial (deltoid) ligament

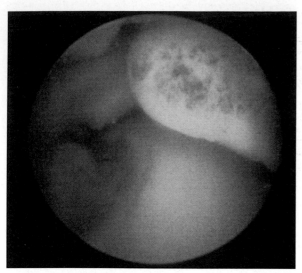

Figure 17 – Chondral damage seen at arthroscopy

SUBTALAR INSTABILITY

A difficult entity to diagnose which is really a component of a lateral ligament injury (the CFL torn) from inversion. Special stress X-rays (Broden - 45° int rotation and 20° caudal tilt) or I.I. may help. Treat as above with CFL reconstruction (as part of Bröstrom operation) for chronic cases.

SPRING LIGAMENT SPRAIN

The mid-foot is prone to twisting injuries with pain localised to the medial arch from sprain of the calca-neo-navicular ligament (spring).

CUBOID SYNDROME

Pain and tenderness over the cuboid in the region of the peroneal (exerting) tendons. S-ankle the foot.

SYNDESMOTIC ANKLE INJURIES (HIGH ANKLE SPRAIN)

(DISTAL TIBIOFIBULAR DIASTASIS)

Previously unrecognised but a probable cause of ongoing painful **"ankle sprain",** though probably occurs from an external rotation injury in the professional athlete. There is marked swelling on both sides of the ankle with tenderness over the interosseous membrane. Suspect where an ankle sprain takes a long time to settle down; perform the squeeze test or abduction/external rotation tests (Fig. 18) and check a mortise-view. Also perform an X-ray (>1 mm reduction in the medial clear space or <10 mm overlap) (Fig. 19). Late X-rays show calcification of the ligaments. Treat in NWB art for 4 weeks or later with diastasis screw fixation and ligament repair where refractory.

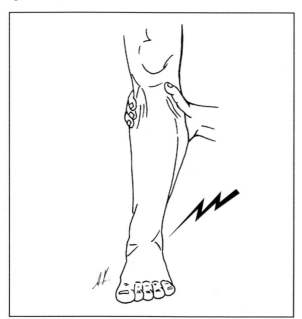

Figure 18 – Squeeze test is used to demonstrate a disruption of the ankle syndesmosis (pain just above the ankle joint), also the abduction-external rotation test is useful

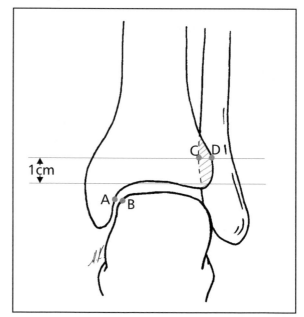

Figure 19 – Syndesmodic injury (high ankle sprain). Where there is >1 mm reduction in the medial clear space (AB) or <10 mm tibio-fibular overlap (CD)

SINUS TARSI SYNDROME

The tunnel beneath the talar neck and upper calcaneus can be a source of pain from overactivity and inversion injury. It may be related to the strained ligament of the tunnel (talo-calcaneal ligament). Distinguish from lateral ligament strain. Treat with NSAID, activities (for hyper-pronation) and possible steroid injection and seldom surgical excision of contents.

PERONEAL TENDON INJURIES

The peroneal tendons work hard. They evert the foot (which wants to drift into equinus) and maintain the transverse/longitudinal arches. They are poorly anchored with a weak holding retinaculum. Forced dorsi-flexion of the ankle in skiing or football can produce tenosynovitis tendinitis tear, partial or complete (peroneus brevis) or dislocation of these tendons. There is marked tenderness with reproducible subluxation. X-rays may show a rim fracture (Fig. 20). Strapping may help, otherwise decompression, repair, tenodesis to (peroneus longus) or early stabilisation in the groove (because of high recurrence rate). Graduated return to sport over 4-6 weeks avoiding "cutting" procedures or sprinting for 6 weeks.

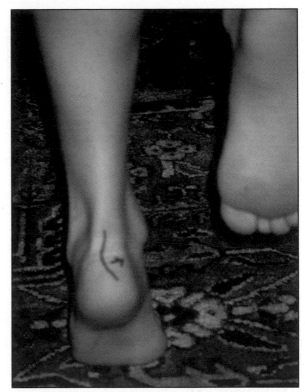

Figure 21 – Single heel raise. Test diagnosis tibialis posterior tendon problems (pain/hesitation = tenosynovitis/ partial tear; not able to lift heel = complete tear)

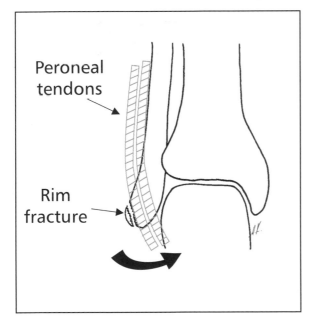

Figure 20 – Rim fracture may be associated with subluxation or dislocation of the peroneal tendons

TIBIALIS POSTERIOR TENDON INJURY

These occur in middle-aged women who are unfit as a result of **chronic degeneration.** The pathology is inflammation (tenosynovitis) or rupture (partial or complete). They experience pain and tenderness along the tibialis posterior tendon with difficulty lifting the heel off the ground in the single heel raise test (Fig. 21). An ultrasound may secure the diagnosis. The arch is flattened and foot pronated. They require NSAID, a medial arch support (for tenosynovitis and partial ruptures), and debridement/tenosynovectomy for refractory cases. Reconstruct complete tears (use the FDL).

TIBIALIS ANTERIOR INJURY

Spontaneous rupture may occur but is unusual. There is localised tenderness and weakened dorsiflexion. Surgical repair is important (either direct repair or tendon/extensor transfer).

TENDO ACHILLES INJURY

Injuries of this region are common and difficult to treat. Overtraining will produce an inflammation around the TA (**peri-tendinitis**), in the tendon (**tendinitis**) or by the tendon (**retro calcaneal bursitis** and **retro-achilles bursitis**). The "painful arc sign" may help to make the distinction (Fig. 22). Certain athletes are at risk (excessive training, poor hindfoot shoe support, on cambered surfaces).

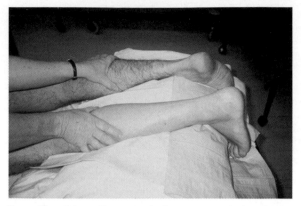

Figure 23 – Simmond's test simply demonstrates whether the TA is intact (squeeze the calf, if the foot does not move, the TA is ruptured)

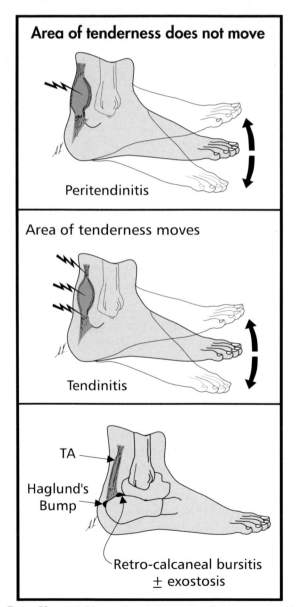

Figure 22 – Painful arc sign. With peritendinitis the area of tenderness does not change with movement of the foot; with tendinitis it does. Retro-calcaneal bursitis is easily localised in front of the bottom of the tendon

A violent contraction of the gastrocnemius-soleus unit may rupture (partially or completely) the TA. Patients report having been hit or kicked in the calf during the push-off phase of running or racket sports. Partial tears are difficult to diagnose; ultrasound imaging is helpful.

Complete tears will invariably have pain, swelling, and a palpable gap (prior to swelling). Do not be fooled by the patient being able to plantarflex (from intact long flexors). Simmond's test is easy to perform and diagnostic (Fig. 23).

Treatment: of TA problems is outlined (Fig. 24).

A tear of the medial head of the gastrocnemius is common in middle-aged tennis players (tennis leg).

Rehabilitation: Cross-train (swim) during surgical recovery with slow re-introduction to pre-injury sports over 3 months.

TREATMENT – TA INJURIES	
Tendinitis/peritendinitis	Rest, NSAID, heel raise, ultrasound, massage (stretching). Rarely surgery with debridement.
Retro-calcaneal bursitis	As above but consider surgery. Earlier with excision of associated retro-calcaneal exostosis. Rarely surgery for retro-achilles bursitis.
Haglund's bump (postero-superior prominence of calcaneus)	Shoe modification, NSAID gel, heel raise or excise.
Partial tendon rupture	May require surgical excision of scar and granulation tissue.
Complete tendon rupture	• Almost invariably surgically repair (open technique). • Later repair is difficult and may require fascial or tendon augmentation.
Warning: Avoid steroids. Exclude Reiter's syndrome, Infection, Gout, Tumour	

Figure 24 – Treatment of TA problems

FRACTURES OF THE FOOT AND ANKLE

Fractures of the ankle are common and require precise treatment to avoid later osteoarthritis (1 mm displacement causes 40% decrease in tibiotalar articulation). They are variously classified (Fig. 25) and are usually from a fall with supination (or pronation) of the forefoot and eversion (or inversion) of the hindfoot. Well-fitted shoes with ankle support will eliminate such injuries. The immediate pain, swelling and deformity is obvious, never hesitate to X-ray. A **displaced** fracture almost always requires open reduction and internal fixation (Fig. 26), a **non-displaced** <1 mm, careful follow-up (6 weeks in cast) with X-ray review to detect early displacement. **A markedly displaced ankle fracture** should be reduced in Casualty to avoid skin problems (blisters/nervosis) (Fig. 27). Exclude a Maisonneuve fracture by careful examination (with X-ray) of upper fibula (Fig. 14). Post-operatively support the ankle in an S-Ankle splint for 6 weeks (NWB) and return to sports at 3 to 5 months.

Residual ankle pain after bony union may be residual traumatic synovitis (**Fergel** lesions) which requires NSAID) or arthroscopic excision.

CLASSIFICTION OF ANKLE FRACTURES	
BEST	**Weber** (position of fibular fracture) A: at/below joint line B: at joint line C: above joint line
LOGICAL	**Lauge-Hansen** (Direction of damaging force) • supination/adduction • supination/external rotation • pronation/adduction • pronation/external rotation
SIMPLE	**Henderson** • lateral malleolus • medial malleolus or combination

Figure 25 – Classification of ankle fractures

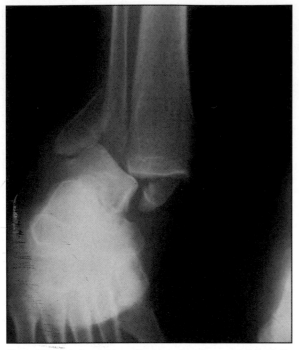

Figure 26 – Displaced **biamalleolar ankle fracture** of footballer (need surgical fixation)

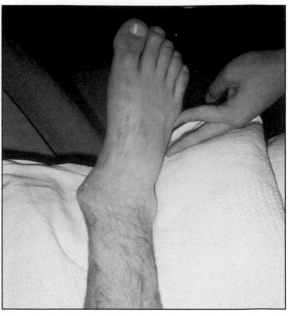

Figure 27 – A clinically displaced ankle fracture should be immediately reduced in casualty to minimise skin, nerve and vascular damage

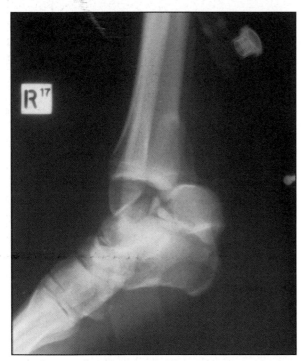

Figure 28 – Fracture of **talar neck** with gross displacement needs urgent reduction/fixation (avascular necrosis will be inevitable)

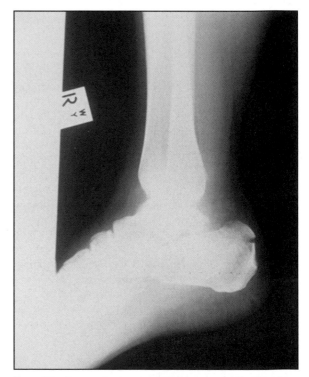

Figure 28 – Fractured calcaneus with comminution is difficult to treat and associated with many complications

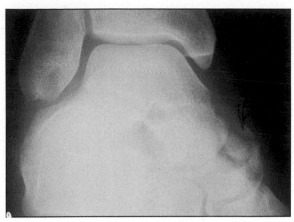

Figure 30 – Fractured navicular with comminution from a horse-riding fall (surgery necessary)

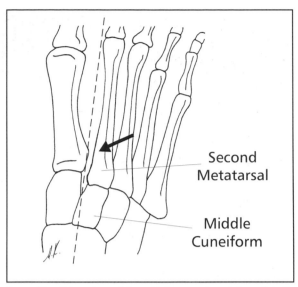

Figure 31 – Disruption of the mid-foot can be subtle and easily overlooked leading to eventual mid-foot collapse and osteoarthritis. The base of the second metatarsal is key to the mid-foot; loss of straight-line alignment of the medial border (of second MT) with medial border of the middle cuneiform means there has been a significant injury

FRACTURES OF THE FOOT

These tend to be under-appreciated. Most can be managed in a below knee fracture walker.

Displaced and intra-articular fractures often require reduction and fixation.

Fractures of the **talar neck** may result in avascular necrosis of the body and so need accurate reduction (Fig. 28).

Fractures of the **calcaneus** can be devastating (widened painful heel, nerve entrapment, tendinitis and later subtalar OA (Fig. 29)). It is best to reduce to restore Bohler's angle (usually requires surgery with bone grafting and early movement).

Navicular fractures can be avulsions, hairline, comminuted or stress type. It is best to reduce and fix the fracture (K-wires) (Fig. 30). Non-union, which is painful, may result.

Mid-foot (tarsometatarsal) fractures (Lisfrane) can be subtle and easily missed (Fig. 31). Careful WB X-rays are important in the diagnosis of mid-foot pain following injury.

Mid-foot pain following injury. Reduction and fixation (with K-wires) is useful.

Avulsion of peroneus brevis (base of 5th MT) and proximal diaphyseal fracture of the 5th MT (Jones' fracture) may take a long time to heal and eventually require surgical fixation (Fig. 32).

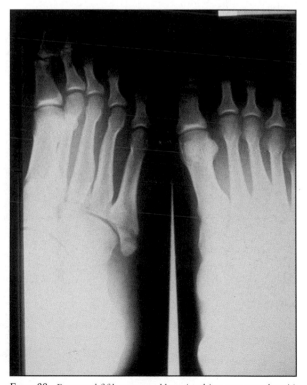

Figure 32 – Fractured fifth metatarsal base (avulsion peroneus brevis) are slow to heal

Most other fractures of the MT shafts and phalanges require reduction and seldom surgical fixation.

Dislocated **MTP** or **PIP joints** need prompt reduction otherwise they become irreducible and a source of severe pain (Fig. 33).

NERVE ENTRAPMENTS

These are not uncommon about the foot and ankle, difficult to diagnose and treat. Many are related to poor (e.g. ski boot) sports shoe fit or hard surfaces. Several have been described (Fig. 34).

All entrapments are diagnosed by localised tenderness over entrapped nerve at level of entrapment. Positive Tinel's test, Neuralgic pain (at rest or at night) nerve conduction studies are usually unhelpful. Treat with orthotics, NSAID, stretching and massage. Surgically release (and excise neuroma) at level of anatomically located tenderness.

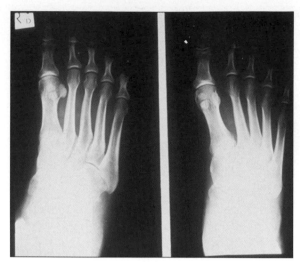

Figure 33 – Dislocated PIP joint of toe is painful and difficult to treat (if left)

COMPARTMENT SYNDROME

Increased pressure within a confined muscle compartment may lead to ischaemia, necrosis, contracture and a useless limb. It's early recognition and prompt treatment is essential. Causes are trauma (with fracture), post-operative and crush injuries (Fig. 35).

The symptoms and signs of an **acute compartment** are well described (Fig. 36). It usually involves the forearm, the lower leg and foot (when

NERVE ENTRAPMENTS	
Type	**Detail**
Tarsal tunnel	Posterior tibial nerve trapped behind medial malleolus under flexor retinaculum. Pain medial foot and sole
Ant. tarsal tunnel	Deep peroneal nerve trapped under inferior ext. retinaculum Pain 1st web space
Jogger's foot	Medial plantar nerve compressed at Knot of Henry. Pain over med toes
Sural nerve	Medial border foot pain
Comm. peroneal nerve	Behind the fibula neck from trauma
Superf. peroneal nerve	Anta-lateral entrapment (12 cm from tip lat mal; distinguish from compartment syndrome)
Saphenous nerve	Injured in thigh (Hunter's canal) or med. knee (post-surgical)
Morton's neuroma	Typically pain between 3rd/4th metatarsal heads from traumatic entrapment causing neuroma (runners) of interdigital nerve. Compression of metatarsal heads reproduces symptoms and patient aware of mobile pebble

Figure 34 – Nerve entrapments about the foot

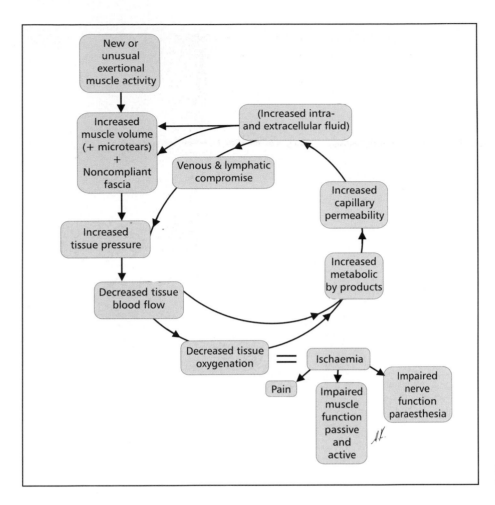

Figure 35 – Pathomechanics of compartment syndrome

DIAGNOSIS COMPARTMENT SYNDROME		
	Acute	**Chronic**
1	# bone present	Pain with sport and slow to resolve
2	Localised tenderness	Tenderness with swelling
3	Pain with active (usually not possible) and passive movement	
4	Paraesthesia	Paraesthesia
Pallor / paralysis / pulselessness are **late signs** where diagnosis has already been missed		

Figure 36 – Diagnosis of acute vs chronic compartment syndrome

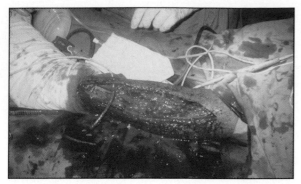

Figure 37 – Cricketer with anterior compartment syndrome of leg (after 12 hours play). Required fasciotomy and later debridement of necrotic muscle (delayed presentation >6 hours)

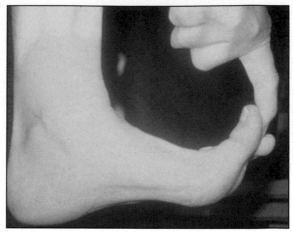

Figure 39 – Plantar-fasciitis – subcalcaneal pain exacerbated by dorsi-flexion of the big toe (windlass effect)

DIFFERENTIAL DIAGNOSIS OF CHRONIC COMPARTMENT SYNDROME	
Problem	**Action**
Stress # bone	See bone scan
Periostitis (shin splints) (pain over postero-medial distal tibia)	Maybe compartment problem of tib post or periostisis of soleus muscle. Do bone scan, consider fasciotomy, orthotics for hyper pronation, massage.
Popliteal artery entrapment	Calf claudication with reduced pulses (when knee extended, foot dorsiflexed).

Figure 38 – Differential diagnosis of chronic compartment syndrome

compartment pressures exceed 40 mmHg). Measuring intra-compartmental pressures is fraught with problems of accuracy and **should not** over-ride clinical judgement. Treatment is to externally split POP/bandages to skin and, if necessary, internally release the compressed compartment (fasciotomy Fig. 37, within 4 hours).

Chronic compartment syndrome (exertional) may be subtle in presentation and results from prolonged training (runners, court sports athletes). The muscles are overworked, swell and a vicious cycle is triggered. The extensor and flexor compartments are usually involved with crescendo pain and tenderness relieved by rest. There may only be paraesthesia with exercise. The differential diagnosis is important (Fig. 38).

Treatment is activity modification, massage, exclude footwear or surface problem, NSAID, orthotics (medial wedge for posterior compartment), cross-training (cycling) and fasciotomy (sometimes, 80% successful).

Here it is useful to carefully measure intra-compartment pressures before/during/after exercise (resting pressure >15 mmHg or delay in fall after exercise of >20 mmHg/over 3 min). Then consider a careful fasciotomy of the compartment involved with mini skin incisions and wound closure.

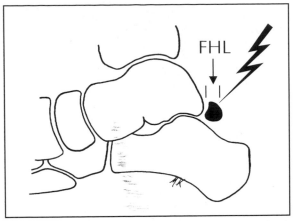

Figure 40 – OS trigonum is the ossicle behind the posterior talus; it may be asymptomatic, fused, fractured, absent or big. Do not confuse with FHL tendinitis. (Pain on resisted flexion big toe)

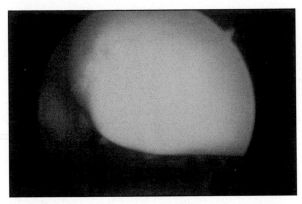

Figure 42 – Arthroscopic view of tibio-talar spur at **time of excision**

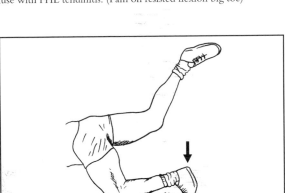

Figure 41 – Turf toe forced dorsiflexion of the 1st MTP joint

PLANTAR FASCIITIS

Common and crippling subcalcaneal (usually medial) heel pain. Related to hyperpronation and pes cavus (Fig. 39). There is localised tenderness; a positive wind lass effect (dorsiflexing the big toe exacerbates the pain). X-rays may show a heel spur (ignore it). Exclude stress fractures, nerve entrapment (medial branch of the **lat. plantar nerve**) and Reiter's syndrome.

Treat with NSAID, stretching and a soft silicone heel cup. Seldom is surgery (release) helpful.

OS TRIGONUM

This ossicle behind the posterior talus (medial tubercle of the posterior process of the talus) may be the cause of pain with plantar flexion in ballet dancers. It can be asymptomatic, fused, fractured, absent or big. X-rays confirm its presence and examination its problem. Treat with injection (not steroids) or excise. Do not confuse with FHL tendinitis (Fig. 40).

TURF TOE

This is caused by a forceful dorsi flexion of the 1st MTP joint in American football on a hard surface (artificial turf and flexible shoes - Fig. 41). X-rays may show a disruption of the plantar volar plate complex. Exclude stress fracture, sesamoiditis, entrapment of FHL. Treat with RICE, taping, custom shoes and sometimes surgical repair of the disruption.

TIBIO-TALAR SPURS

Osteophytic spurs may form on the adjoining surfaces of the lower anterior tibia and talar neck. There is impingement pain with dorsi flexion. Arthroscopic excision is useful (Fig. 42).

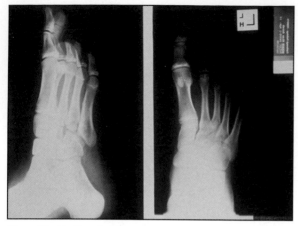

Figure 43 – **Freiberg's disease** is a not uncommon cause of severe forefoot pain in young females

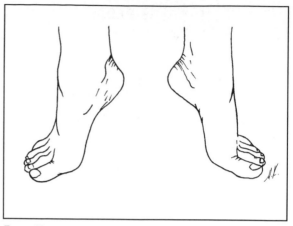

Figure 44 – **Hallux valgus** deformity is increased in the demi-pointe (ballet) position

METATARSALGIA

Forefoot pain beneath the metatarsal heads (with callosities) is vague in nature and related to impact sports. There may be claw toes and/or pes cavus. Exclude a neuroma, stress fracture, Freiberg's infarction. Treat with stretching, NSAID, transverse arch supports (HAPADs) and rarely a closing wedge osteotomy (where a single (usually the second) metatarsal is involved).

FREIBERG'S INFARCTION

This is an osteonecrosis of the second metatarsal head typically in teenage females and with excruciating pain. X-rays may show increased density, or collapse of the metatarsal head (Fig. 43). Symptomatic treatment, debridement synovectomy or limited resection of the distal 2nd MT head.

HALLUX VALGUS

Common in the community from improper shoe size; seen in dancers and catchers from acute injuries (dislocation of 1st MTP joint) or chronic repetitive injury. Ballet dancers and sprinters are poor surgical candidates (post-operative stiffness is debilitating here) and all other avenues must be exhausted (delay surgery as long as possible) (Fig. 44).

HALLUX RIGIDUS

A stiff and painful 1st MTP joint from micro-trauma, osteonecrosis or OA. Seen in push-off sports where long, narrow pronated feet (long 1st MT). Require stiff sole, HAPAD or cheilectomy (excision of painful dorsal osteophytes).

SESAMOIDITIS

Localised pain usually below the 1st MTP joint which may be part of a FHL tendinitis/tethering; seen in dancers. Exclude fracture, stress fracture, OA, dislocation, nerve entrapment and do not confuse with bipartite sesamoid. X-rays (sesamoid views). Treat with metatarsal support, NSAID and rarely shave or excise.

SHORT LEG SYNDROME

A short leg (>2 cm) is prone to injury (stress fractures, MCL knee sprain, patellar subluxation, plantar fasciitis and hyperpronation). The longer leg is prone to ilio-tibial tendinitis. It may be real shortening or apparent (from tilt of tract with tendon contracture - needs stretching). Use partial heel build-up (and/mid-sole build-up).

APPROACH TO THE PERSISTENTLY PAINFUL ANKLE

FOR THE PAINFUL (PERSISTENT) ANKLE CONSIDER THE FOLLOWING ...	
Problem	**Action**
"Meniscoid" synovitis ankle	arthoscopic synovectomy
Avulsion tip fibula	excise
"Asymptomatic" ossicle	excise
Unrecognised fracture ant. process calcaneus	excise
Peroneal or tib. post/tendon problem (synovitis, partial tendon, subluxation)	surgery
Lat. process # talus	fix/excise
Sinus tarsi syndrome	surgery
Subluxation cuboid	
High ankle sprain (± fracture Tilbux)	see text
Impingement inferior band of tibiotalar ligament	arthroscopic excision
Nerve entrapment	see text
Tarsal coalition (children)	excise
Osteochondral fracture/dissecans	arthroscopy
RA or occult tumour	refer

Management

• NSAID – local application • Cross-train
• Water jog • S-Ankle splint
• Gentle PT (low frequency pulsed ultrasound, TENS, WAX)

Figure 45 – Careful consideration of the persistently painful ankle may yield a correctable problem.

16

GUT AND URINARY TRACT

Michael Cox

INTRODUCTION

Most gastrointestinal and urinary problems encountered by the athlete are from blunt abdominal trauma (Fig. 1).

BLUNT TRAUMA

Blunt abdominal trauma is the commonest problem in the athlete. The initial assessment is the same in **all** cases. The mechanism of injury is central to defining the possible injuries. Clinical assessment should exclude severe, life threatening injuries. Routine observations first. (An athlete should **maintain their**

SPORT GASTROINTESTINAL AND URINARY PROBLEMS		
System	**Organ**	**Problems**
Gastrointestinal	Spleen	Haematoma Rupture
	Liver	Haematoma Rupture Hepatic failure (heatstroke)
	Pancreas	Contusion Transection Pancreatitis
	Duodenum	Contusion/ Haematoma Rupture
	Rectum/Anus	Impaling High pressure insufflation
	Small and large bowel	Mesenteric tear Rupture
Genito-Urinary	Kidney	Haematuria Renal failure (Heatstroke) Haematoma Rupture
Bladder		Rupture
	Male urethra	Rupture
	Testis	Rupture Torsion

Figure 1 – Sport gastrointestinal and urinary tract injuries

blood pressure in the presence of a large haemorrhage). **Tachycardia** is a more accurate assessment of the extent of blood loss. **Pallor** indicates marked blood loss. If there is suspicion of significant intra-abdominal injury, start intravenous fluids early whilst continuing to assess. Analgesia after the initial surgical assessment is complete.

SPLENIC TRAUMA

From a direct blow to the left upper quadrant (shoulder in rugby tackle; fall from a cycle) or in association with left thoracic wall injuries (Figs. 2 – 4).

Pain may be localised to left upper quadrant or generalised. Left shoulder tip pain is often present. Pallor, tachycardia or shock indicate a large haemorrhage. Abdominal signs vary from mild left upper quadrant tenderness to marked generalised peritonitis with abdominal distension.

Initial management includes fasting, intravenous fluid resuscitation and nasogastric tube insertion. **An urgent laparotomy** is performed in patients that are shocked or have evidence of ongoing blood loss, persistent tachycardia, falling haemoglobin or progressive abdominal distension.

A **haemodynamically stable** patient is managed non-operatively initially and investigated with a CT scan or ultrasound to diagnose and assess the extent of the splenic injury. **Children and adults** that remain haemodynamically stable can be managed non-operatively with close observation, analgesia and chest physiotherapy. **Operative intervention** is required if there is any clinical deterioration or there is evidence of ongoing blood loss. As **a guide any child requiring more than 25% of their blood volume replaced requires operative intervention.**

When operative intervention is required, **splenic conservation** is attempted rather than splenectomy in order to avoid post splenectomy complications, including overwhelming post-splenectomy sepsis. **Conservative measures** include suture repair, wrapping the spleen in a mesh bag and partial splenectomy. **Splenic injuries** can be graded according to operative findings (Fig. 5); Grade I, II and III injuries can usually be managed conservatively (Fig. 2) although Grade III may require partial splenectomy. Grade IV and V usually require splenectomy (Fig. 3). If splenectomy is performed **immunisation** with pneumococcal, meningococcal and Haemophyllus vaccines within 48 hours is necessary.

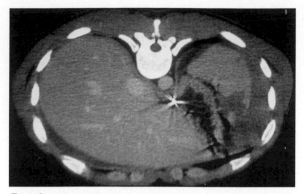

Figure 2 – Splenic trauma managed non-operatively

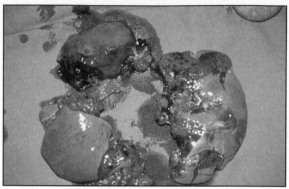

Figure 3 – Splenic trauma requiring surgery. 17-year-old motor cyclist hit a tree. Pale, shocked, urine **clear.** Urgent laparotomy revealed an avulsed shattered spleen and a shattered avulsed left kidney (Fig. 6)

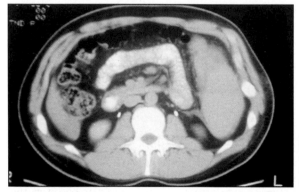

Figure 4 – Splenic abscess. 25-year-old footballer 12 days after blow to upper quadrant with pain and fevers. CT revealed a splenic abscess, that was drained by percutaneous technique

OPERATIVE GRADING SPLENIC INJURIES			
Grade	Injury	Description	Action
I	Haematoma Laceration	Non-expanding subcapsular, <10% of surface area Non-bleeding, < I cm deep	Save spleen
II	Haematoma Laceration	Non-expanding subcapsular, 10 - 50% of surface area. Intraparenchymal < 2 cm diameter I - 3 cm deep	Save spleen
III	Haematoma Laceration	>50% surface area, Intraparenchymal >2 cm diameter Expanding subcapsular or intraparenchymal 3 cm deep or involving trabecular vessels	Save spleen/partial splenectomy
IV	Haematoma Laceration	Ruptured spleen with active bleeding Involving segmental artery or hilar vessels with >25% splenic devascularisation.	Splenectomy
V	Laceration Vascular	Completely shattered spleen Hilar injury with devascularised spleen.	Splenectomy

Figure 5 – Table of operative grading splenic injuries (liver system is similar).

LIVER TRAUMA

Liver trauma is uncommon in low velocity injuries (football), but more common with a high velocity injury (cyclist or motor sports). It is produced by either a **blow** to the right upper quadrant, associated with right thoracic injuries, or a **crush** injury (rolled on by a horse). Hepatic injuries following a **low velocity** injury are usually **minor**, whereas **crush** injuries are often **severe**.

The pain may be right upper quadrant, epigastric or generalised. The initial assessment is to determine if the patient is shocked and has evidence of ongoing haemorrhage. The **shocked patient with a distended abdomen that has not responded** quickly to fluid resuscitation **requires an urgent laparotomy**. If the patient is stable or responds quickly to fluid resuscitation with no evidence of ongoing blood loss a CT scan or ultrasound is performed to assess and grade the injury. Type IV (extensive injury/devascularised segment/deep haematoma >3 cm) injuries invariably require laparotomy and repair. Types I, II and III (capsular tear, superficial injury, deep haematoma <3 cm) injuries can be managed non-operatively initially if the patient remains haemodynamically stable. Any deterioration **requires a laparotomy**. Grade I injuries rarely require operative intervention, whereas grade III injuries require a laparotomy in 40 to 60% of cases. Bleeding may be stopped with suturing, local haemostatic agents or packing. A severe liver rupture (Type IV and V) may require packing and repeat laparotomy and subsequent resection of non-viable liver. Subsequent complications include hepatic abscess and biliary peritonitis.

DUODENAL AND PANCREATIC INJURIES

Injuries to the duodenum and/or pancreas follow a direct blow across the epigastrium with compression of the duodenum and pancreas across the spinal column. The patient may complain of moderate to severe epigastric pain with associated vomiting. As these injuries are retroperitoneal and usually not associated with any significant haemorrhage there are **usually no signs of shock**, no pallor and only minimal epigastric tenderness. A **tachycardia** is often present. As the early signs of duodenal injury may be minimal the **diagnosis may be delayed**. Delay in treatment of a duodenal rupture by 24 hours is associated with a marked increase in morbidity and mortality. When there is a history of a **direct blow** to the epigastrium with **ongoing epigastric pain**; duodenal and pancreatic **trauma must be excluded early**.

Clues to the diagnosis may be leucocytosis, raised serum amylase or loss of the psoas shadow or retroperitoneal gas on a plain abdominal X-ray. A gastrograffin meal will determine if there is any duodenal rupture. A **dynamic enhanced CT scan** with oral contrast will usually define any duodenal rupture and also define any pancreatic trauma which can be graded and managed accordingly (haematoma/serosal tear to duodenal wall rupture or pancreatic duct disruption; laparotomy debridement/repair for latter one or two).

SMALL BOWEL AND COLON

Injuries to the small bowel and colon are **rare** following low velocity injuries, and are more commonly associated with a **very forceful blow** to the abdomen or a deceleration injury.

The injuries include serosal tears, rupture and mesenteric tears. The pain may be central, localised or generalised. There may be associated vomiting and abdominal distension. **Signs** include tachycardia, low grade fever and signs of localised or generalised peritonitis.

Initial management involves fluid resuscitation, analgesia and plain abdominal X-rays. Signs on X-ray include **free air** and **distended** or thick walled loops of bowel. Frequently, the X-rays are unremarkable. A CT scan may detect a bowel injury or blood in the peritoneal cavity that is otherwise unexplained. **The definitive management is laparotomy** and either repair or resection of the affected bowel segment. In the **presence of significant** abdominal signs or clinical deterioration, even if there are no abnormalities on CT scan, a **laparotomy is indicated.**

RECTUM AND ANUS

There are two specific types of anorectal injuries seen in athletes; **impaling** injury and injection of water under high pressure. Impaling is uncommon but involves falling directly onto an object that impales the anus and rectum. The injury may involve the anus alone, the rectum alone or both anus and rectum. Diagnosis is from the history. Examination of the perineum may reveal a skin tear, anal sphincter tear or may be normal. Further examination of the anus and rectum is best performed under a general anaesthetic to assess the injury fully. Broad spectrum antibiotics are given. Operative management essentially involves primary repair with or without a diverting colostomy.

Injection of water under pressure is an unusual injury that occurs in sports such as **water skiing**

where a fall astride allows water to be forced into the rectum under considerable pressure. This causes a **"blow out"** injury at the rectosigmoid junction. Patients present with a history of the fall followed by lower abdominal pain. This is a **tachycardia, fever and signs of peritonitis** in the lower abdomen. Diagnosis is with a gastrograffin enema, where the leak is demonstrated, usually at the recto-sigmoid junction. Management includes fluid resuscitation, analgesia and broad spectrum antibiotics. Operative management depends on the extent of the injury and degree of faecal contamination. The rectum requires debridement and may be repaired and a diverting colostomy formed. If the injury is severe, the rectum is debrided, oversewn and an end colostomy created. Colonic continuity is restored 3 to 6 months later.

KIDNEY

The history of the injury is a blow to the loin or front of the abdomen. There is usually loin pain, although with high velocity injuries to the front of the abdomen the pain is more wide spread, There may be macroscopic haematuria. The findings of examination depend on the extent of the injury. The observations are stable with mild to moderate loin tenderness and microscopic haematuria in association with a minor renal contusion. Patients with a shattered kidney are tachycardic, pale and shocked with marked loin tenderness and macroscopic haematuria. The absence of haematuria does not exclude a renal injury, particularly an injury to the vascular pedicle (Fig. 6).

Initial management involves resuscitation where necessary and analgesia. Imaging of the kidney is required either with an intravenous pyelogram (Fig. 7)

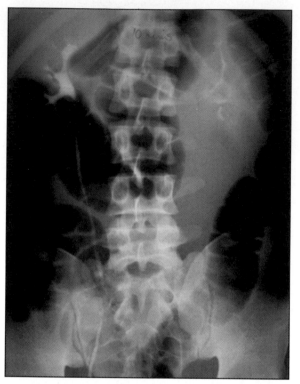

Figure 7 – Kidney trauma. 29-year-old soccer player was hit in the left loin with a knee. IVP reveals free extravasation of contrast from the collecting system

or an enhanced CT scan (better; as allows assessment of the spleen and liver as well). **Most injuries are minor** and include a contusion or small cortical tear with a subcapsular haematoma. These injuries can be managed **non-operatively**. **More extensive** injuries involving the pelvicaleal system or kidneys with multiple lacerations usually require **operative** intervention. If the patient is haemodynamically stable then referral to a urologist for definitive management is required. Those injuries requiring surgery may be repaired or managed with a partial nephrectomy. An **unstable patient** with a **renal injury** requires **urgent** surgery and often a nephrectomy.

BLADDER

Rupture of the urinary bladder occurs following a **blow** to the lower abdomen when the **bladder is full** or in association with a severe **pelvic fracture.** This is associated with lower abdomen pain, often an inability to void, and macroscopic haematuria. There is lower abdominal tenderness and there may be a fullness that is dull to percussion. When the diagnosis is

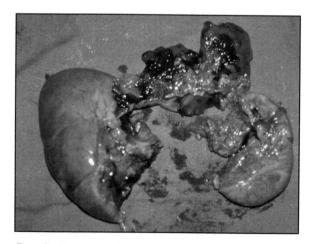

Figure 6 – Shattered, avulsed kidney (details Fig. 3)

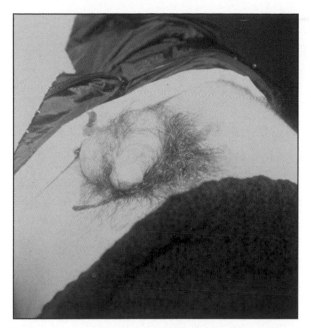

Figure 8 – Ruptured membranous urethra in a skier who straddled a waist high ski pole and shattered his pelvis. Note tell-tale blood at urethral meatus

suspected a urinary catheter should be inserted and broad spectrum antibiotics administered. Macroscopic haematuria is invariably seen. Diagnosis is with a **retrograde cystogram** with either pre-peritoneal or intraperitoneal extravasation of contrast. Management is operative repair and prolonged catheter drainage.

MALE URETHRA

The membranous urethra is injured in a **fall astride** and presents with perineal pain, inability to void and blood at the **urethral meatus** (Fig. 8). There is often a perineal or scrotal haematoma, marked perineal tenderness and blood at the urethral meatus. **Do not insert** a urethral catheter. Management is to perform a **retrograde urethragram** to assess the injury. If there is **no** urethral disruption, a catheter is carefully inserted. If there is **urethral disruption** but there is a delay in urological management, a **suprapubic** catheter is inserted with broad spectrum antibiotics.

SCROTUM AND TESTIS

A direct blow to the scrotum is a painful and not infrequent sports injury. The majority of blows do not produce a serious injury. Occasionally there may be a scrotal haematoma or rupture of the testis. This presents with persistent pain and swelling following a

blow to the scrotum. An ultrasound of the scrotum distinguishes between a scrotal haematoma, which can be managed non-operatively and a testicular rupture that requires surgical exploration. A ruptured testis is explored in order to ensure the testis is viable and to repair the injury (Fig. 9).

Torsion of testis may be intermittent, incomplete or complete (Fig. 10). Intermittent, incomplete torsion presents with episodic, unilateral testicular pain during exercise (relieved by scrotal manipulation), exclude horizontally lying testis which requires bilateral orchidopexy. Complete testicular torsion presents with sudden severe testicular pain that does not settle (often with a history of minor trauma). Swollen tender testis. Urgent surgical exploration required. Do not waste time imaging the testis (high false negatives).

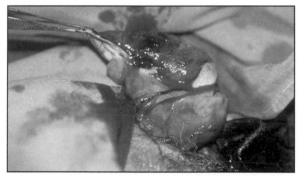

Figure 9 – Testicular rupture.
An 18-year-old man presents after being hit in the scrotum whilst fielding in an indoor cricket match. Urgent exploration (after an ultrasound) revealed a large testicular rupture, with a viable testis that was debrided and repaired

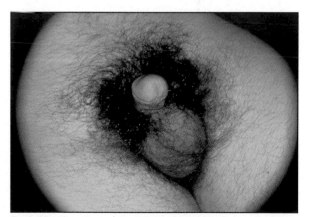

Figure 10 – Torsion (complete) of the left testis in a skier after skiing the moguls

UNCONSCIOUS PATIENT

The clinical assessment of the abdomen in the uncon-scious injured patient is **difficult** as many of the **clinical signs are absent** due to the unconscious state. Clearly if the patient is **shocked with abdomi-nal distension** or other evidence of an abdominal injury an **urgent laparotomy** is required. When the **unconscious patient is haemodynamically stable** without any overt evidence of an abdominal injury, an abdominal injury must be excluded by either a diagnostic **peritoneal** lavage or an abdominal **CT** scan. A CT scan is often preferred as the patient requires a CT of the head to assess the head injury. A CT can also determine the degree of injury, particularly to the liver or spleen, allowing a decision of non-operative management to be made whereas a positive diagnostic peritoneal lavage requires that a laparotomy be performed, even though the injury may be minor. If the patient is **deteriorating from a head injury, then time should not be wasted** performing a CT of the abdomen and a diagnostic peritoneal lavage is performed.

HEATSTROKE, HEAT EXHAUSTION

A severe episode of heatstroke may be associated with **renal failure** secondary to acute tubular necrosis. This may be prevented by rapid, early aggressive fluid resuscitation of the heatstroke patient. However, once established, it requires careful management in a high dependency unit and may require a brief period of haemodialysis prior to recovery of the renal function.

Hepatic dysfunction or even acute hepatic failure may occur in association with heatstroke. This usually starts 24 hours after the episode of collapse and presents with abnormal liver function tests and jaundice. It may progress to fulminant hepatic failure. Treatment is support of the circulation, coagulation and respiration in an intensive care unit.

HAEMATURIA

Macroscopic haematuria may occur after strenuous exercise and is often recurrent in an individual. It is usually of no significance, but if it is of concern to the athlete can be investigated with urine microscopy, culture and an intravenous pyelogram (invariably normal).

Part III

Special Circumstances

17

THE FEMALE ATHLETE

Grace Bryant
Cindy Mak
Kerwyn Foo

INTRODUCTION

Women now compete in many sporting and recreational activities. They participate for various reasons, from an interest in "keeping fit" to the seriously competitive.

Nearly 50% of the Australian Olympic Team in 1996 were female. The female athlete was initially excluded from participating in the modern Olympics. Baron Pierre de Coubertin considered "women's sports against the law of nature".

Most sporting endeavours were considered too gruelling for females. In the 1928 Olympics 11 females started the 800m race, 5 dropped out during the race, 5 collapsed at the finish line and the remaining competitor collapsed in the dressing room. The event was considered too strenuous and dropped from the programme. It only returned in the 1960's. Despite this negative feeling and the fact women were actively discouraged to train, women continued to fight for their right to compete.

Today there are many opportunities provided to women in sports and they are now encouraged to participate in regular physical activity.

Australia in recent years has produced many world

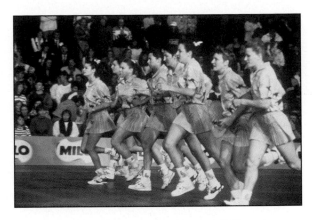

Figure 1 – World Champion Australian Netball Team (courtesy Country Wide Photographic Services)

class athletes, including Dawn Fraser (swimming), Kay Cottee (yachting), Yvonne (Goolagong) Cawley (tennis), Michelle Martin (squash), Michallie Jones (triathlon), Shelley Taylor-Smith (marathon swimming) and the Australian Netball Team (Fig. 1).

With increasing numbers participating in sport, a number of concerns specific to the female athlete have been identified.

Anatomical and physiological differences do exist between men and women (Fig. 2).

ANATOMICAL AND PHYSIOLOGICAL DIFFERENCES BETWEEN MEN AND WOMEN

Women

Men

Anatomical

lower centre of mass
smaller body frame
more varus at hips/femoral
anteversion→*greater Q angle*
wider pelvis
greater valgus at elbows, knees

taller
limbs longer relative to height
larger thoracic cavity, lung, and heart size
wider shoulders
longer humerus

Physiological

higher body **fat**
more surface area per kg
(affects heat conduction rate)
smaller maximum cardiac output

higher muscle mass
more blood volume/red cells/haemoglobin
higher VO_{2max}

Figure 2 – The basic physiological and anatomical differences between men and women

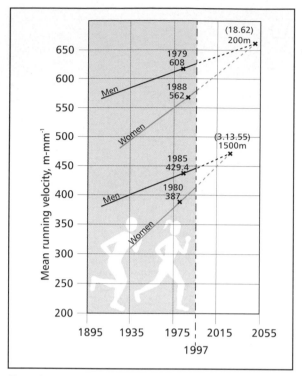

Figure 3 – Men's and women's world records are converging (as women's progression is more rapid). Predicted times for 200 m and 1500 m. Women may overtake men

It is not known whether women's performances will equal men's in every event. They already lead in endurance swimming and are gaining in running events (Fig. 3).

GYNAECOLOGIC CONCERNS

MENSTRUAL CRAMPS

Dysmenorrhoea (menstrual cramps) is abdominal pain associated with uterine contractions or ischaemia during menstruation, and is caused by prostaglandin release by the endometrium. It may adversely affect training or competition. In most women, the symptoms are mild but can be quite disabling in some with the severe painful cramping occurring on day one or day two of the menstrual bleed. It can also be associated with a heavy flow.

There is no reason to avoid exercising at any time during the menstrual cycle. Exercise may actually have a beneficial effect in relieving the incidence of the cramps either because of the exercise related hormonal effects on the uterus or the increased release of Beta endorphins.

If the symptoms are mild, simple analgesics or even nothing is appropriate. If the symptoms are moderate or severe then antiprostagladin medication such as naproxen sodium or ibuprofen are helpful in reducing symptoms by limiting the release of the prostaglandins. They are most effective if taken 24 to 48 hours before the onset of the menses. The oral contraceptive pill (OCP) is also effective in reducing severity of symptoms.

PRE MENSTRUAL TENSION

Pre menstrual tension (PMT) relates to a group of symptoms beginning at ovulation and improving with the onset of menstruation. Symptoms are both emotional and physical (Fig. 4).

These may affect daily activity as well as athletic activity. Regular exercise may decrease the severity or eliminate PMT. This may result from neuro-transmitter changes that decrease the pulse frequency of gonadotrophin releasing hormone (GNRH) or an increase in central Beta endorphin. The PMS symptoms may return if athletic activity is reduced by injury or reduced training. Athletes tend to be particularly distressed by the symptoms associated with fluid retention.

Treatment of PMS is aimed at preventing ovulation and the development of the corpus luteum. OCP's can be effective but unpredictable as some women report an increase in symptoms. Pyridoxine (Vit B6) 200 to 600 mg per day for up to 2 weeks has been used to decrease the fluid, breast tenderness and depressive symptoms. A diuretic agent can also reduce the fluid retention, however it increases the risk of dehydration. For athletes that undergo drug testing for their sporting organisation, diuretics are on the banned list produced by the International Olympic Committee and should not be prescribed.

SYMPTOMS OF PMT	
Emotional	**Physical**
mood swings	headaches
anxiety	fluid retention
depression	bloating
irritability	breast soreness
insomnia	breast enlargement
alteration in libido	appetite changes
	fatigue

Figure 4 – Symptoms of pre-menstrual tension.

CONTRACEPTION

The needs of the female athlete are similar to the general population. The choice of suitable agent should consider her coital frequency, fertility plans and medical history. Athletes who have menstrual irregularity or amenorrhoea should still use contraceptive methods as the condition may resolve spontaneously and can result in an unexpected pregnancy.

Mechanical barrier methods are popular choices. The diaphragm must be left in place for at least 6 hours after the last sexual encounter. It may still be in place at times of training or competition. This should pose no problems but, if uncomfortable, the athlete should be fitted with a small size which will be equally effective as a contraceptive.

The use of condoms should be encouraged for "safe sex" acting to prevent the transmission of sexually transmitted diseases like genital herpes, genital warts, hepatitis B and HIV. The effectiveness of a condom as a contraceptive device is increased with the concurrent use of a spermicidal gel or cream.

Intra uterine devices (IUD's) impose a slight risk of pelvic infection and as such may alter future fertility. They are therefore not recommended for those who wish children later. The IUD is a good choice for female athletes who have regular sex and have completed child bearing and are willing to take a small risk of infection. Women with more than one partner have a somewhat higher risk of acquiring such infections. IUD's may be associated with more cramping and heavier bleeding, either of which may affect performance.

"Natural" methods of contraception (rhythm method, basal temperature and mucus status) are widely used. In female athletes with menstrual irregularities these methods are unreliable.

ORAL CONTRACEPTION

Oral contraceptive pills (OCP) are commonly used for contraception. Most OCP's contain a combination of oestrogen and progesterone. There are many preparations available in monophasic, biphasic and triphasic formulations. The low dose OCP frequently used now has less side effects than the older preparations. Side effects include a potential for weight gain and fluid retention, breakthrough bleeding, alteration in carbohydrate metabolism, adverse changes in clotting factors and platelet functions.

The use of OCP can have some beneficial effects (Fig. 5). They can help decrease premenstrual symptoms and decrease breast volume changes that occur in the second half of the menstrual cycle. OCP use can also decrease menstrual flow and thus reduce menstrually induced iron deficiency. OCP's can regulate the menstrual cycle, decrease dysmenorrhoea and act as a hormonal replacement and thus preserve bone density in women with chronic amenorrhoea. Studies have shown some reduced incidence of endometrial and ovarian cancers, benign breast lesions, pelvic inflammatory disease, ovarian cysts and ectopic pregnancy in women who take OCP.

The effect of OCP on athletic performance is as yet undetermined. Further studies are required, but apart from subtle changes in some cardiorespiratory and metabolic variables, no significant effect on athletic performance has been found.

Contraindications to the use of OCP occurs in 2-3% of the female population. These include pregnancy, smokers over 35 years of age, undiagnosed abnormal uterine bleeding, previous thromboembolic event, breast cancer, oestrogen dependant cancers, active liver disease, intestinal malabsorption disease, uncontrolled hypertension, diabetes with vascular complications and arterial vascular disease.

BENEFITS AND DISADVANTAGES OF OCP USE IN ATHLETES	
The Oral Contraceptive Pill	
BENEFITS	DISADVANTAGES
Reduced dysmenorrhoea	Water retention
Manipulation of the menstrual cycle for competition purposes	Altered glucose metabolism (by the progestin component)
A source of oestrogen for amenorrhoeic athletes	Possible decreased VO_{2max}
May reduce the risk of iron deficiency anaemia (via reduced blood loss)	

Figure 5 – Benefits and disadvantages of OCP use in athlete

MANIPULATION OF THE MENSTRUAL CYCLE

For athletes who feel that their performance is affected during the premenstrual or menstrual phase and wish to avoid their menses, monphasic OCP's can be used to manipulate the onset of menses so they do not occur during a major athletic competition or event.

The OCP can be stopped 7 to 10 days before the event to induce a withdrawal bleed early. The OCP can then be started at the end of menstruation or after the athletic event. If there is a delay in starting the next packet of OCP, ovulation may not be suppressed so additional barrier methods of contraception are advised for the first 2 weeks on recommencing the OCP.

Alternatively, the athlete can skip the 7 day sugar tablet interval and continuing into the next packet thus preventing the withdrawal bleed (menstruation).

For those female athletes not on OCP's, a bleed can be induced 10 days prior to the athletic competition by taking progesterone for 10 days, finishing 10 days prior to the event.

MENSTRUAL HYGIENE

Previously, social attitudes were to avoid training or competition during menstruation. Some cultural beliefs and taboos still exist. It is now known that no ill effect will occur if the athlete continues to participate during menstruation. Tampon use is popular amongst athletes and allows exercise to continue, including water sports.

BREAST

The breast is mainly composed of fatty tissues and contains no muscle. Its size and shape is primarily determined by genetic factors. The breast may increase in size with response to hormonal stimulation gaining up to 40% in the premenstrual period. There is no medical reason to wear a brassiere while exercising and many small-breasted women do not but generally large-breasted athletes are more comfortable wearing one. Excessive movement of the breasts is best prevented with a specialised sports brassiere with limited movement in all directions but which is still comfortable to wear during exercise and rest. It should be individually fitted and should be made with firm, mostly non elastic material that has good absorptive ability. There should be no seams or ridges across the nipples and hooks or fasteners covered. Certain contact sports may be require that the provision for padding be designed into a bra. Plastic "cup" protec-

tion can be required in collision sports like football and martial arts.

The nipple is composed mainly of muscle fibres that respond to cold and tactile stimulation. **Runners' nipple** occurs when the tissue is irritated by rubbing against clothing during activity, particularly in cold weather conditions. It is actually more common in males. It can be prevented by taping across the nipple, applying petroleum jelly, wearing a seamless brassiere, and wearing appropriate clothing. Trauma to the breast is not common but a direct blow can result in a contusion. The bleeding and swelling can be reduced by ice, analgesia and compressive support. The athlete should be reassured that there is no evidence that breast trauma is associated with development of breast cancer.

MENSTRUAL CYCLE AND PERFORMANCE

Early study results are inconsistent with regard to the effect of particular menstrual phase on athletic performance. World records have been set in any phase of the menstrual cycle.

Athletes though, tend to report feeling that their worst performances are during the premenstrual phase or at the time of the menstrual phase.

Studies now have a more scientific basis, with hormonal measurements of serum progesterone to confirm the luteal phase. These are limited and small in number. It is still conceivable that the hormonal alterations of an ovulatory menstrual cycle may impact on some aspect of athletic performance, especially at an elite level or for an individual athlete. Further research is proceeding.

EXERCISE AND THE MENSTRUAL CYCLE

Disorders of the menstrual cycle and their relationship to exercise has been extensively reviewed. Incidences reported range from 5-50%.

Types of irregularities:

- Delayed menarche
- Menstrual dysfunction

This appears to occur along a continuum of progressive severity:

1. luteal phase deficiency
2. an ovulatory cycle with normal oestrogen levels
3. secondary amenorrhoea - low oestrogen levels

DELAYED MENARCHE

In Australia the average age of menarche, (the onset of menses) is 12 to 13 years. This occurs 1 to 2 years after the puberty growth spurt occurs.

In the pre-menarche years, a combination of factors including intense exercise and low body weight may affect the hypothalamic axis, resulting in a delay in the onset of menarche. A genetic component is also considered to be present. The development of the breasts and the onset of menses is delayed but not the development of pubic hair.

Two groups of high performance athletes with delayed menarche exist. Those who exercised intensely prior to menarche and those who did not.

Some studies suggest delayed menarche confers an athletic advantage with the inherited tendency for a slower rate of maturation resulting in a delayed closure of epiphyseal growth plates (longer legs, narrow hips, relatively less body fat). Girls with this physique may be socialised into intense training.

OLIGOMENORRHOEA AND SECONDARY AMENORRHOEA

Oligomenorrhoea - irregular menses

Secondary amenorrhoea - the cessation of spontaneous menstruation for 6 months or more after normal menstrual cycle established.

Incidence varies with different population:

• 5% general population

• 10-20% athletic population (overall)

• 50% endurance athletes.

The diagnosis of exercise-induced amenorrhoea is made by exclusion. It is associated with a reduction of pulse frequency of LH and lower levels of oestrogen and progesterone.

The menstrual cycle has endocrinological coordination by the hypothalamus, pituitary and ovarian follicles. When menstrual dysfunction occurs, the aetiology is not one, but multiple causes, with the hypothalamic-pituitary-gonadal axis playing the key role. Endocrine changes and alteration of the axis occurs with training, diet, stress and other factors not fully clarified (Fig. 6). Other causes of amenorrhoea are listed (Fig. 7).

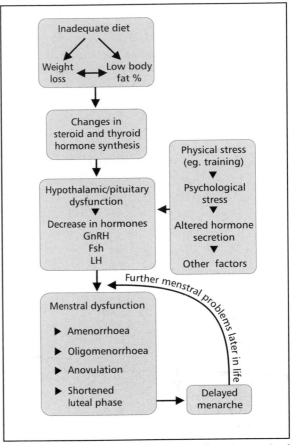

Figure 6 – Proposed factors for the mechanism of exercise-associated amenorrhoea

MOST COMMON CAUSES OF SECONDARY AMENORRHOEA

Pregnancy

Psychological stress

Anorexia nervosa/athletica

Polycystic ovaries

Thyroid disorders

Drug use

Medications

Other medical conditions
- pituitary tumour
- hypothalamic exercise induced

Figure 7 – Most common causes of secondary amenorrhoea

Recently, researchers have further investigated luteal length by studying the hypothalamic - pituitary - adrenal axis. Catecholamines, cortisol and Beta endorphins are all elevated with exercise. Prolactin, LH and FSH are lower in strenuous activity. They speculate that the catecholamines elevated by exercise may interact to suppress LH release of the hypothalamic - pituitary axis.

Overall, reviews suggests that the decreased activity of the GnRH pulse generator in the hypothalamus is the likely cause of decreased gonadotrophin release leading to amenorrhoea. This inhibition of the GnRH pulse generator may occur with activation of the adrenal axis, which is inevitable with strenuous, prolonged exercise.

Factors that may contribute are:

Level of Exercise

There appears to be a relationship between the incidence and severity of menstrual dysfunction and the level of exercise (total amount and intensity).

Strenuous activity may disrupt the menstrual cycle. On decreasing the level of exercise, the menses return and disappear again if intense exercise is reintroduced.

It is thought that exercise, as a form of stress itself or by action of hormones released during exercise (e.g. endorphins, cortisol) affects the hypothalamic - pituitary - axis.

Low Body Fat

An association exists between low levels of body fat and menstrual irregularity. It was previously thought by researchers that a critical percentage of body fat was required for both onset and maintenance of menses. This has now been disproven. Much individual variation exists for their critical level. If the body fat level is increased, the menses tend to return.

Restricted Diets

Nutritional deficiency, including low caloric intake and inadequate nutrient intake is thought to be a factor contributing menstrual irregularity. This may be a direct effect or result from the decreased levels of body fat that occur with such practices.

Stress

Psychological stress can present from many sources. From the sport, relationships, travel, work, school and family. These can be real or perceived expectations and stresses.

Immaturity of the Reproductive System

Menstrual irregularities are more common in the young. The "immature" system is more susceptible when the previously discussed factors are present. That is, those with a history of delayed menarche, irregular menses and no prior pregnancy are more vulnerable.

CYCLE PHASE DYSFUNCTION

ABNORMAL LUTEAL PHASES

Any condition affecting menstrual function appears to affect the luteal phase first.

The luteal phase is the time from ovulation to the onset of the menstrual bleed. It is usually 14 days long and associated with high levels of both oestrogen and progesterone. With luteal phase deficiency it is shortened to less than 10 days duration and a lower than normal progesterone level. These are common in athletes and often not recognised as the female may have a cycle of normal length due to associated lengthening of the follicular phase.

Luteal phase defects are associated with decreased luteinizing hormone (LH) pulsatility.

ANOVULATORY CYCLES

With continued progression, anovulation can occur despite normal oestrogen levels. This is associated with changes in LH pulsatility and consequently lower than normal progesterone levels during the luteal phase. These are very common in the athlete and often missed because the athlete is unaware of any menstrual change.

There appears to be a direct relationship between the levels of exercise and luteal phase defects. Even at recreational training levels of 20 - 30 km/wk, subtle hormone changes associated with a short luteal phase occur.

The main effect of this is infertility and subfertility.

Also, theoretically, in the environment of low progesterone levels, inadequate endometrial protection, endometrical hyperplasma and increased risk of adenocarcinoma can occur. This has not been reported clinically.

SIGNIFICANCE OF MENSTRUAL DYSFUNCTION

There are two major problems that can occur as a result of menstrual dysfunction:

• reduced fertility and reduced bone mass

The female athlete triad of amenorrhoea, eating disorders and osteoporosis is also reflected.

FERTILITY

The incidence of infertility in the general population is 3%. Whilst exercising intensely, the female athlete has an increased incidence of decreased fertility. Whether ovulation is occurring can be assessed by taking the basal body temperature and looking for the rise in temperature that occurs at ovulation. The presence of premenstrual tension and mid cycle pain are other indicators that ovulation has occurred.

If pregnancy is desired, the athlete is recommended to decrease the level of their activity and to increase their body fat level. If ovulation does not occur or menses return, referral to a gynaecologist is recommended for assessment and management and probably initiation of ovulation by pharmaceutical means.

The amenorrhoeic female should not assume they cannot fall pregnant and should be encouraged in the use of contraceptive methods.

Consequences of menstrual irregularity:

• Reduced bone mass

Initially, menstrual dysfunction in athletes was thought to be totally reversible on decreasing or stopping training and that no short or long term health risks occurred. It is now known that a hypoestrogenic state contributes to significant bone mineral loss. In the young, adequate oestrogen and calcium levels have a significant role in the development of the peak adult bone mass.

Adolescent amenorrhoea and the related low level of oestrogen predispose the women to reduced bone mineral accretion and even bone loss regardless of calcium intake. The loss is similar to that which occurs after menopause, with trabecular bone being more affected than cortical. The rate of loss is rapid in the first 2-3 years following the loss of oestrogen (about 4% loss rate per day). During subsequent years the loss is at a slower rate. On resumption of their menses, the athlete may not completely replace this loss and thus may develop premature osteoporosis or have an increased risk of osteoporosis.

The bone mineral density in oligo/amenorrhoea athletes has been found to be lower than eumenorrhoeic athletes.

Moderate level exercise, especially weight bearing exercise, has a positive effect on bone. This can be mediated through the skeletal loading and dynamic pull of muscles or the bones. However, in athletes with low oestrogen levels, this can offset the beneficial effect the exercise has on bone mineral content and despite the exercise the density can be reduced.

Also, in women with amenorrhoea there is a higher prevalence of lower extremity stress fractures.

THE FEMALE TRIAD

The female triad refers to the interrelationships of disordered eating, amenorrhoea and osteoporosis (Fig. 8).

The true prevalence of the triad is not known due to under-reporting of symptoms or denial of any problem existing.

A relationship exists between disordered eating and intense athletic activity. This is particularly seen in sports where physical appearance is important, those where leanness is desirable and those using weight classifications. These sports include gymnastics, figure skating, endurance running, rowing and weight lifting.

Disordered eating behaviours can range from mild to severe. The severe eating disorder anorexia nervosa is strictly defined. 0.5-1% of the population fulfil the criteria. However, unnecessary dieting as well as binge

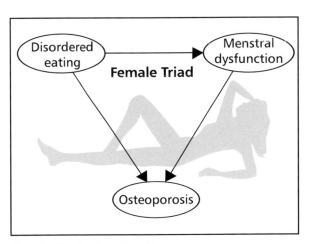

Figure 8 – The Female Athlete Triad

TYPES OF EATING DISORDERS			
	Anorexia Nervosa	**Bulimia Nervosa**	**Eating Disorder not otherwise Specified**
Diagnostic criteria	**A.** Refuses to maintain body weight at or near normal (for age/height)	**A.** Recurrent binge eating - consuming large amounts in a single period, with loss control	Disorders of eating that do not meet criteria for a specific eating disorder. Examples: • Anorexia Nervosa criteria with regular menses; or weight loss, but in normal range
	B. Intense fear of gaining weight/becoming fat, even when underweight	**B.** Recurrent inappropriate compensatory behaviour to prevent weight gain (purging*)	• Bulimia Nervosa with lower frequency/ duration
	C. Disturbed way of evaluating own body weight or shape with denial of seriousness	**C.** Binge and compensation ≥2/week for 3 months	• Binge eating without inappropriate compensation
	D. Amenorrhoea (in post menarchal females)	**D.** Self-evaluation distorted	• Inappropriate compensation after small amount of food
	*Purging – self induced vomiting, misuse of laxatives, diuretics, enemas.		**Nonpurging –** other methods such as fasting and excessive exercise.

Figure 9 – A spectrum of eating disorders exists. The primary disorders are anorexia nervosa, bulimia nervosa and eating disorder not otherwise specified (NOS). These are defined in the Diagnostic and Statistical Manual of Mental Disorders (DSM-IV).

eating and purging ("disordered eating") are much more common (Fig. 9).

Suspicion of the existence of disordered eating is important. It is possible to differentiate between primary and secondary disorders. A clinical feature of both is that there is a strong exercise component expressed by intensive or highly ritualised daily activities.

In primary conditions, exercise is a method for expression of the disorder whilst in secondary, the disordered eating is a result of participating in competitive athletic activities. A low weight is seen as ideal for optimum performance.

Concerns about weight arise and subsequently unhealthy weight control practices may occur (Fig. 10). These practices include self-induced vomiting (bulimia), laxative abuse, use of diet pills and diuretics.

Eating disorders can result in semi-starvation and dehydration. This results in decreased performance and impaired general health. These disordered patterns may involve a whole team or individuals and

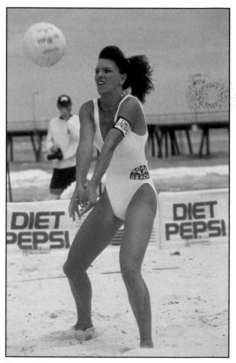

Figure 10 – There is an increased incidence of disordered eating where there is a large focus on body image and thinness as a desirable feature (beach volleyball). (*Courtesy of Country Wide Photographic Services*)

may be the result of pressure from coaches, parents, fellow competitors or the individual. Body image distortion and anorexic-like behaviour may occur during training but resolve when the season finishes.

MANAGEMENT

Recognition and prevention are the mainstays of care for the female athlete in this situation. Awareness of the signs of disordered eating (like going to the toilet immediately after eating and coming back "moist" eyed) awareness of weight loss, changes in eating habits and excessive preoccupation with food and weight.

Management of eating disorders is difficult. The females may have distorted body image (think they are fat when they are thin), be excessively thin, amenorrhoeal and may present with a stress fracture. Management may require a specialist multidisciplinary approach.

TREATMENT OF MENSTRUAL DYSFUNCTION

Before initiating treatment for any menstrual dysfunction, the cause of the condition must be determined.

A thorough clinical assessment is required to exclude other causes, for one should not assume that the menstrual irregularity is the result of the participation in sports. All other potential causes of menstrual dysfunction, including pregnancy, must be excluded. These include gynaecological conditions like polycystic ovaries, endocrine conditions (pituitary, thyroid), psychological stress (grief, depression etc) and medications (post OCP).

DELAYED MENARCHE

If no menstruation has occurred by 16 years of age investigations should be considered. A thorough examination and detailed history is essential to exclude any genetic, gynaecological, neurological or endocrine disorders (e.g. pituitary, adrenal, thyroid).

EXAMINATION/HISTORY

- Weight changes
- Secondary sexual characteristics
- Virilizing changes
- Medications
- Pregnant
- Psychological stress
- Family history – if delayed menarche or chromosomal disorders
- Assess visual fields and visual activity
- Pelvic examination (if not sexually active a transabdominal ultrasound)
- Blood tests – initial tests should include prolactin, TSH, urine pregnancy test (if sexually active)

A progesterone challenge test of a 5 day course of medroxyprogesterone acetate (Provera) will result in a withdrawal bleed if adequate oestrogen is present. More specifically, sufficient gonadotrophins are being produced to stimulate the ovaries, the ovaries have functioning tissue that develops into follicles and the follicles can produce oestrogen that results in endometrial growth and the ability to bleed. This usually occurs within 5 days of ceasing the tablets but can be up to 14 days. If no bleed occurs, then a low level of oestrogen is present or no uterus or an obstructed genital tract.

The next test is FSH/LH levels. High levels are associated with ovarian failure or resistance and further evaluation for chromosomal abnormality or immune disorders is required. Very low levels of less than 10 IU/litre can be associated with pituitary or hypothalamic causes or tumour. Delayed menarche secondary to intense exercise is characterised by low FSH and LH.

After determining no structural or endocrine abnormality is present, the delay can then be attributed to the exercise level. The athlete and her parents can be reassured and advised that by reducing the exercise intensity or frequency and/or slightly increasing the body fat, menstruation will probably result. If no change occurs in 6 months or the athlete is unwilling to change exercise level then replacement of oestrogen in the form of the oral contraceptive pill (OCP) or hormonal replacement therapy (HRT) is advised, as evidence shows that bone mineralisation loss is maximum in the first 2-3 years of the hypo-oestrogenic state.

OLIGIO/AMENORRHOEA

A thorough clinical assessment as described previously is essential.

Investigations should include a pregnancy test, prolactin, thyroid function tests, oestrogen, FSH and LH. With exercise induced amenorrhoea, a low oestrogen level and low LH and FSH is present.

Alternatively, a progesterone challenge test can be performed before LH/FSH as described for delayed menarche. Bone density studies are indicated if the amenorrhoea has been present more than 1 year or after stress fractures are present.

TREATMENT

The oestrogen levels need to be improved for bone health. The athlete should be advised that if the level of exercise is reduced and an increase in percent body fat occurs then generally the menses spontaneously return within 1 to 2 months. If they do not wish to reduce their exercise load then oestrogen replacement is advised. This should begin as early as possible as bone mineralisation loss is maximum in the first 2 to 3 years of amenorrhoea and with resumption of menses or oestrogen replacement, replenishment of the lost bone mass may occur. If the low oestrogen levels have been present for more than 3 years the oestrogen may not restore the loss but works towards preventing further loss. Oestrogen replacement can be in the form of OCP or HRT (conjugated oestrogen 0.625 mg for day 1 to 25 and medroxy progesterone acetate 5 mg day 14 to 25). Oestrogen replacement is contraindicated in certain clinical situations e.g. hypertension, abnormal liver function tests, past history of deep venous thrombosis, and cancer of the breast or endrometrium. Adequate calcium is also important in hypoestrogenic females for bone mass.

LUTEAL PHASE DYSFUNCTION

ANOVULATORY CYCLES

An early form of menstrual dysfunction is anovulation. Anovulation can occur despite normal oestrogen levels. This is associated with changes in LH pulsatility and consequent lower than normal progesterone levels during the luteal phase. These are very common in the athlete and often missed because the athlete is unaware of any menstrual change. An investigation to see whether an abnormality exists is to take the basal body temperature. At ovulation, the temperature increases by 0.2 to 0.6 degrees Celsius and remains throughout the luteal phase. If the next menses occurs less than 10 days after the rise then luteal phase inadequacy probably exists. No treatment is required unless the woman wishes to become pregnant.

PARTICIPATION OF THE PREGNANT ATHLETE IN CONTACT AND COLLISION SPORTS

Female athletes are increasingly seeking to continue sporting activities once pregnant (Fig. 11). Exercise programs should be individualised. Generally exercise is able to be continued and should be encouraged, at a mild to moderate level, during pregnancy as long as the pregnancy is uncomplicated.

GUIDELINES

Generally pregnancy is not a time to commence a new sporting or strenuous programme other than a mild one. Pregnancy itself is a training state. Maintenance of fitness should be the goal.

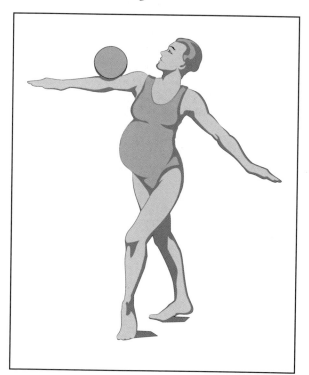

Figure 11 – Pregnant athlete. Individualised exercise programs are fine for uncomplicated pregnancies as long as the exercise is at a mid to moderate level

Guidelines currently available are generally conservative and aimed at the recreational athlete who wishes to gain health benefits both physically and mentally (Fig. 12). Higher levels of exercise activity may be safe for females already conditioned to aerobic activities when they become pregnant. The competitive athlete who wishes to maintain reasonably high levels of exercise should be counselled individually. Discomfort usually forces them to reduce training at about 6 months gestation or some change to water based exercises.

SUMMARY OF RECOMMENDATIONS OF PARTICIPATION OF THE PREGNANT ATHLETE

- Pregnant women are advised not to commence a new competitive sport during their pregnancy.
- Pregnant sportswomen should consult closely with their doctors whilst continuing with sporting participation especially if playing high risk contact or collision sports.
- The pregnant sportswoman should advise their coach, trainer or fitness leader of their pregnancy so that training can be modified accordingly.
- Pregnant sportswomen need to be aware that participation in contact or collision sports carries risks for herself and the unborn child.
- Under the supervision of her doctor the pregnant sportswoman with high levels of fitness and a normal pregnancy may continue participation into the second trimester in non contact and limited contact sports.
- Pregnant sportswomen should avoid overheating (body core temperature > 38°C) especially in the first trimester.
- If any medical or obstetric complication should occur, the sportswoman should consider changing to lower risk activities e.g. non contact sports like swimming and walking as the pregnancy advances.
- Pregnant sportswomen should not attempt to increase the level of their training or exercise at any stage during pregnancy.

Pregnant sportswomen need to pay special attention to:

- a thorough warm up and cool down
- consumption of adequate fluids before, during and after participation
- regulation of intensity (heart rate) at times of maximal exertion so that it does not exceed 140 beats per minute for more than 15 min.

With permission: Reprinted from Guidelines issued by the Medicine and Science for Women in Sport committee of the Australian Sports Medicine Federation May1994.

Figure 12 – Guidelines for participation of pregnant women in sport (from Australian Sports Commission 1994)

No one type of exercise is recommended. Walking and jogging are popular in early pregnancy. Cycling has the advantage of being non weight bearing but in later pregnancy an exercise bike would be recommended due to the altered balance and the risk of falls. In aerobic classes certain exercises may need to be modified like avoiding exercising supine. Low impact classes are recommended. Water exercises are popular also.

PHYSIOLOGICAL CONCERNS

Physiological changes occur throughout pregnancy and these may expose the fetus and/or mother to increased dangers.

Factors to consider:

- Overheating
- Level of exertion
- Risk of injury
- Health status
- Stage of pregnancy

OVERHEATING

Research on animals suggest that maternal core temperatures greater than 39 degrees Celsius are associated with neural tube defects in the fetus. The malformation is a result of the failure of the neural tube to close at about 25 days post conception. In humans, illness induced hyperthermia in the first trimester has been associated with fetal growth retardation, intra uterine death and neural abnormality. There is little evidence that exercise causes such problems. Studies and anecdotal cases of exercising females do not report any increase in congenital anomalies.

However the pregnant female should be advised to avoid hyperthermia. She should not train or compete during the hottest times of the day. She should maintain adequate fluid intake both before, during and after activity. Light, absorbent, loose clothing helps cooling. If exercising indoors it should be well ventilated and cool. The pregnant female should avoid the use of spas and saunas. Moderate exercise in a normal environment results in minimal increases in body core temperature.

Increased maternal plasma volume (up to 50%) during pregnancy may help to maintain optimal fetomaternal heat transfer and dissipation.

LEVEL OF EXERTION

A high level of fitness throughout pregnancy does not appear to either positively or negatively affect the birth outcome. However, women are generally advised not to increase their level of activity once pregnant. Pregnancy is generally not a time to begin a new sport.

High intensity training or competition greater than 80% of maximum heart rate may affect fetal oxygen supply although this has not been conclusively shown in humans. There have been reports of changes of fetal heart rate during exercise (tachycardia and bradycardia) and also reports of fetal bradycardia on ceasing maximal intensity exercise. The uterine blood flow is increased during pregnancy but is decreased during exercise due to shunting from "splanchnic organs to exercising muscles". However, blood flow to the uterus is maximum at the area of placental attachment and therefore there is reduced hypoxic effect on the fetus.

Observed birth outcomes following circumstances of altered fetal heart rate have been normal but it is recommended that the pregnant athlete should avoid maximal intensity exercise and they should exercise at moderate levels of less than 75% of maximum heart rate. The total duration of the session should be about 45 min incorporating an adequate warm up and cool down, three or four times per week and the period of higher activity within the session should be no longer than 20-30 min.

There is a theoretical risk of premature labour associated with maternal exercise due to increased levels of circulating noradrenaline and this may result in increased uterine irritability and premature labour. This is not observed in practice.

RISK OF INJURY

Redistribution of body weight and centre of gravity can alter the athletes sense of balance and this can lead to an increase in falls. The uterus rises out of the pelvis after the first trimester (3 months). A blow to or fall upon the abdomen could damage the placenta. This could have disastrous consequences. Later in pregnancy there is also a greater risk of damage to the fetus itself from direct impact during sport. The athlete should err on the side of caution whilst exercising.

With water skiing, a fall may force water up the vagina and result in an increased risk of miscarriage or intra-uterine infection. Water skiing should be avoided.

Scuba diving is associated with an increase in nitrogen bubbles and linked with an increased risk of teratogenicity. Hence scuba diving should also be avoided.

Additionally, the athlete is at a higher risk of ligament and bone injury due to increased laxity of the joints during pregnancy. Lower back pain is common. This results from circulating oestrogen and relaxin. It is generally advised that hyperextension exercises, avoid abrupt changes in direction and ballistic movements are avoided. The incidence of lower back pain can be decreased by attention to posture, avoiding sudden movements and strengthening abdominal and back muscles.

Hypotension can result after standing for long periods of time and exercising supine as the uterus may compress against the blood vessels and decrease blood return. Exercising supine should be avoided or be brief.

HEALTH STATUS CONTRAINDICATIONS TO EXERCISE

Situations exist that may compromise the health of the fetus or mother and exercise should be avoided or modified.

Medical Conditions

- cardiovascular disorder
- respiratory disease
- infectious disease
- anaemia
- endocrine conditions
- obesity/underweight

Poor Obstetrical History

- intra-uterine growth retardation
- prematurity
- greater than one miscarriage

Current Obstetric Status

- hypertension
- uterine bleeding
- premature ruptured membranes
- cervical incompetence
- intra-uterine growth retardation

SYMPTOMS FOR PREGNANT ATHLETE TO CEASE EXERCISING	
pain	obstetric concerns
tachycardia	vaginal bleeding
palpitations	uterine contractions
nausea/vomiting	amniotic fluid
headache	insufficient weight gain
dizziness	decreased fetal movements
dyspnoea	faintness
back or pelvic pain	sudden onset of swelling e.g. ankles/hands/feet

Figure 13 – Symptoms for Pregnant Athlete to Cease Exercising

The pregnant female should be advised and made familiar with the need to discontinue exercise immediately if any unusual symptoms occur (Fig. 13).

STAGE OF PREGNANCY

Different physiological needs and risks occur at different stages. Throughout pregnancy the maternal oxygen consumption increases (16–32% at term when compared to a non–pregnant female). This is mainly related to the increase in body weight. The pregnant female thus finds it gradually more difficult to perform activities.

Practically, concern has been expressed about supine exercise after the fifth month as the enlarged uterus falls back onto the vena cava resulting in maternal hypotension and decreased blood flow to the fetus. Controversy exists whether brief periods are safe and do not put the fetus at risk. Due to the ligamentous laxity associated with pregnancy, ballistic movements are best avoided.

BENEFITS OF EXERCISE

The pregnant athlete generally has improved well-being both physiologically and psychologically rather than specific benefit affecting the pregnancy itself.

If exercise is continued during pregnancy some studies have found that the mother may weigh less, gain less weight and deliver smaller babies than sedentary women. By being fitter they may cope with labour better but no evidence exists that the labour or delivery is shorter or easier.

POST PARTUM EXERCISE

Exercise participation generally declines significantly during the third trimester of pregnancy. When returning to exercise post partum, all forms of previous exercises should be gradually and gently reintroduced.

The changes of pregnancy including weight gain and ligament laxity take weeks to return to normal so care is required especially in the first 6 weeks after delivery.

After a normal vaginal delivery, gentle exercise like walking can be recommenced immediately and gradually increased. Excessive stretching and lifting should be avoided. The woman should be advised to do what is comfortable.

After a Caesarian section, strenuous activity should be avoided for 6 weeks and weight lifting for 12.

Particular attention should be given to adequate hydration and caloric intake in the lactating woman. A good supportive brassiere should be worn for comfort.

MENOPAUSAL ATHLETE

(Fig. 14)

Menopause is the cessation of menstruation. It is defined retrospectively after no menses for twelve months. The ovaries' ability to respond to stimulation by pituitary gonadotrophin starts to decrease 2-4 years earlier and this results in decreased oestrogen production.

These changes occur about 50 years of age. When it occurs at 40 years or younger it is considered premature menopause.

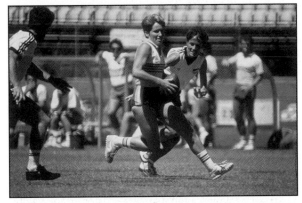

Figure 14 – It is important for the mature athlete to be involved in a variety of sports. (Courtesy of Country Wide Photographic Services)

Symptoms of menopause are related to the lower oestrogen levels. Hot flushes and vaginal dryness are characteristic. Two major concerns in the post menopausal female is the possible development of:

- osteoporosis
- coronary heart disease

OSTEOPOROSIS

Osteoporosis is defined pathologically as a reduced bone mass (osteopenia) resulting in fracture upon minimal trauma. It is the most common metabolic bone disease. It is eight times more common in females than in males. Osteoporosis is a major health problem as it is frequently the underlying cause of fractures in the vertebral column, wrist and hip in post menopause women. Fracture risk is associated with absolute bone density. The lower the bone density the higher the risk. Risk factors for osteoporosis are shown (Fig. 15).

Osteoporosis affects the more metabolically active trabecular bone (spinal) than cortical (long bones). This begins 5 to 10 years earlier in trabecular bone than cortical.

Osteoporosis is preventable and treatable. Factors important in the development of osteoporosis:

1. amount of peak bone mass attained
2. rate of bone loss

OSTEOPOROSIS - RISK FACTORS

Early menopause (e.g. athletic amenorrhoea)

Older age

Slender build (such as runners, gymnasts, dancers, skaters)

Asian or European descent

Family history

Nulliparity

Corticosteroid use

Lack of weight bearing exercise

High alcohol, tobacco and caffeine use

Figure 15 – Risk factors for osteoporosis

The aim would be to acquire as much bone mass as possible in early life and reduce the bone loss in later life.

Bone undergoes a continuous remodelling process with formation and resorption. Peak bone mass is reached at about 25 years of age. Up to this time more bone is being formed than resorbed. This peak depends on a number of interrelated factors - genetics, hormonal status, nutrition, calcium intake and exercise level. Age related bone loss begins at about 40 years of age in both sexes but in women there is an accelerated loss after menopause.

The hormone oestrogen is important in bone mineralisation. A normal level is essential to peak bone mass and to reduce bone mass losses. The bone mineral rate of loss is faster in first few years of the hypoestrogenic state then the rate slows. The initial rate of loss can be up to 4% per year. Osteoporosis and stress fractures can result.

Investigation of osteoporosis is by bone density studies by either dual energy X-ray absorptometry (DEXA) or qualitative computed tomography.

MANAGEMENT OF OSTEOPOROSIS

The greater the total bone mass at maturity the more a woman can afford to lose. Emphasis should be on accumulation of bone in the premenopausal stage rather than a treatment after menopause. With treatment, ideally, it is best to commence intervention early with an aim to decrease the initial rapid rate of bone loss.

Exercise

Moderate weigh bearing exercise has a beneficial effect on the skeleton. Bone loss experienced during disuse can be reversed upon weigh bearing activity. Regular exercise or activity may actually retard the rate of bone loss in the elderly or even increase the bone density. Studies have shown increases in bone mineral content when performing weight bearing exercises to both trabecular and cortical bones. This gain can be lost if the exercise is discontinued.

As well as skeletal loading, the dynamic muscular pull may play a role in stimulating bone density. Women supplementing aerobic exercise with weight training has been found to have higher spinal bone mineral densities compared with sedentary women and those only doing aerobic exercise. Swimmers have significantly greater vertebral and radial bone density than sedentary women despite swimming being considered a non weight bearing exercise.

Calcium Intake

This is essential for the positive effect of exercise and oestrogen on bone health (discussed in nutritional concerns).

Hormone Replacement Therapy (HRT)

The use of HRT is still controversial but most females can preserve bone mineral context of the peripheral and central skeleton and also reduce the risk of cardiovascular disease. The mechanism of action is undetermined though it is considered it may be from a direct receptor-mediated effect on bone metabolism or interference with bone resorption requiring calcium homoeostasis to be achieved by increasing absorption of dietary calcium and decreasing loss.

HRT - conjugated oestrogen 0.625 mg daily combined with medroxyprogesterone acetate 10 mg daily on days 1 to 12 of the calendar month. The progesterone is important to counteract the effects of unopposed oestrogen on the endometrium which is related to a six-fold increased risk of endometrial carcinoma. If no uterus is present, just oestrogen is prescribed. Non compliance usually relates to the incidence of side effects of a withdrawal bleed and PMT. There is an inconclusive relatively slight risk of carcinoma of the breast (1.3 risk) related to HRT.

A decreased frequency of arm and hip fractures by 50-60% and vertebral compression fractures by 80% have been reported if the female takes oestrogen from the perimenopausal period. The role of HRT started late is less clear. If commenced 6 years after menopause there is increased bone mineralisation between 3-5% over 12 months but if stopped, the loss resumes and rapidly reaches the low levels seen before treatment. More research is proceeding.

CORONARY HEART DISEASE

An increased risk exists in the post menopausal period.

Exercise training stresses the cardiorespiratory system. Aerobic exercise is thought to decrease the risk of cardiovascular disease by eliciting a decrease in blood pressure, improving insulin sensitivity and blood lipid results. Many of these changes are related to exercise and associated with a reduction in body fat. Decreased fat may result in increased metabolic rate.

The cardiorespiratory changes seen with aging are partially related to disuse.

Aerobic fitness is associated with a decrease in serum triglycerides and an increase in HDL. This decrease can reduce the risk of ischaemic heart disease.

Studies show regular exercise may protect the female from cardiovascular disease. This has been definitively shown in males. After menopause there is an increased risk of coronary heart disease with females. This results from changes in the lipid profiles that occur after changes in the hormone milieu. HRT has been associated with a decrease in myocardial infarction.

EXERCISE GUIDELINES IN POST MENOPAUSAL PERIOD

There is a need to consider the aims of the patient, and prior participation fitness and activity levels. Are they continuing exercise, returning to exercise after a long period of inactivity or did they never exercise previously?

A preparticipation examination is required with a thorough clinical assessment with attention in the history to any cardiovascular risk factors or coexisting medical conditions that may influence the type and extent of the exercise. The medications being taken must be known. Investigations include pathology screening for Hb, glucose, lipids and ECG. An exercise ECG may also be indicated depending on what was found on clinical assessment.

Generally, a moderate level of aerobic exercise (able to talk to companion whilst doing the exercise) is appropriate e.g. walking, cycling and swimming. Cardiovascular benefit is attained when exercising for about 30 min 3 times per week at a 70% maximal heart rate (determined by 220-age). A good warm up and cool down which includes stretching is important, as is good maintenance of equipment and gear.

Each participant must be made aware of the need to cease exercising immediately if any abnormal symptoms occur (like chest pain, undue shortness of breath) as there is a slight risk of precipitating an ischaemia episode (like angina, myocardial infarction, sudden death). A good evaluation reduces this risk.

NUTRITIONAL CONCERNS

Proper nutrition is important for all athletes, however of particular concern for the female athlete is:

- iron deficiency
- calcium deficiency
- disordered eating (discussed in female triad)

IRON DEFICIENCY

Iron deficiency in female athletes is fairly common. 20-25% of female endurance athletes are iron deficient. Iron is lost each day in urine, trauma and sweat. Further iron is lost with menstruation. The iron stored in the body is small in quantity.

Iron deficiency has been classified into three stages:

1. Iron depletion - depletion of iron stores in the liver, spleen and bone marrow.
2. Iron deficiency erythropoesis - decline in serum iron levels with an increase in total iron binding capacity.
3. Iron deficiency anaemia - haemoglobin values below 120 g/l.

Stage one iron depletion is the most commonly found iron deficiency and it can present with decreased performance and no other symptoms. It may also be associated with tiredness and lethargy. Athletes have a lower rate of lactate clearance and tire more quickly during physical activity.

Evaluation includes iron studies. S. Ferritin reflects the status of iron stores. If the level is below 20 mg/l then iron stores are absent. Anaemia is reflected by a low haemoglobin and hematocrit. This is less common in the athlete.

MANAGEMENT

Menstruating athletes need 15 mg iron per day. Generally only 10-15% of iron intake is absorbed. Vitamin C enhances the absorption. Vegetarian diets are generally low in iron. With poor absorption. Iron supplements may be required. Commencing the OCP to reduce menstrual losses may be appropriate in some athletes.

CALCIUM

Calcium along with oestrogen and exercise is important for bone health and helping prevent osteoporosis. Lifetime calcium intake is important for bone health. Definite benefits on peak bone mass may have established in children and young adults. In the elderly, calcium supplementation alone is not effective in maintaining bone density but in combination with oestrogen it is effective.

In the amenorrhoeal athlete, a study has shown a high calcium diet results in site-specific increases in bone mineralisation.

DAILY CALCIUM REQUIREMENTS	
(Adapted from Australian Sports Medicine Federation Nutrition for Sportswomen)	
Daily calcium requirement (mg/day)	**Appropriate for-**
1000	Girls (12-15 years)
800	Girls (16-18 years)
800	Menstruating women
1000	Post menopausal women
1200-1400	Pregnant or lactating women
1500	Amenorrhoeic athletes

Figure 16 – Daily calcium requirements

Calcium rich foods include dairy products, fish and green leafy vegetables. The daily intake recommended is summarised (Fig. 16).

The bioavailability of calcium supplements varies. The absorption of calcium carbonate and phosphate salts is depressed in the gastrointestinal tract with alkaline pH. Therefore they are best taken after a meal when the gastric juices, which are more acidic, have been stimulated.

OTHER ISSUES

MUSCULOSKELETAL INJURIES

Some injuries occur more commonly in women than in men, due to anatomic and physiologic differences. Anterior cruciate ligament injuries are especially common. However, most injuries are sports-specific rather than gender-specific.

Shoulder injuries

Rotator cuff strain occurs when the arm is forcefully or repetitively placed overhead and pronated (Fig. 17) (***See Chapter 10***).

Knee injuries

Patellofemoral pain is more common in females (Fig. 18). The wider pelvis and increased Q angle at the knee are considered to contribute. Athletes most prone have laterally placed patellae (***See Chapter 14***).

Anterior cruciate ligament injury is common. Risk factors include limb laxity, insufficient restraint of the cruciates by the hamstrings, notch size, limb alignment, skill level and fall-break patterns (***See Chapter 14***).

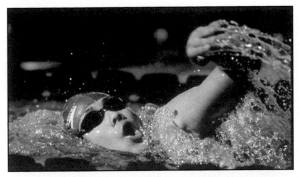

Figure 17 – Rotator cuff problems start when the arm is repeatedly placed overhead and pronated (as in free style; World Champion Chinese Swimmer, Bin Lu)

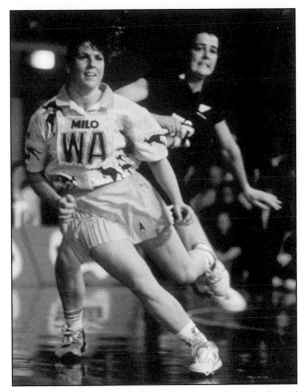

Figure 18 – Females have increased incidence of patello-femoral pain for biomechanical reasons (*Courtesy of Country Wide Photographic Services*)

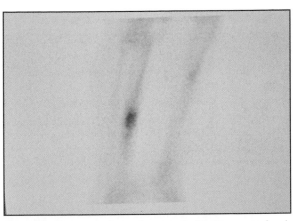

Figure 19 – Bone scan of stress fracture of mid tibia seen in female athlete (X-ray was normal; bone density was reduced)

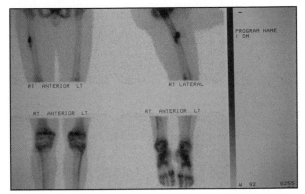

Figure 20 – Stress mid-femur in amenorrhoeic skeletally immature athlete

Iliotibial band (ITB) tendinitis

Thought to develop because the ITB has a greater span in women (due to a wider pelvis and greater prominence of the greater trochanter). Pain occurs from friction of the ITB as it passes over the greater trochanter (*See Chapter 14*).

Ankle impingement

Occurs in sports which require excessive ankle motion (gymnastics, dancing and diving). Forced plantar flexion in these sports predisposes to irritation of the posterior ankle capsule, trauma of the os trigonum and posterior tibial tendinitis (*See Chapter 15*).

Foot disorders

These include bunions, corns, and calluses. Improper shoe wear is the primary cause. Ballet dancers are prone due to the fit of their toe shoes (*See Chapter 15*).

Stress fractures

There is four-fold increased stress fracture risk in amenorrhoea athletes. These are more prevalent in the cortex of long bones (Figs. 19 & 20). It is unknown whether bone density is the link between increased stress fracture and menstrual dysfunction. Other factors involved are diet, training level and muscle strength (*See Chapter 15*). Athletes using oral contraceptives have fewer stress fractures than non-users in some studies

Prevention takes into account menstrual and dietary factors. Calcium and other nutritional deficits should be corrected. Hormonal therapy may be necessary.

Spondylolysis and vertebral body apophysitis

Occurs in gymnasts, divers and skaters. Caused by flexion-extension motions of the spine (Fig. 21) (*See also Chapter 9*).

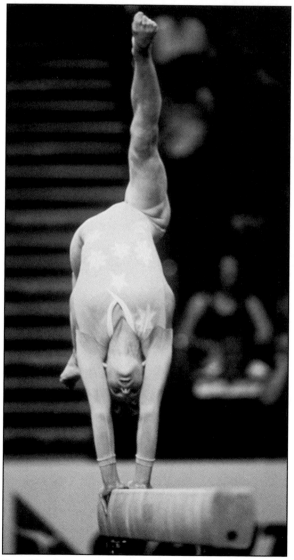

Figure 21 – Gymnasts are prone to spondylosis and vertebral body apoplysitis from repeated hyper-extension

GENITAL INJURIES

Vulval injuries may be sustained when falling astride. Either bruising or lacerations can result. Forceful vaginal drenching is a concern when falling whilst water skiing. Appropriate ski pants are recommended to prevent this.

RELATIONSHIP BETWEEN EXERCISE AND CANCER

Breast and endometrial cancers are associated with early menarche, later menopause and genetic factors. Athletes tend to have late menarche and earlier menopause than non athletes. Thus, does exercise help to protect against certain cancers?

A study of the lifetime rate of cancer of the reproductive system and breast showed lower incidence in athletes than non athletic controls.

Hormone replacement therapy has a very low long term risk of increased endometrial and breast cancers.

PERFORMANCE ENHANCING DRUGS

Female athletes using performance enhancing drugs, especially anabolic steroids, are exposed to particular risks (Fig. 22). Many of these changes are irreversible and have serious consequences. They are banned in national and international competition.

SPECIFIC RISKS OF ANDROGEN USE BY FEMALES
Effects of anabolic steroid use in females
increased size clitoris
lower pitched voice
increased body and facial hair
baldness
fluid retention
higher blood pressure
higher risk of stroke, heart attack, and liver disease

Figure 22 – Specific risks of androgen use by females

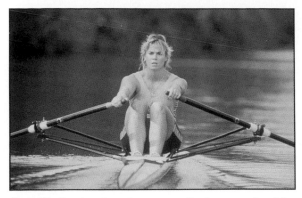

Figure 23 – Rowing, dependent on co-ordination, strength and fine motor skills is particularly suited to the female athlete

GENDER VERIFICATION

The differences between the sexes (Fig. 2) and the differences in performance (Fig. 3) have led to competition between sexes to be segregated. The issue arises of confirming a competitor's sex. The ancient Olympics achieved this by a direct means - men competed naked. In Budapest at the 1966 European Athletics Championships, women paraded nude before a panel of gynaecologists. Since then, a variety of means has been used to verify gender of those competing in women's events. Besides men masquerading as women, there are several intersex conditions that pose problems.

Direct physical examination has fallen into disuse, being considered degrading. Modern techniques used include Barr body detection in cells, polymerase chain reaction (looking for SRY gene on male DNA), but no test is without weakness. It is necessary to ensure strict confidentiality when dealing with personal issues such as gender.

THE FUTURE OF THE FEMALE ATHLETE

Women today participate in far more sporting events than ever before. New challenges to sports medicine arise with each new event. Much data is available on established sports (swimming and running), but less on newer events such as rowing (Fig. 23) and body-building (Fig. 24).

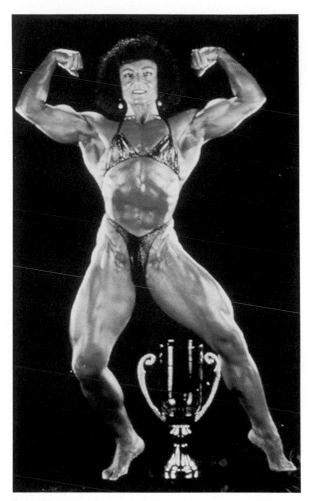

Figure 24 – Female body building promotes endurance, discipline and self-esteem (Miss Universe, 1993)

Performances in female sports continue to improve at a rapid rate. This is due to increases in participation rates, competitive opportunities and better coaching.

However, the problems of the female triad remain a challenge to sports physicians. The question of how to maximise performance without compromising health is vital. The solution lies in a training programme based on sound scientific principles. Such training should result in greater endurance and power, when practised with the discipline required to achieve excellence.

18

THE CHILD ATHLETE

Peter Gray

INTRODUCTION

Sport benefits children. They become fitter (higher VO_2 max) and stronger (greater strength). Their participation in competitive and recreational sport is increasing. However injury may occur. It is important to be aware of the nature and cause of injuries, so that the benefits of sport and exercise can be maximised and injuries minimised.

Children are **not** small adults and have their own physiological and developmental parameters (Fig. 1). They are less metabolically efficient than adults, but can significantly improve performance by improved economy of movement and are more prone to heat illness and to disturbances of bone growth from injury.

In general, child and youth sport is safe

A study of 1818 Dutch school children aged 8 to 17 years involved in sport, and followed for a 7 month period, showed the incidence of sporting injuries was 22%, of which 43% were contusions and 21% sprains.

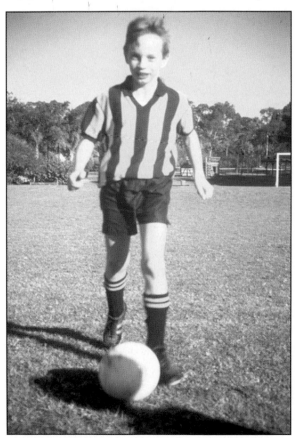

Figure 1 - Children are not small adults. They have their own physiological and developmental agendas

53% of these injuries did not require any treatment, 15% attended a general practitioner, and 16% attended a specialist clinic. 94% did not miss any days school, and only 2% required more than 3 days off school. 64% did not require any time off their sporting activities. 22% were away from sport for a week, and only 7% were off sport for more than 2 weeks.

Other authors' experiences reveal that organised sport is no more or less dangerous than play in other childhood arenas, such as the home, school and the road.

Age, size and maturity of young athletes is a factor. As size and age increase, the speed and violence of collision and contact is greater, resulting in a greater incidence of injury. One needs to be aware of the enormous variability of growth and maturation of children at a similar point in time. Sports programmes that match children according to age alone, misunderstand this variability. Their injury patterns may differ in type and severity from adults (Fig. 2 & 3).

Girls are not any more or less prone to injury than boys, and any **sex difference** relates to the fact that girls usually choose less violent sports.

As one would expect, the incidence of sporting injuries is related to the inherent violence of the sport itself, there being a much higher incidence of injury in football compared to tennis or swimming (Figs. 4 & 5).

Foul play, recklessness and lack of fitness are all major contributing factors to childhood injuries. These are areas that are amenable to influence by **coaches, trainers, parents and teachers.**

A child's readiness for sporting competition is decided by their motor skills level, social sophistication and ability to follow instructions. It is as well to remember that sporting ability **is not** accelerated by early starting.

SOFT TISSUE INJURIES

Soft tissue injuries involving contusions, sprains, and strains are by far and away the **most common** form of injury in the skeletally immature, and tend to be more common in the lower limbs (Fig. 6). **A contusion** is an injury to a muscle belly. **A sprain** is an injury to a ligament. **A strain** is an injury to junctional areas, i.e. bone/muscle, muscle/tendon, or tendon/bone interfaces. These bone tendon injuries have also been variously described as overuse injuries, overload injuries or stress-related injuries.

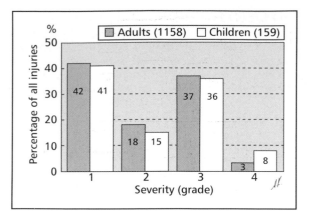

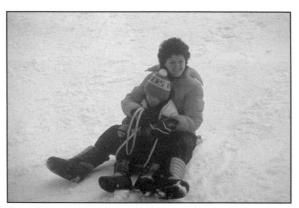

Figure 3 - Bilateral tibial shaft fractures in a 10-year-old skier (small body weight may not release poorly adjusted findings)

Distribution of sites of injury in adults and children

Site of injury	Adult (n)	Adult (%)	Children (n)	Children (%)
Foot and ankle	65	6.0	65	1.0
Lower leg	144	10.0	37	23.0
Knee	353	31.0	48	30.0
Femur	27	2.0	11	7.0
Trunk	71	6.0	2	1.0
Neck and back	37	3.0	11	7.0
Head and face	143	12.0	21	13.0
Upper limb	348	30.0	18	11.0
TOTAL	1158	100.0	159	100.0

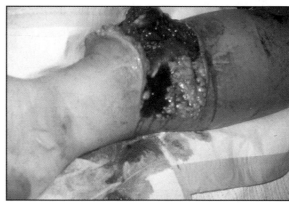

Figure 4 - Open tibial shaft fracture with dead pale and paralysed foot in an 11-year-old (required below knee amputation)

Comparison and frequency of the 5 most common injuries in adults and children

Injuries in adults	%	Injuries in children	%
Knee sprain	25.0	Knee sprain	28.0
Shoulder dislocation	5.0	Shoulder dislocation	12.0
Shoulder sprain	4.5	Shoulder sprain	9.0
Fractured wrist	3.5	Fractured wrist	5.0
Sprained wrist	3.5	Sprained wrist	5.0
Remainder	58.5	Remainder	41.0

Figure 2 - Children's skiing injuries (after Sherry, 1987). More likely to involve the lower limb, with a greater number of shoulder dislocations and are generally more severe in nature

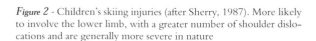

Figure 5 - Tobogganists are prone to lower limb and back injuries

```
┌─────────────────────────────────────────────┐
│  ███ DEFINITIONS OF SOFT TISSUE INJURIES ███ │
│                                               │
│     • Contusion                               │
│          Injury to muscle belly               │
│                                               │
│     • Sprain                                  │
│          Injury to ligament                   │
│                                               │
│     • Strain                                  │
│          Junctional injury                    │
│                                               │
└─────────────────────────────────────────────┘
```

Figure 6 - Definition of soft tissue injury

CONTUSIONS

Soft tissue contusions are probably the most common injury in the paediatric athlete. The initial response to an injury is a haematoma associated with inflammation. This is then followed by muscle regeneration. When a muscle fibre is injured, the peripherally placed satellite cells, which lie between the basement membrane and the sarcolemma, retain some stem cell potential and are mobilised. These are the myoblasts that fuse to form new myotubes. The regenerating myotubes are very similar to embryonic myotubes, and these myotubes possess the cellular components necessary for formation of contractile protein. In a child with an intact basement membrane, complete healing can be expected. With the more severe injury or advanced age, less complete forms of repair with formation of increased amounts of connective scar tissue occurs.

Treatment of contusions is straightforward. Initially rest, ice, compression and elevation are employed. Isometric quadriceps exercises are commenced as soon as the patient is able. Once quadriceps control has been regained, active range of movement is instituted. Shadow weight bearing is allowed, and once the patient has recovered 90 degrees of knee flexion, progressive resistance exercises can begin. Physical modalities such as ultrasound, heat and interferential may be pleasing to the patient, but do not influence the rate of recovery.

It is important to avoid passive stretching of the muscles in any form, as tearing a healing muscle unit can produce more connective scar tissue. Such connective scar tissue can interfere with the muscle's ability to contract efficiently and move through a normal range of motion. A return to sports is dependent upon the demonstration of full strength and full range of motion of the injured limb.

MYOSITIS-OSSIFICANS

Myositis-ossificans traumatica is an unfortunate sequela of severe muscle contusion. Myositis–ossificans refers to the phenomenon of new bone formation in muscle following injury. The quadriceps and brachialis have long been documented as the favoured sites of this condition. It appears most often in the second and third decades, but a lesion in a 5-year-old following a motor vehicle accident has been reported.

Symptoms include pain, swelling and progressive loss of movement. Heterotrophic bone is visible radiologically at about 3 weeks or can be detected earlier on bone scan. The treatment involves rest followed by active mobilisation. Passive mobilisation is **definitely contra-indicated.** NSAID can be beneficial by suppressing new bone formation.

OVERUSE INJURIES

Overuse injuries are the result of unresolved submaximal stress in previously normal tissues. With increasing participation of younger athletes in sport, such injuries are now becoming more common. Apart from the intrinsic demands that such sport places on children, there are **anatomic considerations** for such injuries in children (Fig. 7).

- Firstly, growing bone has a looser periosteum and tendinous attachments than mature bone. This means less force can produce traction overload.

- Secondly, the epiphyses and the apophyses are weak links in the bone-tendon-muscle unit, as they are susceptible to tensile overloads.

- Thirdly, the differential growth patterns in the length of bones relative to muscles, results in decreased flexibility in the large muscle groups of the upper and lower extremities and back. This tightness affects muscle strength by interfering with the normal length-tension relationships. A tight and weak muscle is the most susceptible to overload injuries.

Overuse complaints usually produce a mechanical type of pain (increases with activity and diminishes with rest). The pain may only be precipitated by strenuous sports activity, by limited sports activity, or occur with day-to-day activities (Fig. 8).

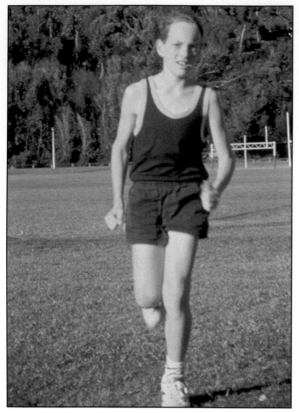

Figure 7 - There are anatomical reasons for overuse injuries in children (looser periosteal/tendinous attachments; epiphyses/apophyses weak links; decreased flexibility)

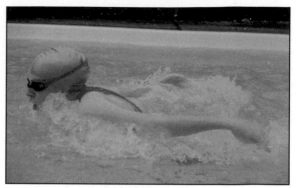

Figure 8 - The most common significant factor is the training programme (butterfly stroke places strenuous forces across the subacromial space of the shoulder)

TREATMENT OF OVERUSE INJURIES

- Identifying the risk factor
- Modifying the factors
- Control of pain
- Undertake progressive rehabilitation with emphasis on restoration of full flexibility, endurance and strength
- A maintenance programme to prevent new injuries or a recurrence of the previous injuries

Figure 9 - Treatment of overuse injuries

Precipitating factors may be anatomic, environmental, or training factors. Anatomic factors may be due to malalignment, fixed deformity, dynamic deformity, or a congenital development condition. Environmental factors include equipment, playing surfaces and weather/altitude. The most common significant factor is the training programme.

Physical examination should include an assessment of the alignment of the involved limb (both angular, rotatory and longitudinal alignment). One needs to assess the range of motion within the joints and the flexibility around the joints. Ligamentous laxity needs to be assessed. Local tenderness with increased warmth and swelling are common manifestations of tendinitis, apophysitis, bursitis or stress fractures.

Investigations may include X-rays, bone scans and ultrasound.

Treatment of overuse injuries involves five phases (Fig. 9).

Patient, parent and coach education remains a significant component of management of overuse problems and focuses on training abuse and improper equipment.

The long term effects of chronic submaximal stress in skeletally immature athletes are still unknown.

FRACTURES

Fractures represent about 20% of sport-related injuries in the skeletally immature, and tend to be more common in the upper limb. They should therefore **always be suspected** and need to be excluded. When **deformity** is present, the diagnosis is easy (Figs. 4 & 10). In the **absence of deformity**, swelling, loss of function and localised bony tenderness are diagnostic. In the presence of bony tenderness, an X-ray is essential to plan appropriate management.

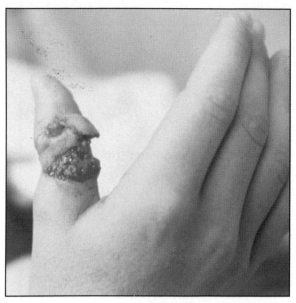

Figure 10 - Open thumb crush injury in a 9-year-old. Growth plate injury is very likely

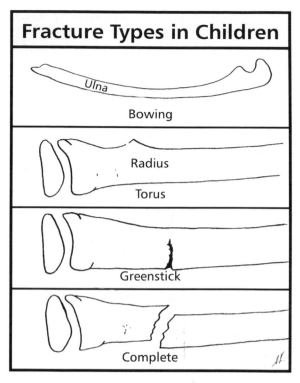

Figure 11 - Fracture types in children - bowing/torus/greenstick/complete

SEQUENCE OF OSSIFICATION

Bone ossifies from a cartilaginous anlage. The **primary** centre of ossification is in the diaphysis, and most of these are present at birth. The **secondary** centres of ossification, the epiphyses and the apophyses, appear at variable times after birth. Epiphyses occur at the end of long bones and are involved in longitudinal growth of the bone. **Apophyses** are at the sites of origin or insertion of major muscles or tendons, and are involved in circumferential bone growth.

Fractures in the skeletally immature can occur through the diaphysis, the metaphysis, the physis or the epiphysis. Young bone is more porous than adult bone due to larger Haversian canals. As a consequence of this, when a force is applied to immature bone there is a longer plastic deformation phase before the bone fails. Thus **four different fracture patterns** can occur in the diaphysis and the metaphysis; namely, the torus or buckle fracture, plastic bowing, greenstick fracture, and the complete fracture (Fig. 11). The type of fracture produced depends upon the duration of, and the force, applied.

Anatomical realignment of fractures is obviously desirable, but during the healing process immature bone exhibits a greater degree of **remodelling** than is possible in the adult.

Following an angulated fracture at the end of a long bone, the physis exhibits a spontaneous ability to change its inclination towards a normalisation of the inclination of the epiphyseal plate. There is, however, an upper limit of angulation that can correct. In practical terms, with regard to the distal radius, complete normalisation will take place after residual angulation of 20 degrees or less. This process is exponential not linear, and at least 2 years of growth remaining is required for almost complete normalisation.

The correction of angulation depends on longitudinal growth. Therefore, the closer the deformity is to the physis, and the longer the remaining growth, the more complete the correction.

PHYSEAL FRACTURES

Fractures occurring through the growth plate have a peak incidence at the age of 12 to 13. This coincides with the period of rapid growth. The separation usually occurs through the zone of cartilage transformation between the calcified and uncalcified cartilage. There

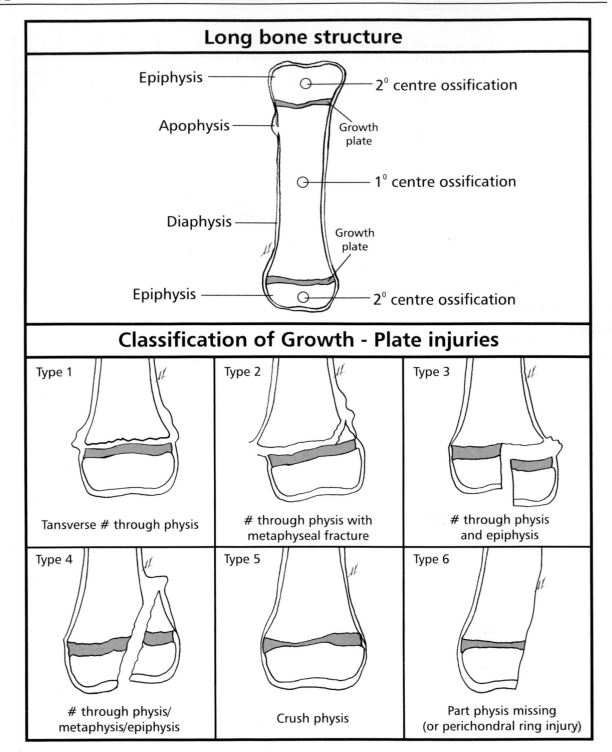

Figure 12 - The Salter-Harris classification of Growth Plate fractures
is a guide to treatment and prognosis

is a high turnover of cells in this region, and the bone here has less resistance to shear and tensile forces than the adjacent bone.

To assist in planning treatment and advising on prognosis, the **Salter-Harris** classification is helpful (Fig. 12). This classification does exclude a number of less common events, and Peterson has formulated yet another classification of epiphyseal fractures which is more encompassing, in particular Type VI lesion when the physis is missing (or perichondral ring injury).

Type I injuries are usually the result of shearing or torsional forces, or avulsion forces in the case of an apophysis. The commonest site of injury is the **distal fibular physis.** Localised bony tenderness is diagnostic. The radiograph usually appears normal. An ultrasound may demonstrate periostial elevation. These injuries require 3 weeks of cast immobilisation. Movement and function return quickly, and complications are extremely rare.

Type 2 injuries most commonly involve the distal radial epiphysis with posterior displacement, and are frequently accompanied by a chip of bone off the ulnar styloid. Anatomical reduction is ideal, but as previously discussed, up to 20 degrees of angulation can remodel. Five to six weeks of immobilisation in a well moulded, short arm cast is required.

Children who present late with Type 1 or Type 2 fractures in an unacceptable position, are best left alone. These fractures heal quickly and attempts at closed manipulation may result in further growth plate damage. Late corrective osteotomy may be required if remodelling fails to correct the deformity.

The most commonly seen Type 3 fracture involves the distal tibial epiphysis (Tillaux fracture). Open reduction to anatomically restore the articular surface is essential. Growth disturbance is not a problem following this fracture, as the fracture occurs just prior to physeal closure.

The most commonly seen Type 4 fracture involves the lateral condyle of the humerus (Fig. 13). This injury requires open reduction and internal fixation. Left untreated, this intra-articular injury will produce joint stiffness and deformity, secondary to mal-position of the fracture. This can be associated with a non-union and progressive valgus deformity of the elbow. Ultimately a tardive ulnar palsy can occur. With anatomic reduction and internal fixation, the long term consequences are minimal.

Pure type 5 injuries are rare. Variable degrees of crush to the growth plate can accompany any physeal fracture, and it is for this reason that physeal plate fractures should be followed up during periods of growth to ensure that growth arrest and deformity has not occured.

The site most at risk of physeal injury and formation of incomplete or complete bony bars is the distal femur (Fig 14). (Lombardo and Harvey reported on 34 cases of distal femoral physeal fractures, and noted that one third developed varus deformity, and one third had a leg length discrepancy greater than 2 cm.)

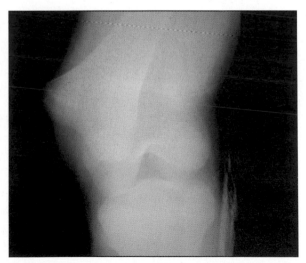

Figure 13 - Lateral condylar # elbow displaced in 5-year-old which requires surgical reduction and fixation

Figure 14 - Growth plate injuries of the distal femur are most prone to growth disturbance (with formation of complete/incomplete bony bars)

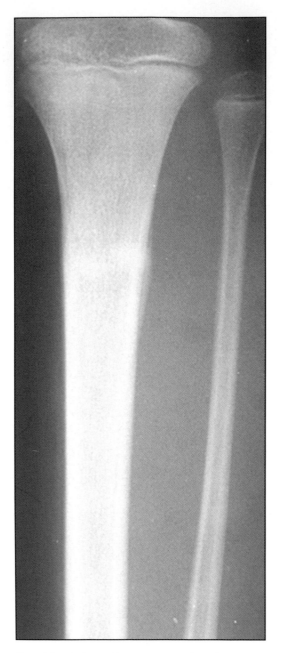

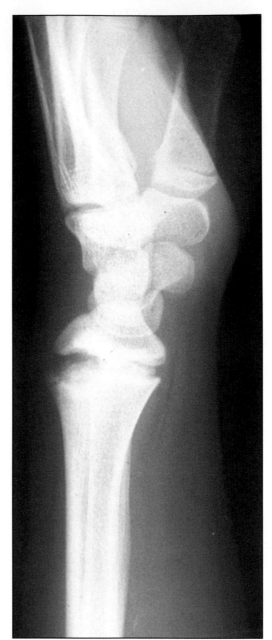

Figure 15 - Tibial stress fracture may not always be apparent on X-ray

Figure 16 - Stress physiolysis of distal radius (reported in gymnasts)

PATHOLOGICAL FRACTURES

Childhood fractures can also occur in pathological bone (such as unicameral bone cysts).

STRESS FRACTURES

Stress fractures do occur in children, and have a direct relationship to age (children have fewer fractures than adolescents, who have fewer fractures than adults). 9% of these fractures occur in children less than 15 years of age, 32% in 16 to 19-year-olds and 59% in those over 20 years. The tibia is the most common site of fractures, accounting for approximately 50% of stress fractures (Fig. 15). Upper extremity stress fractures have been reported, namely in the diaphysis of the ulna, in the non-dominant arm of the tennis player, caused by the use of a two-handed backhand stroke; mid-humeral stress fracture in a 15-year-old tennis player due to excessive service and overhead strokes; stress fractures have been seen around the elbow in throwing athletes; and stress fractures have been seen in the distal radial epiphysis of gymnasts (Fig. 16).

Osteoid osteoma, subacute osteomyelitis, Ewing's sarcoma and osteogenic sarcoma must be differentiated from stress fractures (perform X-ray).

X-rays are usually unhelpful in the diagnosis of these injuries, as in the early phases many stress fractures are radiographically silent. Technecium 99 bone scanning is positive about 12 to 15 days following the onset of stress fracture symptoms (Fig. 17).

Mid-tibial stress fractures have proved difficult to heal, and the majority tend to go on to complete fractures. Once the fracture is complete, non union tends to occur and bone grafting is required to achieve union.

DISLOCATIONS

Dislocations usually involve the patella or elbow. When the patient presents with these joints still dislocated, the diagnosis is easy. However, these dislocations often **spontaneously relocate.** In these cases the diagnosis must be based on clinical evidence, with a high index of suspicion.

The management of patellar dislocation will be discussed later.

Elbow dislocations may be associated with a fracture of the medial epicondyle. The elbow can reduce with

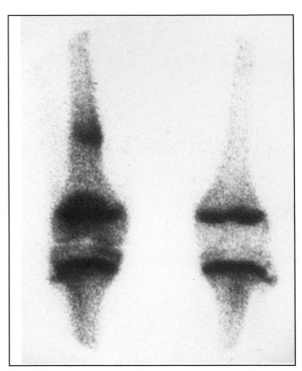

Figure 17 - The Bone Scans (technecium 99) are positive in 12 to 15 days (here stress fracture lower femoral shaft)

this fragment in the humero-ulnar joint. This requires open reduction and internal fixation of the displaced fragment.

The uncomplicated elbow dislocation (Figs. 18 & 19) requires sling immobilisation and ice initially, followed by gradual mobilisation as pain allows. Physiotherapy is **not** required. Return to sport should be delayed **until full elbow extension** has been regained (may take many months).

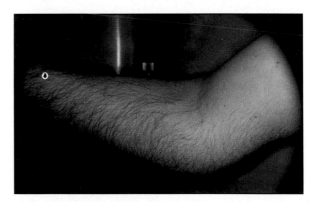

Figure 18 - Dislocation of elbow joint

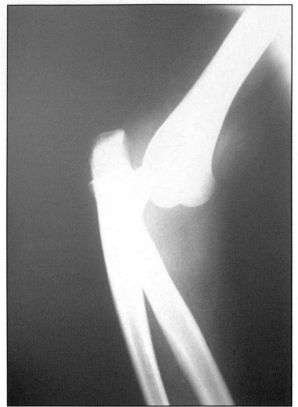

Figure 19 - X-ray showing postero-lateral dislocation of the elbow joint

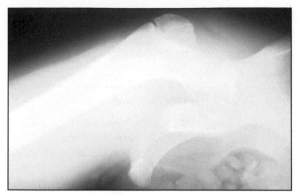

Figure 20 - Dislocation of hip (posterior). An emergency. Immediate reduction is necessary to prevent avascular necrosis

injuries, once a full range of active motion has been restored, then a resisted exercise programme can be commenced, and a return to sport occurs after full strength of the injured areas has been achieved.

Significantly displaced avulsion fractures of the ischium may require open reduction and internal fixation (Fig. 22).

SLIPPED UPPER FEMORAL CAPITAL EPIPHYSIS (SUFE)

This is the **most common** hip disorder in the adolescent. Rarely does the slip occur in association with a discrete injury (an acute slip). Rather there is a gradual micro-fracturing process of the physis under physiological loads (a chronic slip). Occasionally there may be an element of both (an acute on chronic slip).

This condition occurs in about 2 per 100,000 adolescents. It occurs 2.5 times more frequently in boys than girls. The mean age of presentation for boys is 13.5 years and the mean age of presentation for girls is 11.5 years. The condition is bilateral on initial presentation in 10 to 15%, and over time can occur in 25 to 35% of individuals.

The adolescent may present with increasing anterior thigh and knee pain, associated with a limp. The pain may be aggravated by physical activity.

Clinically the leg may lie in **slightly more external rotation** and there is a loss of internal rotation of the hip in flexion (Fig. 23). The diagnosis is usually confirmed on X-ray, but if not, obtain a bone scan (Fig. 24).

HIP AND PELVIC INJURIES

Hip and pelvic injuries are relatively rare in the young athlete (Fig. 20). An all encompassing classification of injuries is presented (Fig. 21).

Of the skeletal injuries, apophyseal avulsion fractures and slipped upper femoral capital epiphysis are the most common.

Apophyseal fractures usually occur during the course of an extreme effort due to a sudden violent muscular contraction. The injury most often occurs in the adolescent athlete between 14 and 17 years of age.

Clinically there would be localised swelling, tenderness and limitation of motion.

The diagnosis is usually confirmed radiologically.

Treatment involves rest and analgesia initially, and movement is then increased as pain allows. As with all

HIP AND PELVIC INJURIES OF THE YOUNG ATHLETE

Skeletal Injuries

- **Apophyseal Avulsion Fractures**
  1. Iliac crest (abdominal musculature)
  2. Anterior superior iliac spine (sartorius)
  3. Anterior inferior iliac spine (rectus femoris)
  4. Lesser trochanter (iliopsoas)
  5. Ischium (hamstring)

- **Growth Plate Injuries**
  1. Slipped capital femoral epiphysis
  2. Salter-Harris physeal fractures

- **Nonphyseal Fractures**
  1. Pelvic Fractures
     (a) Iliac wing fractures
     (b) Acetabular fractures
     (c) Stable pelvic fractures
     (d) Unstable pelvic ring fractures

  2. Femoral Neck Fractures
     (a) Transcervical fracture
     (b) Cervicotrochanteric fracture
     (c) Intertrochanteric fracture

- **Hip Dislocations**

- **Stress Fractures**
  1. Femoral neck
  2. Pelvic

Soft Tissue Injuries

- **Musculotendinous Strains**
  1. Snapping hip syndrome
  2. Iliac apophysitis
  3. Osteitis pubis

- **Contusions**

Figure 21 - Hip and pelvic injuries of the young athlete

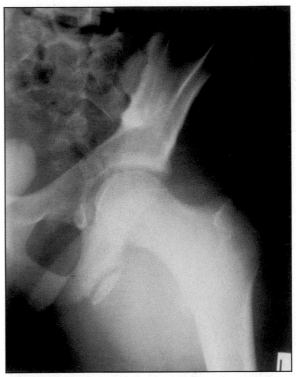

Figure 22 - Avulsion of the ischium in an 11-year-old (not displaced enough for surgery)

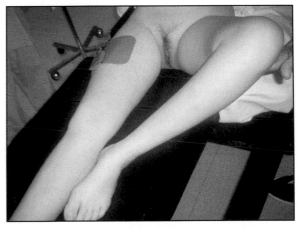

Figure 23 - In SUFE there is knee pain, a limp, and the leg lies externally rotated (rolls into external rotation with flexion)

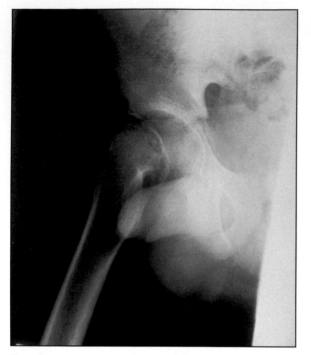

Figure 24 - X-ray of an 11-year-old with a SUFE

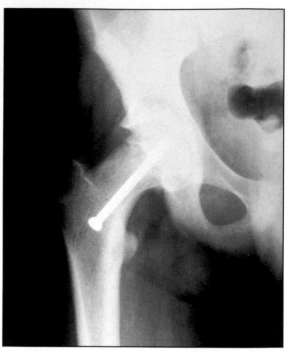

Figure 25 - Treatment of SUFE is a single screw (in situ) to stabilise the epiphysis and encourage early closure of the growth plate

Treatment is operative, with fixation by a single centre canulated compression screw, which stabilises the epiphysis and encourages early closure of the growth plate (Fig. 25).

In the assessment of "sports injuries" in the child, congenital, developmental, infective and inflammatory conditions always need to be considered. Therefore, Perthes' disease, developmental dysplasia of the hip, septic arthritis, and inflammatory synovitis need to be excluded.

THOMSON CLASSIFICATION OF PATELLO-FEMORAL DISORDERS	
• Traumatic	• Overuse
• Malalignment	• Degenerative
• Compressive	• Idiopathic

Figure 26 - Thomson Classification of Patello-Femoral Disorders.

THE KNEE

In the skeletally immature, pain in the front of the knee during or following sports activity, is an extremely **common** presenting symptom to the orthopaedic surgeon.

In an attempt to indicate the complexity of the problem and also to give a basis for rational treatment, Thomson proposed a classification based mainly on mechanical aspects affecting the patello-femoral joint (Fig. 26).

In the **traumatic group,** consider a direct blow to the patello-femoral joint, a traumatic dislocation, a fracture, and meniscal damage.

In the **malalignment group,** idiopathic subluxors and dislocators, and torsional problems, muscle imbalance and bony abnormalities need to be considered.

The **compressive group,** includes "the hamstrung knee" due to excessive tightness of the hamstrings.

The **overuse group** includes Osgood-Schlatter's disease, Sinding Larsen Johansson syndrome, multipartite patellae, and plicae.

The **degenerative group** are usually post-traumatic as a result of osteo-chondral fractures, secondary to patellar dislocation.

In the **idiopathic group** osteochondritis dissecans of the patella, and the small group of idiopathic primary chondromalacia of the patella.

Chondromalacia of the patella is **not a clinical syndrome.** It refers to the morphological change of the articular cartilage lining the retro-patellar surface. It may appear as a bulging, softening, fissuring or fimbrillation of the smooth surface of the articular cartilage, and may progress to surface degeneration. Its diagnosis should be confined to macroscopic, arthroscopic or microscopic observation of the articular surface.

The history and physical examination are very important in the assessment of **anterior knee pain patients.** The character, site, intensity and frequency of the pain, and also aggravating and relieving factors, need to be considered. Catching, popping or giving way, particularly with rotation, suggests patellar subluxation or instability.

On **physical examination,** the lower limbs need to be assessed in regions (Fig. 27). **Firstly above the patella,** looking for muscle weakness or contraction, and looking for excessive internal femoral torsion. **Hip pathology with referred pain to the knee should always be excluded.**

Secondly the patella itself, looking at patellar height (a high patella (patella alta), a low patella (patella baja), or a laterally tilted patella). The laterally tilted patella can also be associated with tight lateral retinacular structures. Excessive lateral patellar mobility with an apprehension sign also requires assessment. An effusion or crepitus suggests the possibility of retro-patellar erosion. Crepitus, however, can be present with a normal retro-patellar surface. Active flexion and extension of the knee allows assessment of patellar tracking.

Thirdly, below the patella, looking for a laterally placed tibial tubercle, a valgus knee, internal tibial torsion, tight hamstrings. Skin changes or alterations in temperature may indicate a reflex sympathetic dystrophy.

PATELLAR MALALIGNMENT

This is a **common source** of sports disability, particularly in sports requiring jumping or rapid changes of direction. The terms "malalignment" and "instability" are commonly used interchangeably. **Malalignment** is an abnormal relationship between the patella and its associated soft tissue and bony surroundings throughout the course of knee motion. **Instability** is usually manifest only at **certain** points within the range of motion when abnormal alignment occurs.

During knee motion the patella follows a course of tilt, flexion and rotation (a toroidal path) (Fig. 28). Stability through this path depends on a complex series of interactions among joint congruity and static and dynamic stabilisers, both local and remote.

Static forces that provide stability include primary knee joint patello-femoral congruity, the menisco-patellar ligaments, the medial and lateral tethers

APPROACH TO THE KNEE	
Above the patella	muscle weakness/contraction, internal femoral torsion
The patella	alta/baja/lateral tilt
Below the patella	lateral tib.tub/valgus/int.tib. torsion/tight hamstrings

Figure 27 - Approach to examination of the child's knee

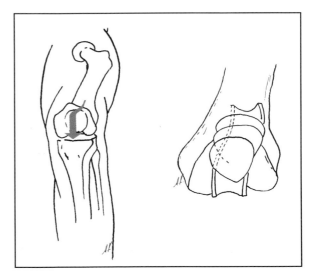

Figure 28 - The patella follows a toroidal path in movement (of tilt, flexion, and rotation)

extending from the ilio-tibial band, vastus lateralis and vastus medialis.

Dynamic forces include the quadriceps groups, specifically the tethering effect of the vastus medialis obliquus. Femoral and tibial rotational abnormalities also affect patello-femoral orientation. The maximum amount of femoral anteversion or tibial torsion that can be compensated for, and tolerated without symptoms, is unknown, but appears to be significant in view of the large number of patients, with femoral and tibial torsion, who are completely asymptomatic.

Anatomic factors purported to predispose patients to patellar instability, include patella-alta, generalised joint hypermobility, increased Q angle, increased femoral anteversion, increased external tibial torsion, abnormal ilio-tibial band attachments, genu-valgum, genu-recurvatum, femoral condylar hypo-plasia, or dysplasia of the patella, or a combination of these. However, no one of these factors is always present in cases of patellar instability, and in some situations none of these factors are clinically obvious.

PATELLAR SUBLUXATION

Patellar subluxation is a transient event in which the median ridge of the patella moves over the lateral edge of the lateral femoral condyle in predisposed patients when pivoting or twisting on a flexed knee. There is a popping sensation, anterior knee pain, and pain over the medial aspect of the knee (stretching of the medial patellar retinaculum). These patellae reduce spontaneously, and as the patella returns to the femoral sulcus, shear stresses are placed on the median ridge and medial facet of the patella, resulting in chondral fractures (with or without the release of chondral debris). This debris then acts as a synovial irritant and can produce an effusion.

The history is very important as the physical examination may reveal an apparently normal knee, or an effusion and any number of the factors previously mentioned.

CLASSIFICATION OF PATELLAR DISLOCATION
• Congenital
• Recurrent
• Habitual
• Traumatic

Figure 29 - Classification of patellar dislocation

X-rays of the knee include AP, lateral, tunnel views and merchant views of the patello-femoral joint (the knee flexed to 45 degrees outline the patella). Such views will assess bony contours, and height of the patella, and exclude osteo-chondral fragments.

CT scanning may help.

Treatment initially is non-operative with an intensive quadriceps rehabilitation exercise programme, lateral retinacular stretching and hamstring stretching exercises. The small number of cases that fail to respond to these measures may benefit from arthroscopic lateral retinacular release.

PATELLAR DISLOCATION

Patellar dislocation is classified (Fig. 29).

Congenital dislocation of the patella

The patella has never been located (as in arthrogryposis multiplex congenita, Down's syndrome or familial congenital dislocation of the patella).

Recurrent dislocation of the patella

The patella dislocates intermittently. The onset is usually in adolescence, and may be secondary to the underlying causes described.

Habitual dislocation of the patella

The knee dislocates with every flexion or extension of the knee. Dislocation in flexion needs to be differentiated from dislocation in extension. Dislocation in flexion is secondary to quadriceps contracture, and if one is able to forcibly hold the patella in the mid-line, the knee cannot be flexed more than 30 degrees. Further flexion is possible only if the patella dislocates laterally. Dislocation in extension is usually due to patellar malalignment. In terminal extension the patella moves laterally, such that it lies outside the normal toroidal path of the patella. As the knee flexes, the patella may or may not engage the patello-femoral groove. If it does not, it then tracks laterally until it flicks back into the patello-femoral groove.

Acute traumatic dislocation of the patella

In acute dislocation differentiate the non-contact type from the contact type (was the patella pushed out of place as it came in contact with the ground or another player, or was it pulled out of joint by intrinsic factors related to the previously mentioned anatomical variations) (Fig. 30).

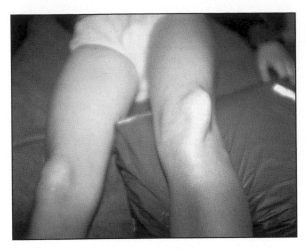

Figure 30 - Acute traumatic dislocation of patella

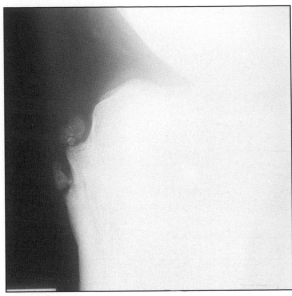

Figure 31 - Osgood-Schlatter's Disease. A micro-avulsion of the patellar tendon (here there is fragmentation of the tibial tubercle)

Treatment is surgical (60% show evidence of osteo-chondral or chondral fractures). Arthroscopic lavage and debridement is required to remove any debris. If there is no significant effusion or pain, and full range of movement, chondral damage is unlikely and an active physiotherapy programme can be commenced. Following surgery, an intensive quadriceps rehabilitation exercise programme is needed along with hamstring stretching. Cast or splint immobilisation should be avoided.

Surgical reconstructive procedures for the management of patellar instability consist of:

- Proximal realignment by means of lateral release, medial reefing or combined lateral release with medial reefing.

- Distal realignment by means of the patellar tendon or tibial tubercle transfer or semi-tendinosis tenodesis.

- A combination of above.

MULTI-PARTITE PATELLA

The bipartite variant is the most common (also three or even four segments). Often an incidental X-ray finding. The reported incidence of bipartite patella ranges from 0.2–6%. It is uncommonly bilateral, and there is a strong male dominance of 9 to 1. There is pain in the supero-lateral quadrant of the anterior knee.

Examination reveals asymmetry with an alteration of the contour of the supero-lateral quadrant (enlarged with associated tenderness). Seen on X-ray.

Treatment includes modification of activity, physiotherapy with lateral retinacular stretching and quadriceps strengthening, a short period of splint immobilisation. If symptoms persist then surgical excision is necessary.

OSGOOD-SCHLATTER'S DISEASE

This is not a disease. It is a micro-avulsion of the patellar tendon from the anterior portion of the developing ossification centre of the tibial tuberosity, due to repeated traction injuries (Fig. 31). The growth plate remains intact.

It is an extremely common source of sports disability. Boys are more commonly affected (girls present between 11 and 13, boys between 12 and 15), and it is five times more common in adolescent athletes. Bilateral in 20 to 30% of cases.

Diagnosis is based on symptoms and physical signs. The pain is usually activity-related (in association with running and jumping sports). There is swelling and

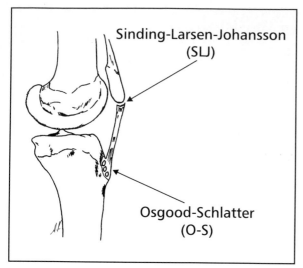

Figure 32 - Sinding-Larsen-Johansson Syndrome is a traction apophysitis of the lower pole of the patella (upper end of patellar tendon; whereas Osgood-Schlatter's is of the lower end of the patellar tendon)

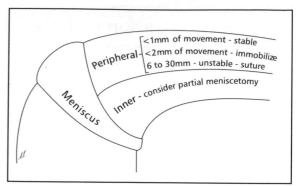

Figure 33 - The treatment of meniscal injuries in children depends upon the site and size of the tear

prominence of the tibial tuberosity, associated with localised tenderness and significant hamstring tightness.

X-rays show soft tissue swelling with fragmentation of the tibial tubercle.

Treatment aims to relieve pain and swelling (ice, oral analgesics, anti-inflammatory agents and physiotherapeutic modalities). Quadriceps strengthening and hamstring stretching are important, as is activity modification but complete denial of sports participation is unnecessary (very occasionally a short period of cast immobilisation is needed).

A painful sequestrum within the patellar ligament may need to be excised.

SINDING-LARSEN-JOHANSSON SYNDROME

This is an apophysitis of the inferior pole of the patella, occurring in pre-teen boys (Fig. 32). It is activity related and associated with jumping and running sports. There is point tenderness over the inferior pole of the patella and there are varying amounts of calcification or ossification of the inferior pole of the patella.

It should be distinguished from an acute patellar sleeve fracture (complete separation of the patellar tendon from the inferior pole of the patella). A sleeve fracture of the patella is defined as an extensive sleeve of cartilage that is pulled off the main body of the bony patella, together with a bony fragment from the distal pole. In such situations the patient would be unable to perform a straight leg raise, and radiologically there would be evidence of a patella alta. This lesion requires open reduction and internal fixation.

Treatment is similar to that for Osgood-Schlatter's disease (symptomatic, with modification of activities, quadriceps strengthening and hamstring stretching).

THE MENISCUS

An increase in the incidence of meniscal injuries in children has resulted from an increased awareness and from the greater number of children participating in organised and unorganised sports.

The exact incidence is not known. Injuries of the lateral and medial menisci occur with equal frequency, but if discoid meniscal injuries are eliminated, the medial meniscus is more often injured. The mechanism of injury is (as in adults) a decelerating contact or non-contact force causing a compressive load with rotation.

There is pain, giving way, stiffness, swelling and occasionally locking. One third of patients have no significant findings on physical examination. In children there is a poor correlation between the physical findings and arthroscopic findings. The younger the child, the poorer the correlation.

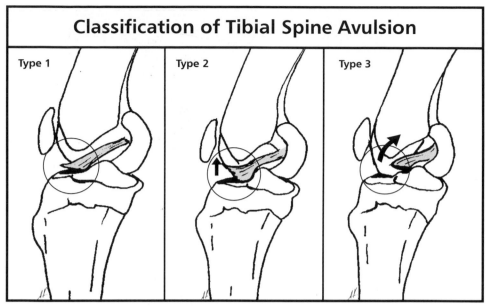

Classification of Tibial Spine Avulsion

Type 1   Type 2   Type 3

Figure 34 - Classification of tibial spine avulsions

The treatment depends on the site and size of the tear (Fig. 33). Peripheral meniscal tears of less than 1 cm are stable (less than 2 mm of motion when probed) and heal with 4 to 6 weeks of immobilisation.

Tears between 6 mm and 30 mm are unstable (occur in red/red or red/white zone), and may heal because of the improved vascularity. Such tears are suitable for meniscal suture followed by 4 to 6 weeks of immobilisation. Meniscal lesions not amenable to meniscal preservation require partial meniscectomy. Following partial meniscectomy an intensive quadriceps exercise programme is undertaken, and no sport for at least 4 to 6 weeks. Following meniscal repair or meniscal healing, at least 4 to 6 months of graduated rehabilitation is required.

THE DISCOID MENISCUS

The incidence of the discoid meniscus varies worldwide from 3–5% in Anglo-Saxons, to 20% in the Japanese. The cause is unknown; as a discoid configuration is not seen in any stage of fetal development.

A symptomatic discoid lateral meniscus causes a snapping sensation over the lateral aspect of the knee. Otherwise they are incidental findings at arthroscopy.

When symptomatic, treat by excision of the unstable part and reshape to a normal crescentic shape.

ANTERIOR CRUCIATE LIGAMENT

The most common anterior cruciate ligament (ACL) injury in the child is an avulsion of the tibial spine. Myers and McIver describe three grades of tibial spine avulsion (Type I fractures non-displaced; Type II some elevation; Type III elevation with displacement and rotation) (Fig. 34).

Associated tears of the medial collateral ligament may occur. Treatment depends on the grade. Type I and Type II injuries require casting with the knee in 15 to 20 degrees of flexion for 6 weeks; Type III requires open reduction and internal fixation (Fig. 35).

These injuries are associated with stretching of the anterior cruciate ligament prior to bone failure (knee laxity is identified by an increase in the Lachmann's sign, but functional instability is not a problem).

Insubstance tears of the anterior cruciate ligament in the skeletally immature are being seen (previously thought to be rare as the tensile strength of ligaments is greater than that of the growth plate; also the capsular and cruciate ligaments are inserted within the epiphyses of the tibia and femur, only the insertion of the tibial collateral ligament crosses the tibial physeal plate).

Anterior cruciate injuries treated non-operatively in the child do no better than in the adult. Treatment

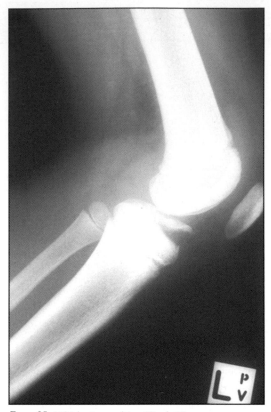

Figure 35 - Tibial spine avulsion (Grade II)

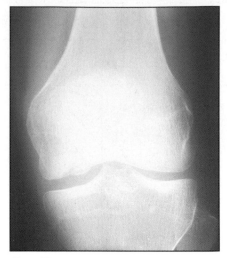

Figure 36 - Osteochondritis dissecans of the knee in the typical location

remains controversial (as the surgical procedure must avoid damage to the physeal plates if there is significant growth remaining). Opinion differs as to when the growth plate can be breached. Some treat as in an adult if the child is within 2 years of skeletal maturity or there is less than 1 cm of growth remaining.

If significant clinical instability exists below this age range, then reconstruction using tubularised ilio-tibial band to provide both a lateral extra-capsular reconstruction and an intra-capsular reconstruction via the over the top position is successful.

OSTEOCHONDRITIS DISSECANS OF THE KNEE

A lesion of uncertain aetiology, rare under the age of 10, with a male predominance of 3 to 1, and a 20% incidence of bilaterality. Eighty percent involve the lateral aspect of the medial femoral condyle, 20% involve the posterior aspect of the lateral femoral condyle.

The patient presents with pain on activity and occasionally a clicking sensation.

There is usually little on physical examination.

X-rays (AP, lateral and tunnel views) usually define the lesion (Fig. 36). MRI may provide information on fragment healing or risk of separation.

The aim of treatment is to prevent fragment separation with its associated risk of early knee osteoarthritis (Fig. 37).

The main prognostic factor is age (Fig. 38) which also guides treatment.

The **childhood group** usually heals spontaneously, and should be followed radiologically until union.

The **immature group** can be observed for 12 months, and if they remain symptomatic and the lesion is radiologically ununited, then arthroscopic Herbert screw fixation is recommended. For those patients under observation, complete cessation of sport is not justified. Activity modification within the limitations of symptoms is all that is required.

The **junctional group** require immediate screw fixation, as there appears to be a greater chance of healing prior to growth plate closure. If the lesion has not separated, then screw fixation alone can be performed. If the lesion has separated, then open surgery with bone grafting and fixation is required.

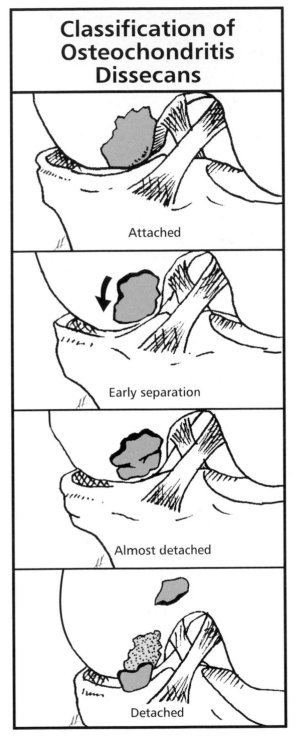

Classification of Osteochondritis Dissecans

Attached

Early separation

Almost detached

Detached

Figure 37 - Classification of osteochondritis dissecans by degree of separation and so guide to treatment

CLASSIFICATION OF OSTEOCHONDRITIS (THOMSON AND GRAY)		
• **Juvenile**		**Age**
Childhood		10-13
Immature	(epiphyses open)	13-16
Junctional	(epiphyses closed)	16-18
• **Adult**		
Mature	(epiphyses closed)	>20

Figure 38 - Classification of osteochondritis dissecans by age; which is the main prognostic parameter

In the adult, open surgery with grafting and fixation is recommended, or if a loose body is already present, then removal.

ANKLE AND FOOT INJURIES

Ankle and foot pain, secondary to congenital and developmental abnormalities are not uncommon and often sport is the precipitating event. Consider the following conditions but do not forget acute injuries:

TARSAL COALITION

Tarsal coalition is a bony or fibro-cartilaginous connection of two or more of the tarsal bones due to failure of differentiation and segmentation of the primitive mesenchyme. Calcaneo-navicular and talo-calcaneal coalitions are the most common.

The age of presentation is 8 to 16 years. A family history may exist (autosomal dominant with incomplete penetrance).

There is gradual onset of hindfoot pain, aggravated by running over uneven ground.

Clinically there may be peroneal spasm resulting in valgus of the hindfoot with pes planus deformity. Significant limitation of sub-talar joint motion is present.

Calcaneo-navicular coalitions can be diagnosed on a X-ray using a 45 degree oblique view. Talo-calcaneal coalitions are difficult to see on X-ray but are well imaged on CT.

Treatment is initially symptomatic with rest and modification of activities. Relieving plaster casts may be required. Those who fail to respond to these measures may require surgery.

Calcaneo-navicular coalitions are treated by resection of the bar with interposition of the extensor-digitorum brevis muscle. The results are very good.

Talo-calcaneal coalitions may be amenable to surgery. The size of the coalition that can be resected is unknown (up to 50% of the involved facet). In the symptomatic patient with an unresectable coalition, and arthritis in the talo-navicular joint, triple arthrodesis is necessary.

ACCESSORY NAVICULAR

Adolescents present with pain and tenderness over the medial border of the foot, aggravated by running or jumping sports or rubbing footwear.

Clinical examination reveals a cornuate prominence on the medial side of the navicular, which may be tender and show pressure from footwear.

An X-ray will confirm the presence of an ossicle at the medial border of the navicular (controversy whether a stress fracture, or a separate centre of ossification).

Treatment is an arch support and modification of footwear. Acute pain, aggravated by weight bearing may require six weeks of cast immobilisation. Rarely excision of the lesion with tightening of the tibialis posterior tendon is required.

OSTEOCHONDROSES

These are idiopathic disorders of enchondral ossification which occur during the years of rapid growth. Trauma may influence their development, particularly from sport.

FREIBERG'S DISEASE

Freiberg's disease involves collapse of the articular surface and subchondral bone of the metatarsal head (most commonly seen in the second metatarsal, then the third or the fourth) (*See Fig. 43, Chapter 15*). More common in females, and presents between 12 and 15 years of age.

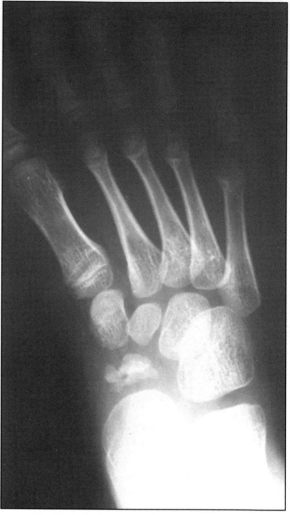

Figure 39 - Kohler's disease with fragmentation of the navicular (almost always resolves spontaneously)

The adolescent presents with pain on weight bearing, particularly during toe off. Clinically there is localised tenderness and swelling.

The diagnosis is confirmed by typical X-ray appearances of initially increased density, followed by collapse with flattening, and occasionally fragmentation with loose body formation.

Treatment consists of rest and the use of a metatarsal dome. Surgery to bone graft the collapsed head, remove loose bodies or realignment with dorsal osteotomy is occasionally required.

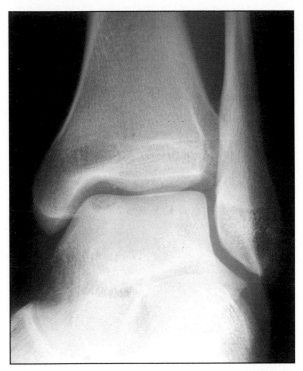

Figure 40 - Osteochondritis dissecans of the medial talar dome (may also occur on lateral dome)

CLASSIFICATION OF OSTEO-CHONDRAL LESIONS OF TALUS (ANDERSON)

- **Stage 1**

  There is subchondral trabecular compression.
  The X-ray is normal.
  The bone scan is hot and the MRI is diagnostic.

- **Stage 2**

  Incomplete separation of the fragment *

- **Stage 2 (a)**

  The formation of subchondral cysts *

- **Stage 3**

  Unattached, undisplaced fragment *

- **Stage 4**

  Displaced fragment *

* Seen on CT

Figure 41 - Classification of osteo-chondral lesions of the talus

KOHLER'S DISEASE

Kohler's disease is regular ossification of the tarsal navicular, resulting in localised pain and X-ray narrowing and increased density of the navicular (Fig. 39). The age of onset of this completely reversible condition is from 2 to 9 weeks. Treatment is symptomatic. Supportive casts for 6 weeks may be required. With time, the bone fully reconstitutes without long-term sequelae.

SEVER'S DISEASE

Sever's disease or calcaneal apophysitis is a common entity in the 9- to 11-year-old age group. The child may present with heel pain, particularly with running and a limp.

Clinically the calcaneal apophysis is very tender. The tendo-Achilles may be tight.

X-rays are not helpful because the calcaneal apophysis is frequently fragmented and dense in normal children.

Treatment depends on the severity of the child's

symptoms, and includes relative rest, calf stretching and strengthening exercises and occasionally the use of a heel raise. It is a self-limiting condition with no adverse long-term sequelae.

OSTEO-CHONDRAL LESIONS OF THE TALUS

Osteochondritis dissecans was used to describe lesions on the medial aspect of the talar dome (Fig. 40). It is now believed that lesions on both the medial and lateral aspect of the talar dome are secondary to trauma. The site of the lesion is the end result of the force applied (lateral fractures produced by inversion and dorsi-flexion, and medial fractures by strong lateral rotation of the tibia on a plantar flexed and inverted foot). Such lesions have been classified (Fig. 41).

The diagnosis should always be considered where persisting ankle pain occurs 6 weeks after an injury.

Investigations include a X-ray and a CT to better define the lesion. If the X-ray is normal, and there is a higher index of suspicion, then a bone scan should be performed. If this is positive, then an MRI scan is useful.

Treatment depends on the stage of the lesion.

Stage 1 and 2 lesions are immobilised in a cast for 6 weeks. Such lesions need to be followed to ensure that union is complete.

Stage 2(a), Stage 3 and Stage 4 fractures may all require surgical intervention, and following arthroscopic assessment, either internal fixation or removal of the lesion may be indicated.

GENERAL WARNING

Treating clinicians need to be always aware that pain and tenderness of a low grade may be the first presentation of a bone tumour in a child (Fig. 42). This needs to be borne in mind when treating overuse injuries and stress fractures. Remember that Ewing's Tumour may mimic osteomyelitis with fever and constitutional symptoms of listlessness.

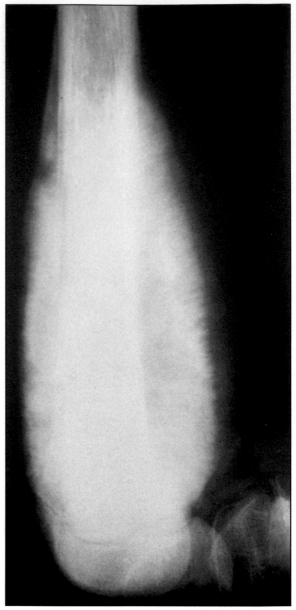

Figure 42 - High grade osteogenic sarcoma of femur

19

THE OLDER ATHLETE

Kerwyn Foo
Cindy Mak

INTRODUCTION

It is difficult to define what an older athlete is. Competitions start at the age of 25 for swimming and at 35 to 40 for athletics. People of all ages regularly compete in marathons.

In prehistory, man rarely needed to consider the ageing process. Life was short and the hunter gatherer did not live long beyond a decrease in ability and performance. In the modern day, athletic performance has become less vital for life, but has remained important into old age. Older people have an interest in maintaining health, and some go further to maintain a competitive edge.

Sports medicine for older athletes is not only about competitive performance. The benefits of exercise are many, but so, unfortunately, are those who do not partake of them. The goal is as much to encourage a healthy active lifestyle as it is to help the older competitor (Fig. 1).

PHYSIOLOGICAL CHANGES OF AGEING

Along with the awareness of our own mortality, we have an understanding that our bodies will age. Ageing is a universal process, causing progressive structural and functional loss. There are theories of why we age. Leonardo da Vinci, after careful anatomical studies, concluded that thickening blood vessels were the cause. Even today, the cause of the ageing process remains unknown.

Ageing causes a decrease in the number, function and regeneration of cells. This leads to structural and functional changes in the older person. Figure 2 shows the physical changes of ageing that are affected by exercise. It clearly shows that the loss of function is due as much to disuse and inactivity as to ageing itself.

Some ageing body systems have implications on the way older people exercise (Fig. 3). Refer to the section **Guidelines for Exercise** (Fig.6) for further recommendations.

In general, functional reserves decrease with age. To attain the same performance, the older athlete must push closer to the body's limits.

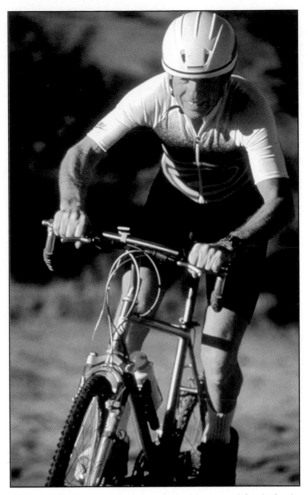

Figure 1 – Senior mountain biking – a healthy active lifestyle for the older athlete

CARE OF OLDER ATHLETE

The aspects to consider are:

- Exercise for older people

- Injuries and problems of older athletes

- Previous sporting activity – ongoing care of athletes as they age

REGULAR EXERCISE SLOWS THE EFFECTS OF AGE ON BODY SYSTEMS		
System	**Ageing Changes**	**Effect of Exercise**
Muscle	• mass and strength lost slowly with ageing • power decreases	• can be minimised with exercise

Bone	• mass loss after age 35,
	  increases after age 55
	• trabecular bone lost before cortical
	• faster loss in post-menopausal women
	• decrease in total body calcium
		• bone loss reduced by regular exercise
		  and good nutrition

Cartilage	• loss of elasticity (may increase osteoarthritis) • greatest risk in knee, hip, ankle, spinal facets if already present	• weight bearing exercise may slow changes • impact may worsen degenerative arthritis

Ligaments and tendons	• lose elasticity with age (increase in
	  sprains and strains)
	• decreased flexibility
	• loss of flexibility and range of motion
	  may increase joint and muscle injury
		• stretching before and after exercise
		  maintains flexibility
		• regular use maintains strength and suppleness

Nervous system	• decrease in conduction velocity and number of neurons/axons • slower reactions and speed • loss of vision and hearing	• reaction times are faster if maintained by use
Cardiovascular	• lower VO_{2max} • less anaerobic endurance • lower cardiac output and maximum heart rate • increased risk of coronary artery disease • slower return of heart rate to resting value • increased vascular resistance	• exercise can maintain VO_{2max} • can stop endurance loss • slows decline in maximum heart rate • aerobic exercise more effective than anaerobic, may decrease risk of CAD
Respiratory system	• decreased compliance • reduced airflow • increased effort of breathing	• regular exercise reduces respiratory changes

Figure 2 – Physical changes of ageing that are affected by exercise

EXERCISE IMPLICATIONS FOR SOME AGEING BODY SYSTEMS		
System	**Ageing Changes**	**Effect of Exercise**
Renal system	• glomeruli loss decreases filtration • loss of total body water (higher risk of dehydration)	• ensure fluids • avoid very hot weather • break up workout
Skin	• thinning of skin decreases thermal insulation • skin becomes more fragile • epidermis looser - predisposes to blisters • reduction in defence to UV radiation	• use sunscreens, hats • well-fitting footwear
Thermoregulation	• reduced heat dissipation	• heat tolerance may be less
Regeneration	• slower healing	• longer rest periods after injury

Figure 3 – Exercise implications for some ageing body systems

EXERCISE PROGRAMMES FOR OLDER PEOPLE

GOALS OF AN EXERCISE PROGRAMME

The ultimate goal of an exercise programme is to improve quality of life. It aims to:

- Improve aerobic capacity
- Increase strength and energy
- Improve balance
- Increase self-esteem
- Improve sleep patterns
- Improve independence
- Provide social interaction and enjoyment

EXERCISE EVALUATION

Any older person starting an exercise programme should be evaluated for risk factors that make them prone to injury or may limit their activity.

HISTORY

The history should include previous and current medical conditions, medication, current nutritional status and previous injuries. Risk factors for coronary artery disease and diabetes mellitus should be identified. A less rigorous exercise program is recommended for those with two or more risk factors.

CARDIOVASCULAR SCREENING

A cardiac stress test should be performed if the patient has one of the following:

- Recent myocardial infarction or coronary artery bypass surgery (Fig. 4).
- Major risk factors for cardiovascular disease (e.g. obesity, hypertension, hypercholesterolaemia, family history, smoking).
- A pacemaker-fixed rate or demand.
- Use of chronotropic/inotropic medication.

At least 70% of the maximum heart rate based on age should be achieved.

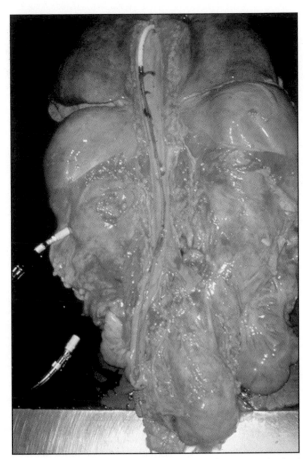

Figure 4 – Balloon pump (in situ at autopsy) has not maintained cardiac output

Stress testing is unnecessary for gentle exercises (non-competitive swimming, walking, bowls).

MUSCULOSKELETAL EVALUATION

The older athlete is more prone to musculoskeletal injury and is slower to recover than a younger athlete. Musculoskeletal evaluation is therefore important.

EVALUATE

Muscle strength – Most injuries to the mature athlete involve the lower limbs. Assessment of knee and ankle injuries is therefore necessary. The athlete should be able to generate enough force to lift at least half of his or her body weight.

Flexibility – The ankle should have at least 10° of dorsiflexion. The hip should have at least a 60° arc of motion. Check for hip flexion contractures, iliotibial band tightness and rectus femoris tightness.

Deformity and joint pain – Check for hallux valgus, genu valgum, femoral anteversion, arthritis and discrepancies in leg length.

SENSORY TESTING

Check for sensory deficits in the limbs, vision, hearing and colour perception.

MET	
Activity	**METs**
Level walking at 4 km/h	3.0
Jogging at 8 km/h	8.4
Swimming, 30 metres/minute	10.0
Tennis	6.0 - 10.0
Soccer	7.0 - 15.0

Figure 5 – Metabolic equivalent units

EXERCISE PRESCRIPTION

A good exercise prescription should include intensity, exercise mode, duration, frequency and progression.

INTENSITY

Intensity is an important variable in exercise prescription. There are several ways to determine intensity levels:

1. VO_{2max} : VO_{2max} represents the ability of an athlete to extract oxygen from the environment and use it to generate ATP during work. Training is induced during exercise at 40-85% VO_{2max}.

2. Maximum heart rate (HRmax): HRmax can be calculated using (220 - age) + 15. Intensity can then be expressed as a percentage of HRmax 55-90%. HRmax is the level recommended by theAmerican College of Sports Medicine to induce training.

3. Metabolic Equivalent Units (METs): A MET represents the VO_2 at rest (35ml/kg/min). The maximum MET level (MML) is the maximum intensity level for an athlete. This can be determined by exercise testing. Optimum intensity recommended is 40-85% MML. The work intensity of different activities (in METS) can be read off pre-existing tables. This allows the athlete to choose an activity most suited to his/her target MET level (Fig. 5).

EXERCISE

Rhythmic activity utilising large muscle groups is preferred. Some weight bearing is also recommended.

DURATION

15-60 minutes continuously at a moderate intensity is ideal.

FREQUENCY

A minimum of 3 to a maximum of 5 days a week (except obese athletes who require a daily low intensity program).

PROGRESSION

Increase intensity, duration and frequency as fitness improves. Aim to keep the heart rate in the desired training range. Only one variable should be increased in any session.

GUIDELINES FOR EXERCISE

The 'Dos and Don'ts' of exercise for mature athletes are shown in Figure 6.

INJURIES AND PROBLEMS OF THE OLDER ATHLETE

INJURIES

Figure 7 shows the aetiology of exercise-related injuries in the aged. Many are running or walking related, with fewer trauma injuries from contact sports. Overuse injuries relate to 70% of injuries seen in the ageing athlete. These tend to progress slowly, be neglected by the athlete and present late. They may be slow to respond and have been self-treated by the athlete.

GUIDELINES FOR EXERCISE IN THE OLDER ATHLETE	
Do's	**Don'ts**
Set realistic goals	High impact activities
Exercise within the limits of the exercise tolerance test	Extremely hot, humid conditions causing dehydration (especially if on diuretictherapy)
Exercise aerobically using large muscle groups (jogging/cycling/swimming)	Extreme cold (causing frostbite, hypothermia, cold-induced angina and bronchospasm)
Incorporate weight bearing activities into the IR programme (for prevention of osteoporosis)	The Valsalva manoeuvre (especially if hypertensive/coronary prone)
Wear appropriate clothing and footwear	High levels of pollution (athletes with chronic airways limitation)
Increase activity gradually	Abrupt changes in amount/ intensity of training
Have rest periods during exercise	Prolonged sun exposure (predisposing to skin cancers)
Warm up and cool down sufficiently	
Treat injuries quickly and adequately	
Exercise with a partner	

Figure 6 – The 'Do's and Don'ts' of exercise for mature athletes

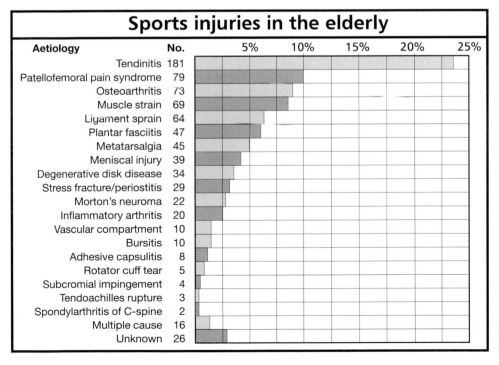

Sports injuries in the elderly

Aetiology	No.
Tendinitis	181
Patellofemoral pain syndrome	79
Osteoarthritis	73
Muscle strain	69
Ligament sprain	64
Plantar fasciitis	47
Metatarsalgia	45
Meniscal injury	39
Degenerative disk disease	34
Stress fracture/periostitis	29
Morton's neuroma	22
Inflammatory arthritis	20
Vascular compartment	10
Bursitis	10
Adhesive capsulitis	8
Rotator cuff tear	5
Subcromial impingement	4
Tendoachilles rupture	3
Spondylarthritis of C-spine	2
Multiple cause	16
Unknown	26

Figure 7 – Aetiology of exercise-related injuries in the aged

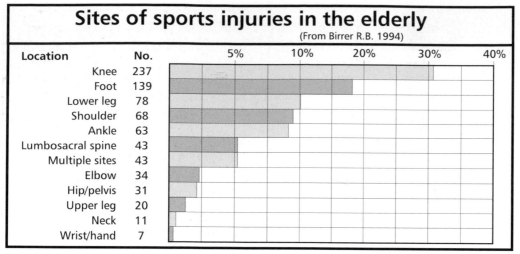

Figure 8 – Locations of injury of the old resemble those in the young, with knee, foot and lower leg being the most common

Locations of injury in the old resemble those in the young, with knee, foot and lower leg being the most common (Fig. 8). The strength and flexibility with age leads to less impact absorption in the lower limb. More knee and foot injuries are the result. Overuse superimposed on tissue degeneration leads to shoulder, tendon and ligament injuries.

Osteoarthritic symptoms are common in older athletes, and may actually be due to another problem. The prevalence of osteoarthritis in the aged can be misleading. **Misdiagnosis** can occur often - injury conditions (such as meniscal tear or extra-articular soft tissue damage) are labelled osteoarthritis, resulting in inappropriate treatment.

DIAGNOSIS

- History - common features are:
  - → aggravation by activity
  - → pre-existing condition
  - → trauma or increased intensity of training.
- Physical examination.

These suffice for 70-84% of injuries in this group.

Investigations that may be useful in the remainder are: X-rays, CT, blood chemistry (bone scan) and arthroscopy.

TREATMENT

Injuries in the older athlete are often managed conservatively.

- RICE
- Decrease activity level 15-25% until symptoms resolve
- Rebuild training level slowly
- Drugs (NSAID and others)
  - → "start low, go slow"
  - → older athletes use many regular medications - beware drug interactions
  - → prolonged therapy may be necessary due to slower healing in the aged
- Physiotherapy (exercises, ultrasound)
- Exercise to build muscle strength (such as quadriceps in knee injury)
- Bracing (in achilles tendinitis, ankle instability)
- Local corticosteroid (*See Figure 17, Chapter 2*).

Only 24% of injuries require surgery.

Specific sports have been studied and the effect of age on injury risk varies (Fig. 9).

OSTEOPOROSIS

Osteoporosis is the condition where the rate of bone absorption exceeds the rate of bone formation. Bone mass begins to decline at the age of 40 in both

| AGE EFFECT ON SPORTS RELATED INJURIES FOR SPECIFIC SPORTS ||
Sport	Age effect on injury risk
Soccer	high acute arm injury risk
Marathon/long distance running	varies from no increased injury to sport most affecting injury risk
Running	no effect
Golf	more overuse shoulder injuries in older golfers
Orienteering	more muscle ruptures in older athletes, more acute injuries
Ball games	increased accident rates

Figure 9 – Age effect on sports related injuries for specific sports

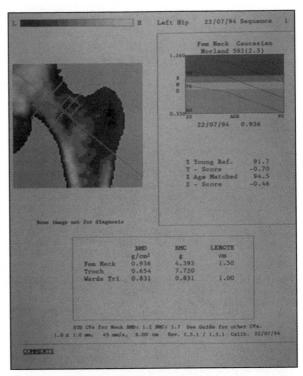

Figure 10 – Decreased bone density predisposes to fractures (here measured on bone density scan of hip region)

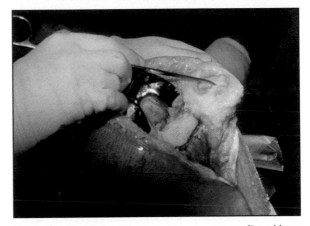

Figure 11 – Osteoarthritis is more common among elite athletes, endurance runners and power sports (osteoarthritis seen here at total knee replacement)

sexes. Bone loss further accelerates in women after menopause.

The ageing process contributes to osteoporosis by slowing the resorption and redeposition of components of the bone matrix (Fig.10). There is also an age-related decrease in total body calcium. The result is an increase in fractures, especially of the hip and vertebral column.

Osteoporosis poses major problems for the older person just beginning an exercise program. He or she should start slowly and cautiously, allowing time for the skeletal system to adapt.

Studies have shown that **regular physical activity** (especially resistance-type activity) and good nutrition can increase bone mineral content in all age groups. Beginning an exercise program, even late in life, can be beneficial to the skeleton. However, an excessive amount of training seems to be detrimental to the skeleton, indicating that an optimal amount of exercise may exist.

ONGOING CARE

Often the older athlete was a younger athlete and trained throughout life. Former athletes may have problems arising from past sporting activity. There are some common consequences from the "past sins" of a training history.

It is possible that increased osteoarthritis is found among former elite athletes (Fig.11). Power sport participants are more likely to have premature osteoarthritis. Endurance running has also been considered as a factor in osteoarthritis. Other arthroses, especially of the hip and knee, seem to be more common in past athletes.

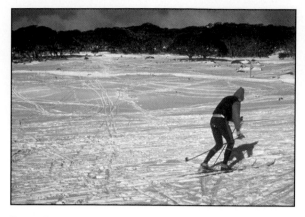

Figure 12 – Old endurance athletes (here cross-country skier) need more carbohydrate and are prone to dehydration

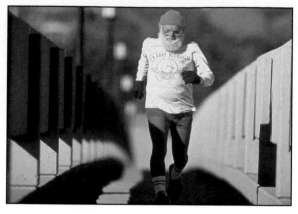

Figure 14 – Short distance running times drop-off more with age than longer distance

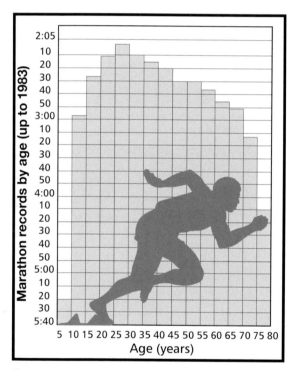

Figure 13 – Peak athletic performance decreases with age (here marathon records by age in the USA)

Soccer players and weight lifters have had more mild lumbar disk changes than non–athletes, but the overall incidence of back pain is lower.

In general, previous injury during a sporting career can return as a chronic condition if the older athlete does not take adequate precautions. Older athletes soon learn that the ageing body is less forgiving than in their youth.

OTHER ISSUES

NUTRITION

Whether to perform competitively or to improve general health, the older athlete's exercise programme requires a good diet.

The older athlete needs to maintain the same mix of food groups as that of younger athletes. If involved in endurance training, carbohydrates need to be increased to 60-70% of the diet (Fig. 12). Adequate protein is essential (vegetarian diets must be well planned).

Vitamin supplements can only be of assistance if the dietary intake is inadequate. Iron is especially important for distance runners. All older athletes must pay attention to calcium intake to support bone mineral density.

Dehydration is more common in the aged. Drinking water prior to, during and post-exercise reduces risk of heat and dehydration (*See Chapter 4*).

ATHLETIC PERFORMANCE

With the advent of masters competitions, older people are increasingly taking up or returning to competitive sport. The age divisions of some sports reflect that peak athletic performance tends to decrease with age

(Fig. 13 & 14). Short distance running, jumping and some throwing events are more affected whilst long distance running decreases less.

CONCLUSION

As the population ages, it becomes more important that the mature members of society remain active and healthy. Encouraging exercise and sporting activity among older people will reduce the social and economic costs of an elderly population in failing health.

Older people use sport for diverse reasons: health, social contacts and also high level competition. The physician must be ready to advise each individual according to their sporting goals and situation. With adequate advice and care, there is little reason why the older person should not continue to enjoy the many benefits of sport.

20

THE DISABLED ATHLETE

Talal Ibrahim
Vincent Lam

INTRODUCTION

Who is the disabled athlete?

The disabled athlete is the person who suffers physical, sensory, or cognitive impairment that interferes with his or her participation in sport (Fig. 1).

HISTORICAL PERSPECTIVE

Early sports participation by the disabled was on an individual basis. The origin of organised competitive sport for the disabled was directly related to the rehabilitation of Second World War veterans with spinal cord injury. It was the renewed interest in sport as therapy in post-war hospitals in the UK and USA that led to the present day state of sport for the disabled.

The development of the first international competition for the disabled was in 1949. The games were held in Austria and this was the first 'World Winter Games' for the deaf. Subsequently, international competitions involving other disabled athletes, amputees and spinal cord injured have been taking place throughout the world. Organisations such as the International Sport Organisation for the Disabled (ISOD) was formed in 1964 and its objective was to co-ordinate sport competitions for all disabled athletes.

The disabled groups considered:

- Sensory: the deaf athlete.
             the blind athlete.

- Physical: the spinal cord injured.
             the amputee athletes.
             the cerebral palsied athletes.

Disabled athletes with the above physical impairments are classified as either wheelchair dependent or independent.

- Cognitive: mentally handicapped.

- Les Autres: disabled athletes who do not fit into any of the disability groups above, such as muscular dystrophy, multiple sclerosis, dwarfism.

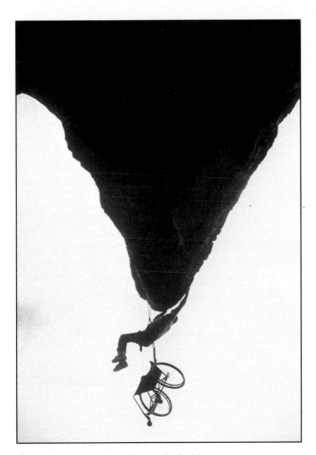

Figure 1 – No limits. Paraplegic rock climbing.

ATHLETES WITH SENSORY IMPAIRMENT

THE BLIND ATHLETE

- Blind athletes have a partial or complete loss of sight. Eligibility for athletic competition is granted only to those individuals who have a visual acuity of 6/60 or less.

- Blind athletes can compete in a wide variety of sports including baseball, bowling, cycling, marathon, racing, track and field, and wrestling. The events include modification of some rules to facilitate participation by blind competitors.

- The only specific sports medicine problem for the blind is related to falls. Falls on the outstretched upper limbs are not uncommon, leading to the same types of fractures and soft tissue injuries as in the able-bodied athletes. Sprains of the knee and ankle ligaments are also not uncommon.

THE DEAF ATHLETE

- The deaf athlete's hearing impairment is often the result of sensorineural deficits caused through cochlear damage. Equilibrium deficits with a loss of balance and co-ordination may compound the athlete's disability if there has been damage to the semicircular canals or vestibular apparatus.

- The deaf athlete is not restricted and able to participate in any sport available to the able-bodied.

- Major dangers arise from a lack of audible warnings and potential slowness in communication. Apart from serious trauma consequent upon these problems, there is **little evidence to suggest** that the injuries sustained by the deaf differ significantly from those of the able-bodied.

- The deaf athletes may compensate by **maximising their visual abilities** through training powers of observation and peripheral vision.

ATHLETES WITH PHYSICAL DISABILITY

SPINAL CORD INJURIES

- When the spinal cord is damaged, there is a loss of motor and sensory function below the level of the spinal cord lesion. The extent of the motor and sensory loss depends upon this level as well as upon the degree of damage of the spinal cord. **Quadriplegia** at the level of the cervical region, **spastic paralysis** at the thoracic region and **flaccid paralysis** at the level of the lumbar region.

- The majority of athletes with spinal cord injury are wheelchair dependent, thus giving them the label **"wheelchair athletes"**.

- Athletes with spinal cord injury compete in many sports, but track and field and swimming are the most popular. Other competitive sports for such athletes include archery, basketball, fencing and marathon racing (Fig. 2).

- The low levels of physical activity in the wheelchair athlete predispose them to:

  - An increased risk of cardiovascular disease by unfavourable modification of risk factors.
  - Diabetes and other medical conditions associated with **obesity.**
  - The development of osteoporosis and renal calculi.

THE CEREBRAL PALSIED ATHLETE

- Cerebral palsy is a group of disorders of impaired brain and motor function with an onset before or at birth, or during the first years of life (Fig. 3). The condition has multiple aetiologies and the most obvious manifestation is impaired function of the voluntary musculature.

- Track and field and swimming are popular sports for these athletes. Participants may be ambulatory or compete in a wheelchair depending on the extent of their motor dysfunction. It should be noted that half the cerebral palsied athletes compete in wheelchairs.

THE AMPUTEE ATHLETE

- Amputee athletes have a partial or complete loss of one or more limbs.

- The amputee athlete usually participates in sport with or without a prosthesis, or in a wheelchair.

- Track and field and swimming have been popular sports for amputee athletes.

- Sport may help to **prevent atrophy** of the stump muscles, **improve circulation** of the stump and **strengthen the remaining muscles** in the affected limbs.

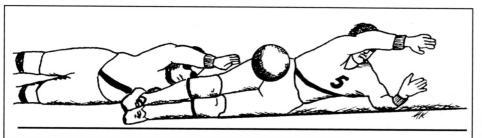

Figure 2 – Paraplegic basketball players without wheelchairs.

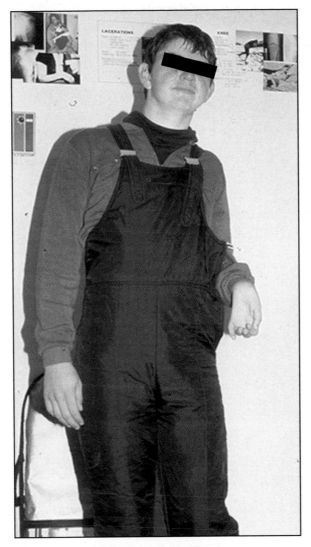

Figure 3 – 16 year old skier with hemiparesis (from MVA at age 5 years

Children's Diseases (after O-Bar-Or)

Children, whether well or ill, can safely participate in physical fitness programmes. In fact, training may improve physical fitness for such diseases as bronchial asthma (but beware exercise-induced bronchospasm), cystic fibrosis (follow for signs of arterial desaturation), diabetes mellitus (improves control) and chronic renal failure (better appetite), muscular dystrophy, mental retardation, obesity and rheumatoid arthritis. There are physical and mental benefits (improved self-esteem), however the exercise prescription **must be specific** to the problem.

ATHLETES WITH COGNITIVE DISABILITY

- Mental retardation specifies as an IQ less than 70 resulting from pathophysiologic processes affecting the cerebrum during the developmental period.
- Mentally retarded athletes are not restricted and are able to participate in any sport available.
- The mentally retarded, prior to systemic training, are often not as physically fit as the general population.
- Approximately 75% of mentally retarded individuals have **one or more** other medical conditions.

LES AUTRES

Les Autres is the French term for "the others". This denotes other locomotor disabilities.

The type of disabilities include:

- Dwarfism.
- Multiple Sclerosis.
- Friedrich's ataxia.
- Limb deficiencies, including absence of arms or legs
- Conditions characterised by muscle weakness related to peripheral nerve damage (Gullian-Barrè Syndrome).
- Arthritis of major joints.

WHEELCHAIR ATHLETE

- Wheelchair athletes are those disabled by spinal cord injury, cerebral palsy, lower extremity amputation or any of the disorders included with Les Autres. The common denominator for these disabled athletes is their **mobility impairment** and **need of a wheelchair** for sports participation.
- Wheelchair locomotion is **not an efficient means** of transportation. The mechanical efficiency of wheelchair locomotion is at best 5%, compared with a minimum of 20% for walking or cycling at similar velocity.

- The **design of sports wheelchairs** is constantly evolving. Recent design modifications are intended to improve the mechanical efficiency of the wheelchair, facilitate a more effective wheelchair stroke and minimise the risk of upper-extremity injuries (Fig. 4).

WHEELCHAIR SPORT INJURIES

- The most common injuries incurred by wheelchair athletes are soft tissue injuries, blisters, lacerations, abrasions and cuts (Fig. 5).

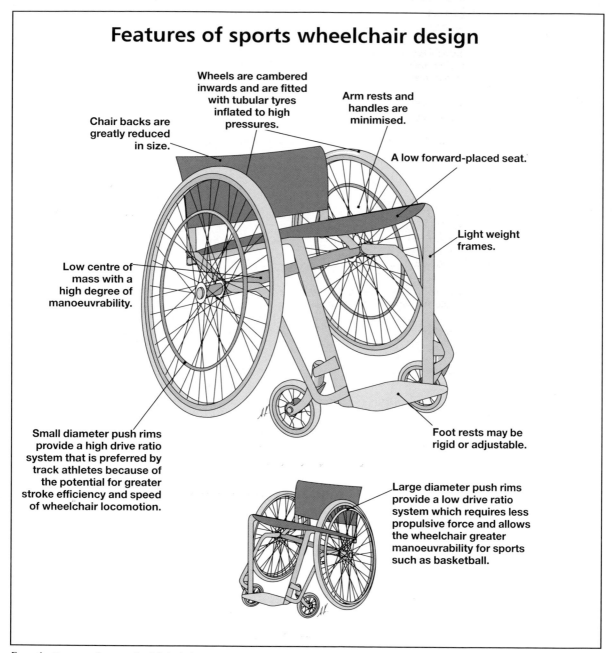

Features of sports wheelchair design

Chair backs are greatly reduced in size.

Wheels are cambered inwards and are fitted with tubular tyres inflated to high pressures.

Arm rests and handles are minimised.

A low forward-placed seat.

Light weight frames.

Low centre of mass with a high degree of manoeuvrability.

Small diameter push rims provide a high drive ratio system that is preferred by track athletes because of the potential for greater stroke efficiency and speed of wheelchair locomotion.

Foot rests may be rigid or adjustable.

Large diameter push rims provide a low drive ratio system which requires less propulsive force and allows the wheelchair greater manoeuvrability for sports such as basketball.

Figure 4 – Features of sports wheelchair design

Region	Type of Injuries	Prevention
Shoulder	Direct trauma: • contusion of muscle, soft tissue • sprains • capsulitis • rotator cuff problems • fractures Non-traumatic: • bicipital tendonitis due to tendon strain caused by overuse and inadequate warm-up	• adequate training in correct technique • strengthening of the shoulder stabilisers • warm-up, cool down and stretching procedures • equipment modification • early reporting and treatment of shoulder pain
Elbow	• as 'shoulder' • lacerations and abrasions	• wearing of clothing on the upper arms • use of tube socks on the rim
Wrist	• as 'shoulder' • lacerations and abrasions	• use of padded push rims • use of gloves and padding over the wrist and heel of the hand
Hand and fingers	• abrasions and lacerations particularly of the knuckles • avulsion of the nails • finger injuries related to the catching of fingers in the spokes of the wheelchair are common	• use of gloves and taping • padded push rims and plastic wheel covers • removal of sharp edges on the wheelchair
Upper back	• muscular spasm related to overuse during maintenance of trunk stability • blistering at the top of the upper back	• postural correction by specific strengthening exercises • wearing a shirt and padding on the back of the wheelchair seat post or the back of the wheelchair
Buttock	• pressure sores and ulcers	• padding or cushion on the wheelchair seat • intermittent lifting from the seat • combination of the above preventive measures

Figure 5 – The sports injuries of wheelchair athletes

SPECIAL MEDICAL PROBLEMS OF WHEELCHAIR ATHLETES

URINARY TRACT COMPLICATIONS

- Neurological control of the urinary tract is usually lost after spinal cord injury.

- Resulting complications of significant risk include bladder and kidney infection, stones, bladder distension.

- Kidney damage secondary to infection alone is the **main cause of death** in spinal cord injury.

PRESSURE SORES

- Pressure sores are one of the most common and costly complications of spinal cord injury. Skin breakdown is usually caused by prolonged pressure and compromise of the blood supply to affected tissues.

- Wheelchair athletes who sit in the chairs with their **knee higher** than their buttocks are particularly prone to pressure sores. Further risk of pressure sore development is inherent as the athlete's **skin becomes damp** with sweat and other moisture.

- Prevention of pressure sores is important in all persons with spinal cord injury. Such measures include:

  - Intermittent shifting and lifting of the buttocks from the wheelchair's seat relieves pressure.
  - Wearing moisture-absorbing clothing to reduce skin laceration and friction forces.

- Frequent skin checks of the trunk, sacrum, buttocks and legs.

AUTONOMIC HYPER-REFLEXIA (AHR)

- AHR is a particular complication of spinal cord injury above the **4th to 6th thoracic** vertebrae.

- AHR occurs as a result of the loss of central inhibitory control over the isolated distal spinal cord. A generalised sympathetic hyperactivity may be triggered in response to numerous sensory stimuli, for example bladder distension.

- AHR in a person with spinal cord injury presents with sudden hypertension, bradycardia, headache, anxiety and profuse sweating.

TEMPERATURE REGULATION DISORDERS

- Impairment of thermoregulatory function is a significant complication of spinal injury.

- The loss of sensory afferent inputs from the spinal cord and muscles below the level of the lesion may limit hypothalamic responses to exercise and temperature.

- The loss of lower extremity skeletal muscle pump in disabled athletes such as amputees reduces venous return to the heart during exercise and further compromises thermoregulatory responses.

- Wheelchair athletes are generally at a thermoregulatory disadvantage and certain precautions must be taken to prevent the occurrence of hyperthermia and hypothermia.

21

REHABILITATION AND PHYSIOTHERAPY OF THE ELITE ATHLETE

Robert Standen

OVERTRAINING (OVERUSE) INJURIES

The athlete who performs maximally and trains daily is prone to overtraining injuries (Fig. 1). Such injuries are associated with biomechanical "alignment" problems; imbalances in muscle length, power, and hyper/hypomobility of joints. The causes can be genetic, inappropriate training protocols, previous injury or a combination.

It is important:

- **To diagnose the presenting pathology and grade the severity.** Investigation should be thorough so as to return the athlete to competition quickly (consider MRI and bone scans). Accuracy of diagnosis is important. A stress fracture can potentially destroy an elite athlete's career whereas a stress reaction can often be successfully managed with training programme modification.

- **To take a thorough history such as the time of onset of symptoms.** (Longer term symptoms are usually associated with pathological change that is less readily reversible and so requires longer rehabilitation periods; symptom behaviour over the period gives an indication of the chronicity). Was the onset sudden suggesting acute trauma as a result of overstretching of body tissues or contusion? A

longer duration of onset of symptoms may suggest an overtraining injury requiring different management; also consider any changes to training that may be linked to onset of symptoms (remember there is often a delay associated with the onset of pain). Also **changes to extrinsic factors** (such as equipment, training surface, training environment) and **changes to intrinsic factors** (alterations in training programmes) that predispose athletes to injury . Elite athletes training for endurance events will often develop overtraining injuries prior to tapering their training before a major event. Similarly acute injuries in sprinters and weight lifters will occur more often as training intensity is increased, and training volume is decreased, prior to the competition phase of a training cycle. Multi sprint team sports such as football and hockey will have far more overtraining injuries during preseason than when teams are training in endurance with long runs or working with weights in the gym.

- **Ensure an appropriate biomechanical analysis** is conducted to determine the factors requiring modification to return the athlete to maximum performance and minimise chances of re-injury (separate components and examine separately). **Simple tests** conducted in the clinic will give an indication of problems associated with athletic performance (Fig. 2).

- **Video** may be useful to **analyse** sporting gait, make the athlete **aware** of his problem, act as a baseline for treatment reassessment and help determine treatment goals with the injured athlete. Digitised video analysis in the laboratory is necessary for determining vital components for a particular skill. Video analysis of athletic performance in the sporting environment can reveal problems not seen in the relatively artificial laboratory environment (Fig. 3).

Treatment should aim to **minimise rest periods from training** while ensuring that the condition does not worsen (develop training schedules that do not irritate condition). These should be sport-specific, continually monitored and progressed.

It is also important to modify **intrinsic and extrinsic biomechanical problems.** Look at sporting techniques, training programme, muscle retraining, strengthening and stretching, soft tissue techniques, mobilisation and manipulation of joints to restore maximal range of movement and the use of orthotic devices to compensate for bony malalignment problems (less often surgery is required) (Fig. 4).

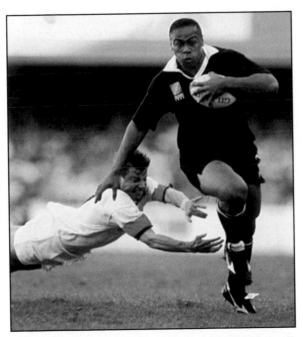

Figure 1 - Elite athlete, Jonah Lomu, in action (NZ All Blacks, 1995)

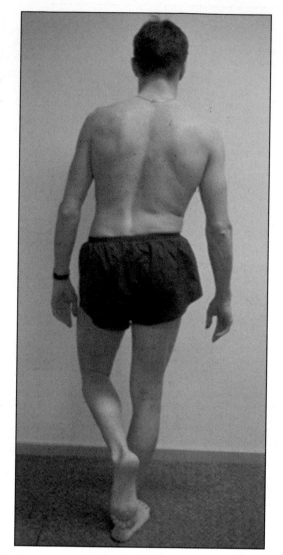

Figure 2 - Test for pelvic stability in the clinic

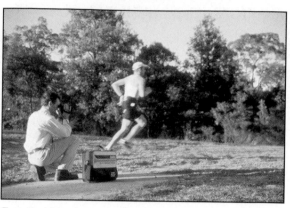

Figure 3 - Athlete being videoed in the field

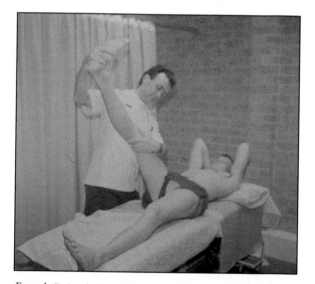

Figure 4 - Patient being mobilised on table (measurement of gastroc-nemius muscle length)

ACUTE INJURIES

(CONSERVATIVE VERSUS SURGICAL MANAGEMENT)

Acute injuries in elite athletes require early intervention and assessment. The decision to manage an injury with **surgery or** with **conservative treatment** may not be clear. An injury that requires surgery for its long-term management may, where possible, be managed conservatively until such time as the elite athlete has an appropriate break in their competitive season. As surgical techniques improve and rehabilitation times are greatly reduced, surgery is considered earlier and for a greater range of acute and chronic conditions in this group. Management of time out from competition and training requires careful consideration when deciding on rehabilitation strategies.

MINIMISING REHABILITATION TIME

Immediately an injury occurs a **short-term plan** should be formulated. Goals of the short-term plan include prevention of further injury, reduction of swelling and diagnosis of pathology. Aggressive investigation and management by a multidisciplinary team is required to minimise time out. Team members include the medical team (Sports Physician, Surgeon, Physiotherapist, Masseurs) and the coaching staff (Coach, Sprint Trainers, Skill Trainers, Strength Trainers, Medical Trainers).

The well-informed athlete must be included in the goal setting process to maximise compliance and minimise behaviours that result in a longer rehabilitation period. Once a diagnosis has been established and the severity determined, **medium and long-term plans** are then implemented.

If **surgery** is indicated then an accelerated rehabilitation period is appropriate. A coordinating professional is vital to ensure coaches, trainers and other team support members are informed of the progress.

Intensive physiotherapy is useful for injuries. These conservative programmes run concurrently with modified sport-specific training programmes and are monitored.

The aims of these rehabilitation programmes are to restore: muscle power and control, proprioception, maximum joint range of movement, off load stress from injured area, minimise loss of cardiovascular condition and gradually return to sport.

RESTORING MUSCLE POWER AND DEFINITIONS

Muscle retraining should simulate the **muscle length** and **speed** required for the athlete's sporting performance. Progression from **closed chain** to more functional **open chain** training is used. **Eccentric** and **concentric** strength balance of **agonist / antagonist** muscle groups is vital. Changes in muscle performance must be measured through rehabilitation (Fig. 5). Know specific strength requirements.

Maximum concentric strength is the maximum load that can be moved once by a subject (referred to as 1 RM, repetition maximum; measured using free weights, weight machines or dynamometers).

Absolute strength is a measure of **eccentric power** (the maximum number of repetitions that can be per-

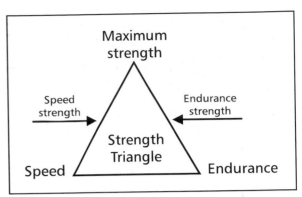

Figure 5 - Strength triangle

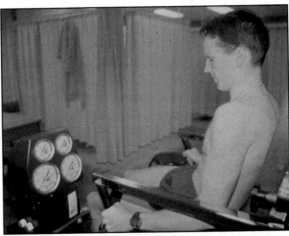

Figure 6 - Athlete using leg press. Leg press and weighted leg press are used early in rehabilitation

formed with an absolute load). Muscles of the same cross sectional area are at greater risk of injury during eccentric muscle loading than with concentric loading, as fewer motor units are used. Running down hill results in a greater incidence of delayed onset muscle soreness **(DOMS)** and **muscle fibre damage** than running up the same gradient. Running uphill will require greater relative use of energy substrates such as glycogen and pyruvate and so production of lactic acid. This is the prime argument current physiologists use to suggest DOMS is not the result of intramuscular build-up of metabolites (such as lactic acid). The **"no pain no gain"** approach to training appears groundless and DOMS suggests muscle damage (Fig. 6).

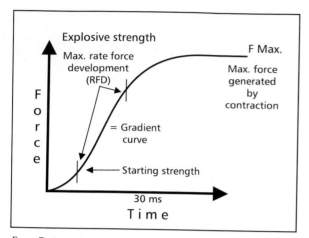

Figure 7 - Force/time graph for isometric contraction showing starting strength, explosive strength and F.Max.

Maximum isometric strength, or maximum voluntary contraction **(MVC),** can be the easiest and most economic measure of maximum strength. Relatively inexpensive equipment such as spring balances can be used to monitor improvement in an athlete's maximum strength following injury.

Relative strength is measured in the same way as absolute strength except the resistance varies as a percentage of the concentric IRM measure.

Strength–endurance. Absolute strength and relative strength give an indication of the strength–endurance relationship.

Speed–strength (power) is determined by mechanical power generated by muscles. Speed-strength gives an indication of the amount of work able to be done by muscles over a time period and how quickly a force can be generated in a muscle.

Explosive strength is the maximum rate at which a force can be generated. It is important in sprinters and in multi sprint sports (soccer and rugby) rather than in endurance events. Speed is improved with specific, rapid, low resistance training and high repetitions (repeated practice at high speed, for example short fast sprints). Training speed-strength requires the combination of strengthening exercises and speed reproducing movements against resistance.

Stretch–shortening Cycle (SSC) determines the 'reactive' or elastic strength in muscles. A high jumper will have a short SSC with a very high stretch load while a vertical jump has a low stretch load and long SSC (Fig. 7).

Training and rehabilitation adaptations. Hypertrophy of muscle fast twitch fibres occurs as the number of glycolytic enzymes increase in response to anaerobic training loads. **Hypertrophy** of **slow twitch fibres** occurs as a result of increased capillarisation of muscle fibres, increased sarcoplasmic proteins, oxidative enzymes and increased mitochondrial numbers.

Selective training of muscle fibres requires very different training programmes. Hypertrophy of fast twitch glycolytic fibres requires 3-5 sets of 5-8 repetitions of 80-85% of 1RM. By comparison, hypertrophy of aerobic slow twitch fibres requires 3-5 sets 15-20 repetitions of 60-70% of IRM. Heavier resistance training is required to select hypertrophy of fast twitch fibres. Athletes using predominantly high intensity, glycolytic muscle fibres require different hypertrophy training programmes from endurance athletes. Cross sectional area is related to muscle strength. Hypertrophy is one way a muscle improves its performance.

Hyperplasia. Whether muscle size is the result of hyperplasia remains controversial.

The changes that occur in **muscle architecture and flexibility** may be the result of muscle training. Sarcomeres are believed to be added to muscle fibres in response to stretching muscle, allowing muscles to generate tension over a larger joint range. So if a muscle is trained at the extremes of its range, sarcomeres will be added to lengthen the muscle.

The **types of collagen** found in the connective tissue in muscle may change as a result of training (more elastic fibre types over relatively fibrous collagen components after training). **SSC** is influenced by these changes.

Neural. Changes in muscle strength are often greater than the proportional changes in muscle cross sectional area. Training brings about improved muscle performance as a result of the more effective recruitment of appropriate muscle fibres (motor units) for a given activity. There is improvement in intramuscular coordination and intermuscular coordination.

The neural control of the secondary stabilising muscles is learned. Training of the antagonist muscle groups so that their protective activation is minimised results in increased muscle performance. This is the rationale of free weight training (as opposed to guided resistance training with machine systems). **Machine systems** do not require co-contraction of antagonists or secondary stabilising musculature. It is less functional and so less relevant to real sport. However, guided machine training can allow safer training of muscles around injured joints or where secondary stabilising muscles are injured or deconditioned (as a result of immobilisation). For these reasons, equipment such as leg presses are used early in rehabilitation prior to open chain dynamic training programmes (Fig. 6).

MUSCLE FUNCTION IN ELITE ATHLETIC PERFORMANCE

Force Production. Kinetic energy is produced by the active component of the muscle unit (the sarcomere), and **potential** energy is produced by changing the relative position of body segments (maximising tension in the elastic components of the body).

FORCE REDUCTION

Excessive kinetic energy not required in a skill must be absorbed by the eccentric activity of the antagonist muscle groups.

Stabilisation. In order to maximise athletic performance and minimise stresses placed on the body, adequate core strength is vital. **Core strength** is associated with the region between the chest and knees, sometimes known as the "power zone".

Core strength ensures optimum postural stability and alignment. The "core" acts as a force couple linking the body segments. Core strength is necessary for controlled athletic performance of all sporting technique and so it is considered vital during rehabilitation of elite athletes.

RESTORATION OF CONTROL AND PROPRIOCEPTION

Damage to the various proprioceptive organs may occur. Damage to the muscle spindle or the joint receptors within the knee can result in a decreased awareness of the body's position in space. There is an associated loss of the body's ability to adequately regulate fine muscle movements around joints. Problems of this nature become more apparent as the speed and complexity of a task are increased.

Instabilities as a result of injuries to joints such as knees and ankles require increased fine motor control to compensate for any dynamic instabilities and to avoid re-injury.

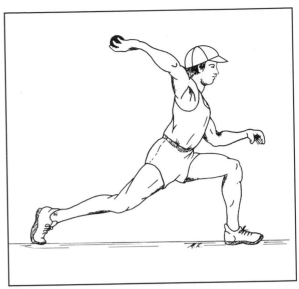

Figure 8 - Rehabilitation for soft-ball pitcher with rotator cuff injury includes jogging, softballs, EMG biofeedback, push-offs, slide board, pitching supervision.

Muscle control must be fully and appropriately trained prior to return to competition. **Proprioception** is probably the **key factor** in the prevention of re-injury following early return to competition.

RESTORATION OF PROPRIOCEPTION

Progressed, sport-specific, dynamic balance exercises that challenge kinesthetic receptors are used as soon as the athlete can begin to move post injury.

Initial training may be static and relatively simple (standing on one leg and catching a ball post ankle ligament sprain) and progressed (Fig. 8).

RESTORATION OF JOINT ROM

Decreased ROM can occur from: relative loss of muscle length from injury and immobilisation; stiffness and/or adhesions in the ligaments, capsule, (excessive scarring of soft tissue structures from injury or surgery); changes in bony alignment; joint congruity; and decreased muscle bulk.

Loss of flexibility may result in decreased ability to absorb force and so excessive loads across the joint should be avoided.

Also consider the adjacent joints. Lumbar spine or knee problems may occur in a runner with a loss of internal rotation of the hip.

Flexibility and power are important to avoid injury.

Treatment includes: sustained stretching of muscles and joints (controversial).

Laboratory testing of the length tension relationship in ligament and tendon suggests that a sustained stretch is the most appropriate.

Stretches may be effective. Cyclic loading of the muscle, tendon or ligament tissue results in an increase in **"slack length"**. Time required to effectively stretch is variable, 10–30 seconds will give good results with the hamstrings or calf. Road cycling teams benefit from regular stretching of the iliotibial band (durations of 2 min) to maximise long-term length changes. The iliotibial band is a large relatively stiff structure. Mobilisation and manipulation of joints accelerates ROM. Mobilisation is directed repetitive pressure placed on a restricted joint (do not exceed the available passive joint range and not at high velocity).

Manipulation is a high velocity technique (associated with a "click").

SOFT TISSUE MASSAGE

Soft tissue massage has been shown to give a short-term increase in the resting muscle length of unexercised muscle and a decrease the incidence and severity of delayed onset muscle soreness (DOMS). Massage can minimise microtrauma and so maximise performance in later competition (timing post exercise is critical to minimise the microinflammatory response).

Massage can increase the circulation to a muscle and improve the clearance of metabolites, the nutrition of muscle fibres and increase muscle temperature (and so flexibility).

OFF LOAD STRESS FROM INJURED AREA

Biomechanical problems distal to the site of injury may slow progress (stiffness of the thoracic spine or tight hamstrings in a pitcher limits trunk rotation and so increases the loads across the shoulder).

MINIMISE LOSS OF CARDIOVASCULAR CONDITION

Loss of aerobic condition will make the athlete susceptible to fatigue and further injury. Modified training programmes must begin as soon as possible.

Endurance training requires overloading muscle with light resistance and high repetitions (water running programmes for lower limb injuries; modified circuit training and interval training).

Peripheral aerobic fitness (increased muscle vascularity and mitochondrial mass) may be lost. Central aerobic fitness (cardiac output) should be maintained.

GRADUATED RETURN TO SPORT

As endurance and speed returns, closely monitor (with physiotherapist and skills coach) to ensure technique is effective in minimising stress on the injury.

MENTAL ATTITUDE

(TO INJURY AND REHABILITATION)

Elite athletes are aware of the need to care for their bodies (sport is the most important facet of their lives, and their source of income). Psychological well-being must also be considered.

Commitment to a rehabilitation programme is vital. The athlete must be focused. There may be a slow return to sport because of concern about second injury with loss of confidence and depression.

Support of trainers and coaches is important as there may be a grief reaction.

"Dangerous attitudes" can decrease the chances of a safe return to sport (Fig. 9). Many elite athletes tolerate high levels of pain in the normal course of sporting performance, making them poor judges of when to stop and rest. "Toughing out" pain can result in relatively minor injury becoming major, with a longer recovery. It is important to know which pains to ignore.

Elite athletes must give 100% to every game in order to be successful and injuries are more likely to occur. Expectations are high (from team, coaches, officials and fans). The culture of some team sports is such that athletes are encouraged to return to sport too soon. The proper recovery from injury is in the best interests of all concerned. Injury in elite athletes is a true crisis. The injured athlete requires appropriate support and patience.

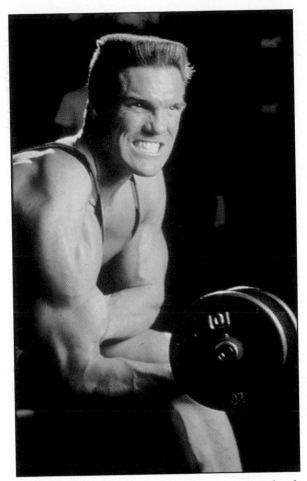

Figure 9 - "Dangerous" attitudes can decrease the chances of a safe return to sport

MODALITIES USED IN PHYSICAL THERAPY

- Cryotherapy (ICE) - 72 hours/reduces bleeding and oedema after injury. Use as cold packs/ice massage/cold hydrotherapy/sprays. Avoid RA conditions, or where cold sensitivity.

- Heat prior to exercise/stretching - old technique/useful for muscle or collagen injury/can be harmful. Use as hydro collator packs/paraffin baths/fluidotherapy/hydrotherapy/contrast baths.

- Iontophoresis (direct current with topical medication).

- Ultrasound (high frequency mechanical vibration)
    - continuous heats
    - pulsed (low frequency)
    - can combine with topical steroid

  Useful for pain and muscle spasm. May help healing. Avoid: where burns, coma, in the groin, near spinal cord, for pregnant or cardiac patients, near growth plates or myositis ossificans.

- Diathermy (high frequency electromagnetic currents). Microwave/shortwave forms.

- Ultraviolet therapy.

- Faradic stimulation. Piezoelectric phenomenon. Relieve pain. Bone and muscle repair. Possible use for muscle training.

- TENS to control pain

- Traction. Useful for LBP.

- CPM (continuous passive motion). May aid cartilage healing.

Figure 10 - Modalities used in physical therapy

MODALITIES IN PHYSICAL THERAPY

Various physical therapies are available to provide symptomatic relief following injury (Fig. 10). However, they should always be used in conjunction with a range of motion exercises and muscle conditioning.

THERAPEUTIC EXERCISES AVAILABLE

Shoulder. Active and passive-assisted ROM (for flexion/external rotation/abduction).

Strengthening - use high repetition, low weight, isotonic exercises with eccentric and concentric muscle contractions.

- Shoulder: shrugs/supraspinatus/abduction, external rotation, throwing programme (Fig. 11).

- Elbow: stretch flexors and extensors/pronation/supination with cricket bat, biceps and triceps curls (Fig. 12).

- Knee: quads, straight leg raise, hip abduction/flexion, hamstring curls and stretches. Exercise bike (Fig. 13).

- Ankle: heelcord stretching (against wall and/or on incline), tib ant strengthening, proprioceptive programme (wobble board), peroneal and tib post strengthening (Fig. 14).

Shoulder Strengthening

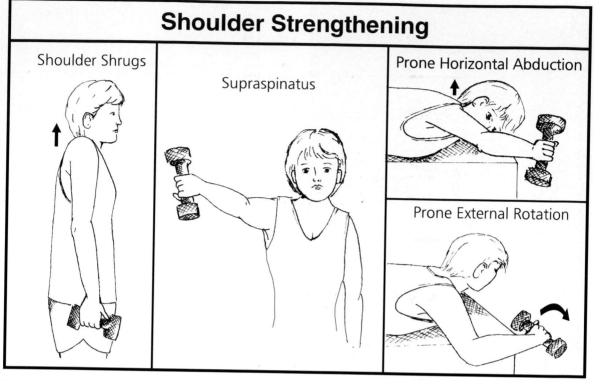

Figure 11 - Shoulder strengthening: shrugs, supraspinatus, abduction, external rotation. Hold for 5 counts, 5 sets of 10, 1 to 5 lb, 3 times a day

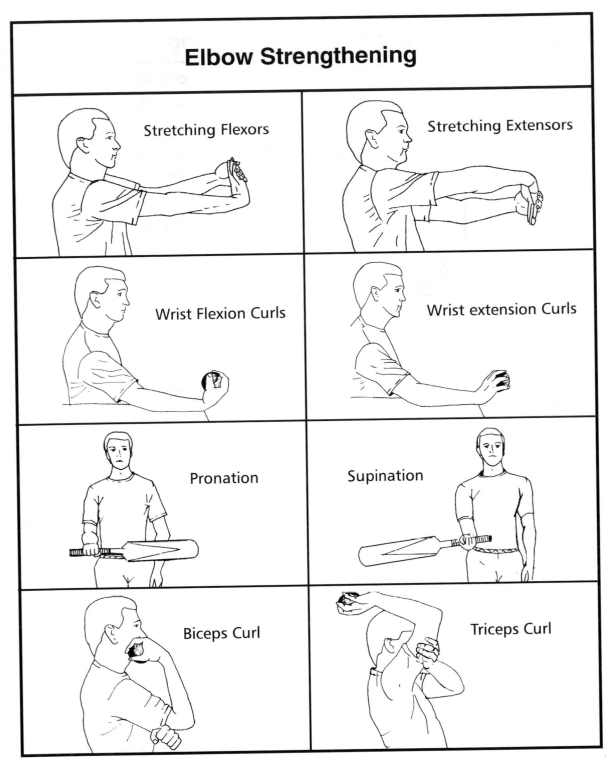

Figure 12 - Elbow: stretching flexors/extensors, flexion/extension curls, rotation, biceps and triceps curls. Hold for 5 counts, 5 sets of 10, 1 to 5 lb, 3 times a day

Knee Strengthening

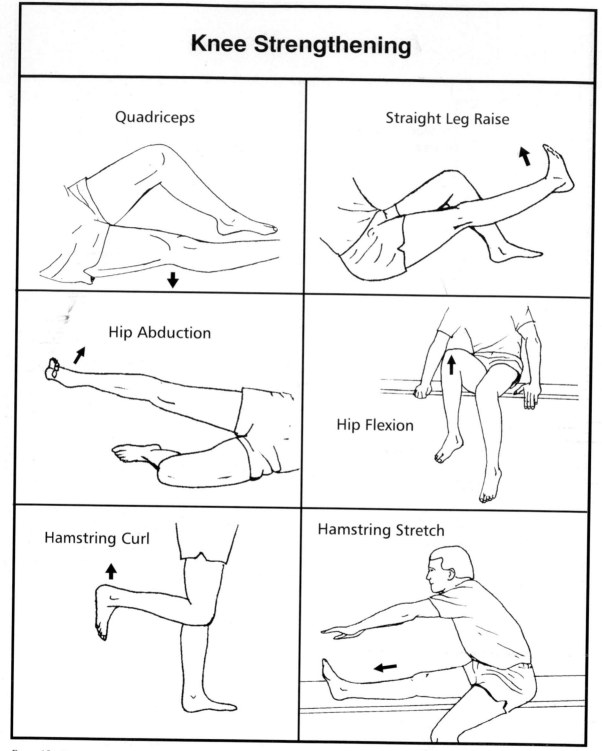

Figure 13 - Knee: quads, SLR, hip abduction, flexion, hamstring curl/stretch. Hold for 5 counts, 5 sets of 10, 3 times per day

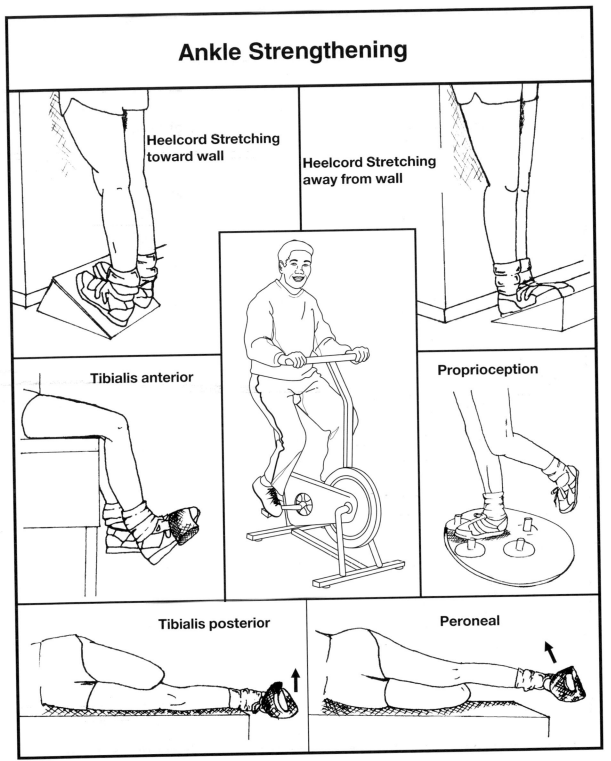

Figure 14 – Ankle: heelcord work, tibialis anterior, proprioceptive, tibialis posterior and peroneal strengthening. Hold for 5 counts, 5 sets of 10, 1 to 5 lb, 3 times per day 'cycle work'

22

PSYCHIATRY AND SPORTS MEDICINE

Phillip Boyce
Vanessa Tung

PSYCHOLOGY AND SPORT

Psychological factors have a major influence on sporting performance. Sport psychology, the province of sport psychologists, deals with the issues of motivation, 'positive thinking' and anxiety control, and the ways that they can be modified to maximise performance. Interpersonal factors, particularly how team members can work together, are also dealt with by sports psychologists.

It should be noted that athletes have no more mental health problems than non-athletes. In fact athletes have a lower incidence of schizophrenia and dementia.

The sports physician is concerned with how psychological factors can influence recovery or lead to injury. They also need to be aware of the common psychiatric disorders, as having such a disorder does not preclude a person from participating in sport and, in some cases, sport may be beneficial to the person's psychiatric illness. They also need to be aware of how some individuals may be attracted to certain sports for psychopathological reasons, i.e. gymnastics and eating disorders, martial arts and personality disorders. Sporting injury can precipitate psychiatric disorder in some individuals and a psychiatric disorder or behavioural disturbance may affect recovery from an injury. Finally, some disorders can be closely related to sporting activities.

ILLNESS BEHAVIOUR

Illness behaviour includes the ways in which given symptoms may be differentially perceived, evaluated and acted upon.

Under normal circumstances an individual will behave in such a way as to facilitate improvement, and not become overly involved in being 'sick'.

ABNORMAL ILLNESS BEHAVIOUR

Behaviours regarded as inappropriate or maladaptive. Abnormal illness behaviours may be two types: 'illness affirmation' or ' illness denying'.

'Illness denying' behaviour can be an important factor in sports medicine as this type of behaviour can lead to injuries being exacerbated or made worst, recovery from injury being delayed – or increasing the potential for long-term damage.

EXAMPLE OF ABNORMAL ILLNESS BEHAVIOUR

- Continuing participation in sporting activities after an injury.

- Not following rehabilitation (physiotherapy) programmes.

- Returning to sporting activities too soon after injury.

- Persisting in inappropriate sporting activities which increase risk of, or delay recovery from, injury.

ORIGIN OF ABNORMAL ILLNESS BEHAVIOUR

Multifactorial in origin; important factors include sociocultural (including the 'team' or the need to be 'macho'), interpersonal and personality.

MANAGEMENT

Counselling is generally needed. This will involve trying to understand the reasons for the abnormal illness behaviour. The risks of their behaviour need to be pointed out, especially where it may involve long-term damage, and assurance that appropriate illness behaviour will speed recovery. The situation may be difficult if a sportsperson fears he or she may be dropped from the team when injured.

In such situations discussion with the coach may, with consent, be appropriate.

ANXIETY, PERFORMANCE AND THE ANXIETY DISORDERS

Underpinning our understanding of anxiety and its relationship to sporting performance and to the origins of the anxiety disorders is the Yerkes-Dodson Curve (Fig. 1).

This shows the relationship between performance and anxiety. As anxiety increases, performance improves. However, when anxiety increases to a certain point (which varies from individual to individual) performance deteriorates rapidly. The aim in sports psychology is to be able to achieve the ideal anxiety level to produce the best performance.

Persons suffering from anxiety disorders, and to some extent depression, have disabling anxiety levels which contribute to their distress.

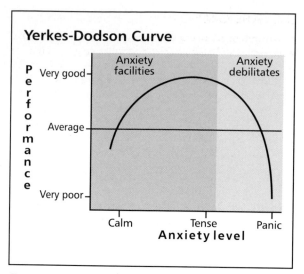

Figure 1 – The Yerkes-Dodson curve shows the relationship between performance and anxiety (drops off after certain variable point)

For some individuals, their anxiety disorder may present as difficulty with performance, especially when the anxiety is in response to pressure on them to perform well. Treating the underlying anxiety disorder will help improve their performance.

ANXIETY DISORDERS

EPIDEMIOLOGY

Between 2 and 5% of the population suffer from an anxiety disorder at any one time. This is slightly more common among men.

ESSENTIAL FEATURES

An essential characteristic of the anxiety disorder is an excess of anxiety which gives rise to troubling and disabling symptoms for the individual. The way the anxiety disorder presents varies according to the type of disorder they have.

SYMPTOMS OF ANXIETY

These groups of symptoms include: symptoms of autonomic arousal; symptoms of muscle tone; symptoms of hypervigilance (psychic symptoms) (Fig. 2).

TYPES OF ANXIETY DISORDER

PANIC DISORDER

Feelings of panic (> 5 symptoms of anxiety) arising in situations in which most people would not normally expect to be fearful, accompanied by fears of going 'crazy' or 'dying' and a need to escape.

SYMPTOMS OF ANXIETY		
Autonomic Symptoms of Anxiety	**Symptoms relating to Motor Tone**	**Symptoms of Hyper-vigilance**
Palpitations	Shakiness	Irritability
Tachycardia	Tremor onset	Insomnia
Cold, clammy hands	Muscular aches	Trouble staying asleep
Sweating	Lump in throat	Easily startled
Blepharospasms	Distractibility	Poor concentration
Paraesthesiae	Restlessness	Feeling keyed up
Dizziness	Easily tired	
Hot and cold spells	Trouble swallowing	
Frequency of micturition		
Diarrhoea		
Nausea		

Figure 2 – Symptoms of anxiety (autonomic/motor/hyper-vigilance).

AGORAPHOBIA

Avoidance of situations where escape may be difficult such as public transport, travelling alone or crowded places for fear of having a panic attack.

GENERALISED ANXIETY DISORDER

Months of excessive and disproportionate anxiety and worry. Accompanied by symptoms of motor tension, autonomic overactivity and hyperarousal.

SOCIAL PHOBIA

Excessive and unreasonable fear of scrutiny and of negative evaluation. Social situations are avoided or endured with considerable anxiety.

OBSESSIVE COMPULSIVE DISORDER

Obsessions: thoughts, images or impulses which repeatedly occur, are intrusive and distressing and do not resist attempts to suppress or neutralise them.

Compulsions: repetitive behaviours which may arise in response to obsessions. They are thought to reduce or prevent harm and reduce anxiety and are excessive and uncontrollable. Obsessive Compulsive Disorder occurs when these symptoms cause interference with everyday life.

LOSS, GRIEF AND DEPRESSION

INJURY AND LOSS

Sporting injuries result in 'loss' for the sufferer. The extent of the loss will depend on the extent of the injury, the disability associated with it, the impact it has on future participation in sport, age and stage of life cycle, personality style and the psychological investment in physical ability. All of these factors need to be taken into account when assessing the psychological impact of an injury.

TYPES OF LOSS

The loss may be temporary or permanent. The loss will generally involve a loss of self-esteem or self concept. An injury can involve a loss of:

- Ability to perform at optimal level
- Function
- Activity
- Interest, recreation or outlet
- Social/contact/social support (mateship)
- Self-esteem

LOSS AND GRIEF

A natural process occurs to help an individual deal with the loss. This involves a series of stages; denial or numbing, protest, despair or depression, and finally resolution or coming to terms with the loss. It is important to distinguish between a depression and the despair associated with loss of function. Recognition and appropriate early treatment of a depression is essential as a depression can become chronic with increasing disability.

In some individuals the sense of loss will be great, especially when involvement in sport has been a major part of their life, and a major source of self-esteem. Often their only recreational activities and social support are linked with sport.

LOSS, LIFE EVENTS AND PSYCHIATRIC ILLNESS

Psychiatric disorders do not generally arise out of the blue, they are usually precipitated by some event, especially for those who have some pre-existing vulnerability. This vulnerability can be genetic (especially for the functional psychoses), biological or, as is most common, psychosocial (Fig. 3).

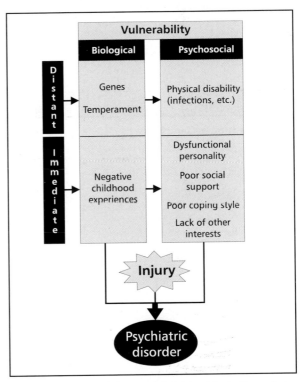

Figure 3 – A vulnerability model for psychiatric illness being precipitated by injury. Injury on its own will not precipitate illness; the individual also has to have one or more vulnerability factors to interact with the negative effect.

They can commonly be precipitated by adverse life events. Sporting injury is an adverse life event and may induce psychiatric illness in vulnerable individuals. The importance of an injury can be the loss associated with it.

MANAGEMENT

Counselling will be necessary for individuals who experience loss. This involves reviewing what has been lost and what it means to the individual, helping her or him adjust to the loss and focusing on new realistic goals and activities to become involved in, so as to restore self–esteem.

A. Anxiety

  1. Have you felt keyed-up and on edge?
  2. Have you been worrying a lot?
  3. Have you been irritable?
  4. Have you had difficulty relaxing?

(If 'Yes' to any **one** of above, go on to:)

  5. Have you been sleeping poorly?
  6. Have you had headaches or neckaches or tightness in the head?
  7. Dizzy; trembly; sweating; diarrhoea; frequency; tingling, etc (autonomic anxiety)?
  8. Been worried about health?
  9. Difficulty falling asleep?

D. Depression

  1. Low energy?
  2. Loss of interest?
  3. Loss of confidence in yourself?
  4. Felt hopeless?

(If 'Yes' to any **one** of above, go on to:)

  5. Unable to concentrate?
  6. Lost weight (due to poor appetite)?
  7. Early waking?
  8. Felt slowed up?
  9. Felt worse in mornings?

A patient can **self-assess** whether they are anxious or depressed.
1 point for each positive answer.

→ Add A-score; add D-score.
   Anxiety states usually score at least 4 on A; depressives at least 4 on D.

Figure 4 – Patients can self-determine whether they are anxious or depressed

In some situations this counselling needs to be extensive, especially when the loss is far reaching such as with a spinal injury.

There are guidelines for patients to determine whether they have an anxiety or depressive state (Fig. 4).

DEPRESSION

EPIDEMIOLOGY

Affects around 5% of the population. Females more than males. Lifetime risk: 15% for males, 25% for females.

CLINICAL FEATURES

A persistent depressed mood and/or loss of interest and pleasure in activities, along with a range of somatic symptoms (disturbance in sleep pattern; appetite and weight change; decrease in sexual drive; loss of energy, fatigue), and/or psychological symptoms (low self-esteem; feelings of worthlessness and guilt; poor concentration; memory complaints; difficulty making decisions; hypochondriacal complaints and self pity) and/or affective symptoms (depressed mood; apathy; irritability; loss of interest in usual activities; loss of pleasure in usual activities and feeling of hopelessness) and/or psychomotor symptoms (psychomotor retardation or agitation).

MANAGEMENT OF DEPRESSION

Mild to moderate depression treated with psychosocial treatments such as Cognitive Behaviour Therapy or counselling.

Moderate to severe depression requires antidepressants in addition to psychosocial treatment. Antidepressants include tricyclic antidepressants, selective serotonin reuptake inhibitors and monoamine oxidase inhibitors.

FUNCTIONAL PSYCHOSES

The functional psychoses (bipolar disorder and schizophrenia) are less common than anxiety or depression, affecting between 0.6 and 1% of the community. Persons suffering from these disorders can successfully participate in sporting activities, particularly those with bipolar disorders who have long periods free of symptoms.

Involvement in sporting and other recreational activities is encouraged as part of the psychosocial rehabilitation for persons with chronic functional psychoses.

BIPOLAR DISORDER (MANIC DEPRESSIVE ILLNESS)

Bipolar disorder is characterised by episodes of either mania or depression with periods of wellness in between. Age of onset is late adolescence, early adulthood.

ESSENTIAL FEATURES OF MANIA

Elevated mood characterised by: mood disturbance (elation, overcheerfulness, and/or irritability); motor disturbance (increased energy, less need for sleep, overactivity); and disturbance of thinking (grandiosity, belief in being special or having super powers).

The episodes of depression are clinically similar to other forms of moderate to severe depression.

Treatment

1. Symptomatic treatment. Antipsychotic drugs for mania, antidepressants for depression.

2. Psychosocial treatment. Education about the illness.

3. Prophylactic treatments. Mood stabilising drugs - lithium carbonate, carbamazepine and sodium valproate. Drug compliance is essential and discontinuation leads to relapse.

SCHIZOPHRENIA

ESSENTIAL FEATURES

Characterised by disturbances in: thinking (the **content** of the persons's thought - delusions and false, fixed ideas out of keeping with the culture - and the **form** of the person's thoughts with a loss of logical associations between thoughts); perception (auditory hallucinations); behaviour (which may be bizarre and unpredictable); affect (either blunted or inappropriate) and volition (apathy and withdrawal).

Chronic schizophrenia is characterised by apathy, social withdrawal and a blunted affect. Symptoms such as delusions and hallucinations can also be present.

OTHER DISORDERS

PERSONALITY DISORDERS

Personality disorder is characterised by the presence of personality characteristics which are relatively constant throughout life and cause the person and/or society to suffer.

Some individuals, particularly those with unstable or antisocial personality disorders may become overly involved in sporting activities for pathological reasons (i.e. martial arts for antisocial personality).

Sporting injury may affect these individuals, with 'acting out' behaviour. Such behaviour includes deliberate self-harm, suicide attempts and risk-taking behaviour. Alternatively they may become depressed or anxious.

EATING DISORDERS

Eating disorders (*See Chapter 17*) most commonly affect women, but men are also affected.

ORGANIC DISORDERS

DELIRIUM

Characterised by clouding of consciousness (fluctuating levels of attention and concentration), disorientation, and confusion. Delirium may arise from: trauma (head injury); infections; metabolic change (electrolyte imbalance, anoxia, alkalosis, acidosis, hypothermia); endocrine disorders and from toxicity (alcohol withdrawal).

MANAGEMENT OF DELIRIUM

Identification and treatment of the underlying cause. Sedation using an antipsychotic medication (haloperidol) is sometimes necessary.

BOXING ENCEPHALOPATHY (PUNCH DRUNK, DEMENTIA PUGILISTICA)

A chronic brain syndrome with psychiatric and physical symptoms. Physical symptoms include: dysarthria; facial immobility and poverty and slowness of movement. In later stages there may be ataxia, a festinant gait, tremor and spasticity.

Psychiatric symptoms: dementia (memory impairment) apathy, irritability and/or disinhibition also present.

The disorder is the result of repeated head injury.

MANAGEMENT

Prevention is the main goal. Symptomatic management may be required

The **issue of drugs in sport** is usually limited to the use of either illegal substances, dosages or applications.

However, the use of regular medications with their side-effects should be considered as they may be responsible for suboptimal performance.

In psychiatry both facets need to be addressed. Stimulants and opioid analgesics are banned. B Blockers are banned in selective sports. **MIMS** publishes the permissability of drugs to be used in competitive sports based on the **IOC Doping Classes.**

Side-effects such as sedation and insomnia, tremors and movement disorders, hypotension, visual and GIT symptoms can affect both performance at competition level and the athletes ability to train effectively.

Figure 5 shows the common side-effects of the major drugs used in psychiatry.

EXERCISE ADDICTION (FITNESS FANATICISM)

An unhealthy reliance upon sport for daily well-being. There is **dependence** (need exercise to feel good to the exclusion of marriage/job/friends), **tolerance** (increasing need), and **withdrawal** (tired/weak 24 hours post exercise cessation).

Usually this behaviour is positively reinforced so problems appear late.

May be related to endorphins and usually presents with overuse symptoms. Commonly seen in running.

Difficult to treat: includes rest, cross-training. Often athletes only stop when they have to because of injury: may lead to overuse injuries, and career/marriage/eating problems.

Exclude (and differentiate from):

Over-training : Seeking a higher level of performance without taking rest (increased basal resting heart rate).

Staleness : Performance not improving (with fatigue, insomnia, weight-loss/mood changes)

Burn-out : Mental fatigue with training

PSYCHOLOGICAL ENHANCEMENT OF PERFORMANCE

Peak performance depends upon having the necessary physical **skills** (preparation and repetition); **emotional skills** (confident, controlled anxiety and determination), and **cognitive skills** (goals defined, visual imagery, concentration, no distractions and high expectations). Athletes may use mental imagery to modify performance.

Common Drugs ▶ / Side-effects ▼	Anti-Pyschotics	Tricylic Antidepressant	SSRI	Reversible	Irreversible	Lithium	Carbamazepine	Sodium Valproate	Benzodiazepam	Stimulants (eg. Amphetamines)
Sedation	✔	✔		✔			✔	✔	✔	
Insomnia			✔	✔	✔					✔
Agitation			✔		✔					✔
Headache			✔		✔					
Movement Dis.*	✔									
Ataxia						✔	✔		✔	✔
Parkinsonism	✔									
Tremor	✔					✔		✔		
Muscle weakness						✔			✔	
Memory						✔				
Dizziness					✔		✔			
Nystagmus									✔	
Diplopia							✔			
Blurred vision		✔		✔						
Dry mouth		✔	✔	✔						✔
Constipation		✔		✔						
Diarrhoea			✔			✔				
Nausea			✔		✔	✔	✔	✔		
Anorexia										✔
Appetite stim.								✔		
Weight gain		✔								
Hypotension		✔		✔						
Photosensitivity	✔									

* Tardive Dyskinesia, Akathisia, Dystonia

Figure 5 – The common side-effects of the major drugs used in psychiatry

APPENDIX

USEFUL CONTACTS

American College of Sports Medicine
Box 1440
INDIANAPOLIS, IN. 46206

American Orthopaedic Society for Sport Medicine
Sports Medicine
70 West Hubbard, Suite 202
CHICAGO, IL. 60610

Center for Disease Control
Division of Injury, Epidemiology and Control
ATLANTA, GA 30333

Sports Medicine Centre
Australian Institute of Sport
CANBERRA ACT 2601,
AUSTRALIA

Sports Council
16 Upper Woburn Place
LONDON WC1H OQP

Medic-O-Games
Olympic Games for Doctors
Talk and Run, Sydney
AUSTRALIA
Contact ,   Fax 61-47-242567
                Email: Sherry@usa.net

Sports Medicine Information
Sports Medicine Division
Department of Orthopaedic Surgery
Nepean Hospital
PENRITH NSW 2750
AUSTRALIA
Fax: 61-47-242567

Email: sherry@usa.net
Sports Medicine and orthopaedic educational web
site. Visit. http://www.worldortho.com

Sports Specific Injuries

SPORTS	COMMON INJURIES
Football	Stingers (traumatic neuropraxia brachial plexus) Head spearing Transient quadriplegia (cervical cord neuropraxia) Shoulder dislocations Clavicle fractures Hip pointers Thigh contusion Turf toe Blocker's exostosis (humeral exostosis) Knee ligament (MCL/ACL) Spondylolysis
Soccer	Subdural haemorrhage (from heading) Shin abrasions Blisters Ankle sprains Groin pain Haematomas
Volleyball	Patellar tendinitis Iliotibial band tendinitis Knee ligaments (MCL/ACL) Ankle sprains Stress fractures TA Morton's neuroma Bursitis (Calcaneal) Rotator cuff tendinitis Mallet finger hand fractures Sacro iliac pain
Wrestling	Infectious diseases (Herpes gladiatorum) Cauliflower ear "Weight cutting" Dehydration Knee injuries Shoulder injuries
Basketball	Ankle sprains Quadriceps contusion Jumper's knee Knee ligaments (MCL/ACL) Heel pain Eye injuries Jones' fractures "Rebound rib" (stress fracture, first rib) Mallet finger
Swimming	Heel pain Exterior tendinitis foot "Breast stroker's knee" (patello-femoral) Rotator cuff tendinitis Multi-directional shoulder instability Low back pain/scoliosis Swimmer's ear

SPORTS	COMMON INJURIES
Track and Field	"Hitting the wall" (lactic acid build-up in anaerobic metabolism) Overuse injuries especially to lower limb Runner's knee (patello-femoral) Jumper's knee (infra-patellar tendinitis) Iliotibial band tendinitis Shin splint Plantar fasciitis "Runner's anaemia"
Baseball/ Softball	Sliding injuries (to leg) Stress # ulna (pitcher) Throwing injuries Little leaguer's elbow (medial epicondylitis) Little leaguer's shoulder SLAP (shoulder) lesions Valgus overload elbow
Gymnastics	Overuse (rotator cuff, spondylosis, wrist impingement, patellar tendinitis, stress #, patello-femoral) Gymnast's wrist ([+] ulnar variance) Stress, overload elbow Sever's disease calcaneus Pars defect (spine)
Golf	Lumbar strain Golfer's elbow (medial epicondylitis) Lateral epicondylitis de Quervain's # Hook hamate Rotator cuff tendinitis "Yips" (dystonia arm) Skin cancer Head injury
Racquet Sports	"King-Kong" arm (over-development of dominant arm) Rotator cuff tendinitis ('dead-arm') Tennis elbow Forearm nerve entrapments Low back pain Abdominal wall sprain Tennis leg Eye injuries
Downhill Skiing	Knee injuries, sprains (MCL, ACL) Skier's thumb (UCL/MCP) Facial lacerations Tibial fractures Shoulder dislocations
Nordic Skiing	Knee sprains (MCL, ACL) Ankle sprains Skier's thumb Shoulder injuries Exercise - induced bronchospasm Cold injuries

SPORTS	COMMON INJURIES
Ice Hockey (most dangerous for non-fatal catastrophic injury)	Cervical spine injuries (# and catastrophic) Concussion Acromis clavicular disruption Goal Keeper's thumb Ankle sprains and fractures Eye injuries
Rowing	Drowning Tendinitis wrists Muscle sprains
Boxing	Head injuries (subdural haematoma, epidural haematoma) Hand fractures Facial lacerations Chronic brain injury (dementia pugilistica)
Dance	Turn-out injuries (Pars stress fractures, hip tendinitis, shin splints, ankle impingement [pointe]) Scoliosis "Snapping" hip Stress fractures Eating disorders
Mountaineering	High altitude illness
Cycling	Neck/back sprain Ulnar neuropathy (handlebar palsy) Pudendal neuropathy Traumatic urethritis Vulval trauma Biker's knee TA tendinitis Metatarsalgia
Martial Arts	Facial fractures Dental injuries Limb fractures and contusions

FURTHER READING

Sports Medicine Secrets. MB Meillion. (Ed). Hanley & Belfus, Inc, Philadelphia, 1993.

Sports Medicine. Colour Guide Series. Churchill Livingstone. E Sherry, 1997.

The Olympic Book of Sports Medicine. A Dirix, HG Knuttgen, K Tittel. Blackwell Scientific, 1988.

The Oxford Textbook of Sports Medicine. M Harries *et al*, Eds. Oxford Medical Publications, Oxford, 1994.

Sports Medicine for the Primary Care Physician. RB Birrer, Ed. 2nd Ed. CRC Press 1994.

The Hughston Clinic. Sports Medicine Field Manual. CL Baker, (Ed). Williams and Wilkin, 1996.

Orthopaedic Knowledge Update. Sports Medicine. LY Griffin, (Ed). Am Acad Orthop Surgeons, 1994.

Science and Medicine in Sport. J Bloomfield *et al*, Eds. Blackwell Science, 1992.

Review of Sports Medicine and Arthroscopy. M D Miller, Ed. Saunders 1995.

ABC of Sports Medicine, G McLatchie *et al*, Eds. BMJ, 1995.

INDEX